introductory
maternity nursing

introductory
maternity
nursing
FIFTH EDITION

Doris C. Bethea
R.N., B.S., M.S.

Formerly Clinical Specialist, Maternity Nursing, and Instructor,
Practical Nursing Program, Porter Memorial Hospital,
Denver, Colorado; Assistant Professor of Nursing,
Union College, Lincoln, Nebraska

J. B. LIPPINCOTT COMPANY
Philadelphia
London · Mexico City · New York · St. Louis · São Paulo · Sydney

Sponsoring Editor: Nancy Mullins
Manuscript Editor: Marjorie Pannell
Indexer: Katherine Pitcoff
Design Coordinator: Anita Curry
Designer: Adrianne Underdonk Dudden
Cover Design: Kevin Curry
Production Manager: Kathleen P. Dunn
Production Editor: Linda J. Stewart
Compositor: McFarland Graphics
Printer/Binder: R. R. Donnelly
Cover Printer: Lehigh Press

5th Edition

7

Library of Congress Cataloging in Publication Data

Bethea, Doris C.
    Introductory maternity nursing.
    Includes bibliographies and index.
    1. Obstetrical nursing. 2. Pediatric nursing.
I. Title. [DNLM: 1. Obstetrical Nursing. 2. Pediatric Nursing. WY 157.3 B562i]
RG951.B4 1989   610.73'678   88-9176
ISBN 0-397-54693-9

Any procedure or practice described in this book should be applied by the health-care
practitioner under appropriate supervision in accordance with professional standards
of care used with regard to the unique circumstances that apply in each practice
situation. Care has been taken to confirm the accuracy of information presented and
to describe generally accepted practices. However, the author, editors and publisher
cannot accept any responsibility for errors or omissions or for consequences from
application of the information in this book and make no warranty, express or implied,
with respect to the contents of the book.
Every effort has been made to ensure drug selections and dosages are in accordance
with current recommendations and practice. Because of ongoing research, changes
in government regulations and the constant flow of information on drug therapy,
reactions and interactions, the reader is cautioned to check the package insert for
each drug for indications, dosages, warnings and precautions, particularly if the drug
is new or infrequently used.

preface

In an age when hosptials are big business and health-care providers are competing for consumer dollars, consumers have more of a say in what maternity services and facilities should be available. As a result of consumer interest, a variety of services and types of facilities are now being offered. One popular demand is for greater involvement by the family in the birth experience. The provisions that have been made to meet this demand are presented in the fifth edition of *Introductory Maternity Nursing*.

Advanced technology has also had a tremendous impact on modern maternity care. For example, as a result of this progress, infants weighing 1000 g or less at birth may survive if given proper care. Infertile couples now have options never before possible, such as *in vitro* fertilization and embryo transplants. With these advances, however, have come legal, ethical, and moral questions as to the appropriate use of this technology. Inclusion of such questions in the text exposes the nursing student to issues that may well affect her practice during her career.

Nursing continues to emphasize the development and utilization of assessment skills by the care-giver. This edition introduces the nursing process and provides basic information that the student can use to develop her skills in identifying the nursing needs of her patients and in implementing appropriate care. The importance of sensitivity and caring on the part of the nurse while providing care is stressed. More than 15 nursing-care plans are included that demonstrate the application of the nursing process to patient care.

The fifth edition of this book includes more material than previous editions on the effects of family relationships on the individual and society, as well as additional material on human sexuality. Acquired immuno-deficiency syndrome (AIDS) is discussed for the first time. The content of this edition has been reorganized to demonstrate more clearly the differences between normal and abnormal presentations. The behavioral objectives listed at the beginning of each chapter and the clinical reviews at the end of each chapter, features helpful to instructors and students in the past, have been retained.

Effort and attention have been directed toward presenting all the material in the text clearly and concisely. It is my hope that both instructors and students of maternity nursing will find this book the answer to their needs for a comprehensive, basic text in maternity care.

Doris C. Bethea, R.N., B.S., M.S.

acknowledgments

I wish to express sincere appreciation to my friends and colleagues who helped make this edition, and previous editions, possible. Special thanks go to Marlene Ringer, Edith Allen, Theda Archer, Ellie Dietsche, She-lin Huang, Annette Rockwell, Barbara Putnam, Margaret Marvin, James Rudolf, Margaret Jo Russell, Laura Savage, Tina Fuhrman, Cheri Yoches, Peggy Eichenberger, Roseanne Versio, Lynne Kelley, Barbara Rhoads, Evelyn Smith, Vivian Evans, Donna Kaemingk, Katherine Christie, Julie Lundgren, Eve Hoygard, Penelope Childress, Leslie Opperman, and Charlotte Sodia. I am also grateful for the generous assistance of David T. Miller, Joyce Mkitarian, and Nancy Mullins of the J.B. Lippincott Company.

I am indebted to the administrations of Porter Memorial Hospital, Denver, Colorado; Swedish Medical Center, Englewood, Colorado; and Lutheran Medical Center, Wheat Ridge, Colorado, for making their facilities available. I would also like to express appreciation to the publishers and organizations who permitted use of illustrations, assessment tools, and other forms included in the text.

Gratitude is expressed to the parents, nursing students, nurses, and physicians who agreed to be photographed for the illustrations.

contents

The Family and Pregnancy 1

the family in modern 1 society

○ Discuss the importance of the family to the individual, to society, and to future generations.

○ Describe the nuclear family and tell how it differs from the extended family.

○ Name two or three evolving life-styles and tell how they differ from the traditional family.

○ Discuss the expectations one may have as a family member.

○ List some problems the single parent might experience and suggest ways of dealing with them.

"What does it mean to have a family?" the television spokesperson asked 10-year-old Jason who was being interviewed on the weekly "Child for Adoption" segment of the mid-day news program. The youngster looked at her shyly and replied, "Having people that love me."

The love that Jason craved is provided by the caring family. Within such a family one develops feelings of belonging, acceptance, confidence, self-worth, and security. A wholesome family provides discipline that promotes responsible behavior and lays the foundation for a productive life. The family is the first school for teaching life skills, moral values, and social interactions. Within the family one develops pride in one's ancestry (roots) and expectations for the future. Members of a family are bound together by ties of love, marriage, blood, or adoption.

During a lifetime, one may belong to many different groups, but none is more important or more influential on one's life than the family. The family is the basic unit of society: What the cell is to the body, the family is to society. The quality and stability of society depend on the families that constitute it. Values, cultures, and sometimes religious beliefs are passed from one generation to the next through the family.

NUCLEAR AND EXTENDED FAMILIES

Traditionally, the family has consisted of the legally married husband and wife, and their children (Fig. 1-1). This group is called the *nuclear family*. In some instances, the grandparents, and possibly aunts and uncles, live in the same household with the husband, wife, and children; this arrangement would be an example of the *extended family*. The extended family that includes grandparents, aunts, uncles, and other relatives living in close proximity is well suited to the communication and transmission of values and ethnic culture from one generation to the next. In the nuclear and extended families the husband's role has traditionally been that of the breadwinner and the wife has been the homemaker. Until recently, the wife usually was not employed outside the home, at least not until the children were grown. However, in today's society with the high cost of living, many wives feel compelled to work outside the home whereas others choose to do so because of their desire for accomplishment through a career.

ALTERNATIVE LIFE-STYLES

Although nuclear and extended families still constitute a large part of society, various other life-styles are now evolving. These evolving life-styles represent a rejection of traditional values and emphasize the right of the individual to choose the way he/she wants to live. They are due to many factors, including the women's liberation movement, the availability of

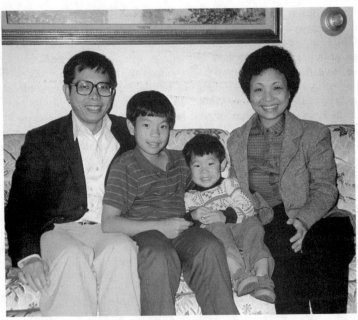

FIG. 1-1. *A nuclear family—father, mother, and two children.*

effective contraceptive methods and abortion, easy divorce, a change in society's view of pregnancy out of wedlock, economic pressures, rejection of the "establishment," and others. Some of the more commonly encountered evolving life-styles are (1) social contract families; (2) common-law marriages; (3) single parents; and (4) commune families.

The social contract family is one in which a man and woman decide to live together but are not legally married. The couple choosing this type of arrangement maintain that their bond of love and trust is more significant and binding than legal bonds authorized by a church or state. Some couples select this life-style because they reject the idea of a civil contract as such; others because of the apparent ease with which they can sever the ties if they so desire; and others seem to want to avoid the unhappiness they experienced in their own family. Partners in this type of arrangement supposedly share equally in all responsibilities of the home: financial, household tasks, childrearing, and so forth. The woman keeps her own name and the couple are very open about their relationship. These couples may use contraception; they may have abortion(s); or they may choose to have children.

Common-law marriages have existed for a long time, but they are mentioned here to differentiate them from the social contract family. In this arrangement, a man and woman decide to live together as a family, but for one reason or another they do not become legally married. This type of life-style is found most often among the poorer socioeconomic group. Except for the absence of legal sanction, this life-style is much like the traditional family in that the husband is the breadwinner, the wife the homemaker, and the wife and children adopt the husband's name. This type of marriage is usually considered legal after the couple have lived together for a specified number of years.

Single parents have always existed as a result of death, divorce, and desertion. However, as a result of changes occurring in society, the number of single parents is increasing. As less stigma is attached to birth out of wedlock, more unwed mothers are choosing to keep their children. Furthermore, some single women who do not wish to marry but who want children are choosing to have children out of wedlock or to adopt them. Some single men are adopting children for the same reason.

The single parent's coping ability may be challenged as she, or he, is faced with the total responsibility of being breadwinner for the family as well as parent. In most instances, part of the responsibility for child care must be shared with others. Child care centers are frequently used for this purpose although the single father, often being more financially secure than the single mother, may employ a caretaker to come into the home. To help ease the financial burden and also to simplify child care, some single parents have arranged to live together with their children in group homes or boarding homes. Four to ten mothers with their children share common dining and living quarters while each mother and her children have their own private sleeping quarters. The children of all the mothers play together and share toys, and they may have one caretaker while the mothers work.

Commune family lifestyles are diverse and may be located in either rural or urban areas. This group of people who choose to live together have common interests, value systems, and goals. They are often antiestablishment and antimaterialist. Some communes have been established as a result of involvement by the members in religious and philosophical causes. Some communes are comprised of monogamous couples with their own private quarters while other communes have group marriage. In still others, the commune functions more like a community than a family, with the members sharing expenses, household duties, and child care. In some communes the children are cared for by all members without regard for biologic parentage; in others, the biologic mother is the care-giver for the first year or two.

Pregnancy is the means by which the family, and therefore society, is perpetuated, or continued. Pregnancy occurs as a result of the sperm from the man uniting with the mature ovum (egg) from the woman, usually following sexual intercourse. After approximately 9 months, pregnancy terminates in the birth of a child. Birth is one of the greatest of all events that occurs among the human race.

CLINICAL REVIEW

ASSESSMENT: Jason, who was interviewed on the television program, was adopted by a married couple who live on a farm. This married couple also has two other adopted children, a 12-year-old boy and a 6-year-old girl.

1. Besides love, what other benefits can Jason receive from belonging to this family? *discipline, moral values, life skills, security*

2. What benefit, if any, might Jason *not* receive from belonging to this family? *ancestory*

3. The type of family to which Jason now belongs is

   a. A social contract family
   b. An extended family
   c. A nuclear family
   d. A single parent family

BIBLIOGRAPHY

Dresen S: The young adult adjusting to single parenting. Am J Nurs 76:1286, 1976

Jensen MD, Bobak IM: Maternity and Gynecologic Care: The Nurse & The Family, 3rd ed, pp 78–95. St. Louis, CV Mosby, 1985

Reeder SR, Martin LL: Maternity Nursing, 16th ed., pp 27–30, 41–48. Philadelphia, JB Lippincott, 1987

the family and pregnancy 2

BEHAVIORAL When the goals of this chapter are reached, the student will **OBJECTIVES** be able to:

○ Discuss the initial reactions of wife, husband, and children to a pregnancy.

○ Describe the possible physical, emotional, and financial effects of pregnancy on the expectant mother.

○ Discuss the three psychological tasks of pregnancy, stating when they occur, what is accomplished, and their significance.

○ Discuss when maternal–infant and paternal–infant bonding begin and tell how each can be promoted.

○ Explain how the expectant father can actively participate in the pregnancy.

○ Explain why the husband may need reassurance during pregnancy.

○ Discuss the possible effects of pregnancy on other children in the family and explain how parents can help them in their adjustments to it.

○ Describe the effects that pregnancy can have on the teenager and her family.

○ Discuss some of the special problems faced by the single parent.

○ List four or five factors that will influence the mother's decision to breast-feed or formula-feed the infant.

○ Describe the characteristics of clothing that promote comfort of the infant.

○ List clothing and nursery supplies that should be available for use in caring for the newborn.

○ List five or six personal items that the mother needs to have ready to take to the hospital with her.

○ List three or four items of clothing that will be needed for the baby when discharged from the hospital.

NURSE AND THE FAMILY

As a member of a family herself, the nurse can easily recognize and understand the importance of the family and its influence in society. She also needs to understand how the family functions in times of crisis, such as when sickness strikes or a family member becomes pregnant. In such instances, the family responds not only according to its culture and religious beliefs but also according to the strength of the bonds or "ties" that hold it together. These bonds are strong in closely knit families, and what affects one member affects all members. The extended family and also the immediate family may be significantly involved.

As the family rallies to protect and support the patient, the nurse may observe large numbers of family members hovering around the patient. When she accepts that they are there because they are concerned and caring, she can use them to promote the best possible care for the patient. Undoubtedly, they know the patient better than the nurse does. By listening to them and by involving them and the patient in the patient's care, she will not only be meeting their needs but she will also find that the patient is more receptive and responsive to her care. The family can thus provide strong support to the nurse as well as to the patient.

In our highly mobile society, a woman may be separated from her family by many miles during her pregnancy. The support that she and her husband would normally receive from them may be greatly missed. This is especially so if they have not had sufficient time to develop close friendships in the new area. In this instance, they may look to the nurse to provide the support they are lacking.

The hospital stay for maternity patients is short. Although the new parents can take advantage of the teaching available, they may not be able to absorb it all and may feel bewildered and insecure when they take their infant home. The nurse can help them to utilize their family, if they live nearby, as a resource and support system. If they have no family living nearby, the nurse can be a resource or refer them to other sources of support.

NUCLEAR FAMILY

INITIAL REACTIONS TO PREGNANCY

The initial reaction to a pregnancy will depend greatly on whether it was desired and planned or whether it was an "accident" and therefore unplanned, and perhaps unwanted.

Wife. When the wife first suspects pregnancy, she may attempt to deny or discount the signs by attributing them to something else. For example, she may tell herself that the amenorrhea is due to fatigue or excitement. If she has nausea and vomiting, she may think that she has the "flu" or that she has eaten something that did not "agree" with her. If the pregnancy is desired, she may be afraid that in her eagerness she is seeing signs that are really not there; if she does not want to be pregnant at this time she may try to postpone her awareness of it for a while. When the symptoms persist and she is convinced of their significance, she may be filled with happiness and joy or she may be dismayed and resentful. She may seek confirmation from the doctor before telling her husband or she may tell him first and then consult a doctor.

Husband. If the pregnancy is planned, the husband receives the news with enthusiasm and elation. He sees it as fulfilling his desire for a son or daughter and he is proud. If the pregnancy is unplanned, he may mask his feelings of disappointment and attempt to be happy in order to provide the support and encouragement that he knows his wife needs, or he may show his disappointment. However, he may be able to discount any obstacles that may be apparent more rapidly than his wife can, and often by his acceptance and understanding he is able to help her make an earlier adjustment to the pregnancy.

Children. The initial reaction of the children in the family to a pregnancy will depend on their ages, their parents' reactions, and how they feel they will be affected. Very young children probably will not experience any feeling toward a pregnancy because they will not comprehend its meaning. However, they may imitate the feeling they sense in the person telling them. Their first true reaction may occur at the time the new baby is brought home, when they may feel jealous and threatened because of the attention it receives from the parents.

Older children will be influenced by how they were affected by a previous pregnancy. A positive attitude in older children can be promoted by parents who are genuinely pleased about the pregnancy and who explain to the children at the beginning how the expected child will fit into the family.

After confirmation of pregnancy, satisfactory adjustments are usually made. Perhaps it is good that a period of at least 9 months elapses between conception and birth so that the necessary adjustments can be made and planning for the anticipated new family member can be completed.

EFFECTS OF PREGNANCY

Pregnancy has far-reaching effects on the family. Whether the family is large or small, rich or poor, each member is affected in some way.

Wife. The woman responds to pregnancy totally—her entire being is affected by it: diet, clothing, appearance and feelings, sexual responses and desires, job, social and recreational activities, rest and sleep, relationships with family and friends, daily life, and long-range plans.

As her internal organs change size and position to accommodate the developing child and her hormone and glandular activity increases in preparation for birth, the pregnant woman's external appearance changes. At the same time her capacity to love and care for others may seem to increase as her thoughts and concerns encompass not only her present family but also the new life that is developing within her. She also experiences a deeper and more meaningful relationship with her husband, who is so much a part of the experience of pregnancy. Thus, as the vital, though temporary, physical growth accompanies the pregnancy so also does the more lasting emotional growth and maturity.

Other emotional changes are also experienced by the woman, such as sudden mood shifts. Moments of depression may occur without any apparent reason. She may burst into tears over insignificant incidents, or she may experience a feeling of elation and well-being previously unknown to her. The pregnancy is constantly with her—she cannot lay it aside even for a few moments—and, realizing this, she may sometimes feel trapped.

If the woman has feelings of insecurity regarding the pregnancy or her husband's love, she may unconsciously seek reassurance by requiring additional attentions and making extra demands of him. For example, she may awaken him at unusual hours of the night to get her some item of food which she craves.

Her attitude and feelings toward sexual relations may change. If she had been tense and unresponsive for fear of becoming pregnant, she may now enjoy sexual activity without fear.

Early in pregnancy she may be annoyed by some of the first discomforts. Later she may suffer any one of them, or a combination (Chap. 8). She may have to make changes in her eating habits, such as relinquishing some of her cherished desserts and eliminating her favorite between-meal snacks, in order to maintain a desired weight. From the first sign of chloasma and the slightest bulge of her abdomen until the last indication of pregnancy has vanished, she is likely to be concerned about her appearance.

Finances may also be a concern of the wife, particularly if the pregnancy is unplanned and occurs at a time when the couple have expenses that require her salary as well as his. Pregnancy can create financial burdens also when the husband is still in school and the couple or family is dependent on the wife's income for support. This is especially true when the pregnancy makes her continued employment impossible and at the same time increases their expenses. Finances can also be a concern if this pregnancy means that the present housing will be inadequate and a larger dwelling will be needed or if the family income was already too meager to provide the minimum essentials.

An unplanned pregnancy may mean that the money that she and her husband have been saving for the future will have to be spent now on doctor and hospital bills, and on needs for herself and the infant. It may also mean postponing or giving up plans for continuing her education, graduating with her class, or qualifying for a coveted job.

As with the planned pregnancy, the unplanned pregnancy is usually accepted by the wife, and as it progresses it becomes more important and her other plans become less important. Sometimes during the pregnancy she will undoubtedly worry about whether or not the baby will be "normal" and healthy, whether labor will be difficult, and above all whether she will be a good mother, able to adequately care for her infant.

In the course of pregnancy, the expectant woman makes many adjustments. Three of these are of such significance that they have been labeled "psychological tasks," and typify the emotional growth the woman experiences as pregnancy progresses. Most women work out these tasks satisfactorily so that by the end of pregnancy they are able and ready to begin their roles as parents. However, if these tasks are not worked out satisfactorily and feelings of anger and resentment are not resolved, the effects on the child and family may be harmful. Usually one of these tasks is accomplished during each of the three trimesters of pregnancy; they may not be clear-cut, but may overlap or merge.

The first task is acceptance of the biologic fact of pregnancy. This task is usually accomplished during the first trimester while the woman's concerns center on her *self* and what is happening to *her*. At this time emphasis is on the pregnancy and how it affects her; there is little awareness of the child and she may have ambivalent feelings about the pregnancy and about becoming a parent.

The second task is acceptance of the fetus as a being separate from herself. This task is accomplished during the second trimester. The woman realizes that she is going to have a baby, and her attention is focused on the child. Maternal attachment to the child is believed to begin during this period as the woman hears the heartbeat and feels the movements of the fetus; the child becomes dear to her. Even though a woman works through this task and accepts the pregnancy and wants the child, there may be times when she would like not to be pregnant and "wishes away" the child. These ambivalent feelings are normal; however, they may be the basis for guilt feelings if the child is born defective.

The third task, accomplished during the third trimester, is for the woman to get ready for the birth of the child and to realize that she is going to become a parent. She needs to prepare to part with the child in the sense that she will no longer be its sole support and protector; others will be able to share the child with her. She is often bothered at this time by her heavy body and the discomforts of pregnancy and there is a strong desire on her part for the pregnancy to end; she is ready to assume her role as a parent.

Husband. In his role as partner in the marital team and as father of the newly conceived offspring, the husband is definitely involved in the pregnancy. He may, as some men do, prefer to limit his role to providing an adequate income for his family, or he may actively participate in the pregnancy. Fulfilling his responsibility as "breadwinner" is important to the health and well-being of his wife, the expected child, and other family members. However, if he sees this as his only function, he may deprive himself of an opportunity to grow emotionally and to strengthen his relationship with his wife by providing companionship and emotional support at a time when she needs and appreciates them most.

The husband who actively participates in the pregnancy is concerned not only with economic security but also with promoting the physical, social, and emotional well-being of his wife and in maintaining a happy home environment. From the beginning of pregnancy until his wife is able to resume all her normal activities following the birth of the baby, the husband fills a most important protective and supportive role that can be filled by no one else.

If the pregnancy results in the wife's having to give up her employment or if it otherwise creates financial pressures, the husband and wife may revise their budget and eliminate or postpone desired but nonessential expenditures in order to live within his income. If these measures are not sufficient to make up the deficiency in income, the husband may seek additional employment.

He is eager that his wife receive competent and complete medical supervision and care throughout pregnancy. He accompanies her on her visits to the doctor, when possible, and becomes acquainted with the doctor and the plan of care. He finds out the anticipated cost of the medical care and makes arrangements for payment. By being interested and informed he is able to help his wife achieve the desired goals of care.

The husband may accompany his wife to classes for expectant parents concerning pregnancy, labor, and the care of the infant. If they plan to have natural or psychoprophylactic childbirth, he learns his part in this procedure and coaches her so that she will be able to cope efficiently during labor. If they plan to utilize a hospital or alternative birthing center, they may wish to visit the facility beforehand. If they have made preparation for it, the husband stays with his wife during labor and birth, thus sharing the experience with her and giving his support at every stage of the pregnancy.

During pregnancy, as at other times, the wife needs to participate in social activities. Social contacts provide mental stimulation and keep both husband and wife in touch with their peer group.

The husband can give his wife encouragement and support in many ways. His interest in each new development of the pregnancy, such as feeling for movements of the baby and trying to hear the baby's heartbeat, reassures her that he wants the pregnancy as much as she does. By such undertakings as preparing his own breakfast and that of the children so that the wife does not have to be around food when she is nauseated, or tying her shoes for her when she cannot bend over, he shows thoughtfulness and concern for her. By complimenting her on her appearance when she doubts her attractiveness, he helps her to feel positive about herself. He may be bewildered at times by her sudden mood changes, but his patience and understanding reassure her of his love. By maintaining his sense of humor at times when she seems to have lost hers, he turns tense situations into pleasant ones.

Reassurance may also be needed by the husband. He may sometimes feel that he is a failure when his efforts to keep his wife happy meet with moodiness and resistance. He may feel unsure of his wife's love because of the limitations of sexual activity during pregnancy. The cause for these restrictions should be explained to him, and his wife must make a real effort in other ways to assure him of her love. There may be moments when the husband feels a twinge of jealousy and may feel "left out" of the situation because of the necessarily close relationship between the developing baby and the mother.

The father, as well as the mother, begins to form attachments to the child during pregnancy as he anticipates parenthood. The more involved he is in sharing the experiences of pregnancy, such as watching and feeling fetal movements and attending childbirth classes, the stronger his attachment to the baby is likely to be.

Occasionally, a husband develops symptoms during pregnancy that are commonly experienced by the expectant woman. For example, about the third month of pregnancy he has nausea and vomiting. Later he has indigestion, heartburn, and backache. When his wife is in labor he develops abdominal pain. These symptoms usually disappear with the birth of the baby. The cause for these symptoms is unknown, but they are thought to be due to identification and empathy with the pregnant wife or to "conception envy" and jealousy of the woman's ability to bear a child, or to a combination of these.

Just as the wife grows emotionally through the reproductive process, so does the husband. As he shares the experience with her and sees a new life come into being as a result of their love, his love for his wife deepens and his capacity for caring increases and strengthens. His life becomes enriched and reaches dimensions that would not have been possible without the experience of fatherhood.

The chances of good pregnancy outcomes and a decreased risk of problems to mother and infant are better when the husband and wife have a loving relationship that includes respect and unselfish concern for each other. To promote this type of relationship they should make a determined effort to spend time together sharing joys, concerns, social activities, and communicating to each other their needs and expectations. Cultivating an understanding, caring relationship takes time, energy, and careful planning. It doesn't "just happen" even though some couples seem more compatible than others, and developing the desired relationship may be easier for them than for others. Regardless of the cost in time and effort, the rewards of such a relationship are well worth it to the couple and to the family members.

Children.   Early in pregnancy the effect on the children may be simply that the father prepares breakfast for them because "Mother isn't well" or breakfast is later than usual for the same reason. They may also find themselves at the baby-sitter's while their mother is keeping her doctor's appointment. Depending on their ages, they may or may not be aware that the pregnancy is the cause of their mother's not feeling well in the mornings or that it is the reason for her trips to the doctor.

As the pregnancy progresses and is discussed in the family, the children will present their opinions on the desirability of a brother or sister. Often the preference of the parents is felt by them and they will express the same desire. They will be eager to tell their playmates and neighbors about the expected new member of the family.

The children may sometimes be affected by the mood changes and fatigue of their mother. She may surprise them by being sharp with them when they have done nothing to warrant this behavior, or she may laugh when they expected a scolding.

Depending on the size of the family, the ages of the children, and the size of the home, changes may have to be made in the children's sleeping arrangements. Such changes may be traumatic to the children and may create feelings of resentment toward the expected child unless they are included in the planning and can be made to feel that the change was their idea. A gradual change over time usually results in a smoother adjustment than does a sudden change.

Parents can help young children (or an only child) get used to the idea of a new baby by showing them a baby, letting them touch it, and letting them see their parents hold and cuddle it.

TEENAGERS AND PREGNANCY

When the single teenager discovers that she is pregnant, she may feel confused, embarrassed, resentful, angry, and scared. She may however feel proud if she views pregnancy as a status symbol. She must make major decisions, the first of which is whether or not to tell her parents and partner. If she decides to tell them, they will probably influence her other decisions, which include whether to stay in school, marry, have an abortion, continue the pregnancy and relinquish the child for adoption, or continue the pregnancy and keep the child. If she does not tell her parents or partner, she may feel lonely and isolated trying to cope with a situation that is overwhelming. Although she needs professional help, she may not know how or where to seek it. She may be too young to understand what is happening and too immature to deal with the situation or to make the necessary decisions.

The ability of the single teenager to cope with pregnancy is influenced by her own inner strengths and personal values and the values of her support group (family and close friends). Although society is now generally more accepting of pregnancy among single persons, the individual may find that her group does not approve. If this is the case, she may experience guilt feelings and loneliness. The pregnant teenager may withdraw from school or, if she continues in school, she may not participate as actively in school and social functions as she did previously. This may be to conceal the pregnancy (if she has not made it known), or because her interest and attention are more involved with the pregnancy, or because she is experiencing the normal discomforts and mood changes of pregnancy. If her friends are unaware of the pregnancy, they may interpret her behavior as disinterest in them and they may include her less in their plans. She may then feel isolated and rejected. Her feelings of loneliness and isolation may cause her to fantasize about the baby with the result that she becomes attached to it before it is born. She may anticipate that it will provide all the love that she needs and wants. She may however be so hurt and angry because she is pregnant that, although she continues the pregnancy while planning to relinquish the child for adoption, she remains detached from the reality of it. If she does not have an abortion, she may feel trapped by the pregnancy because it is ever with her and affects every aspect of her life. If she has an abortion, she may feel relief initially but later she may experience guilt feelings and depression.

Culture and ethnicity affect the acceptance or rejection of pregnancy in the unmarried woman. The black culture, for example, incorporates the child into the existing family system without stigma. The grandmother often becomes the primary caregiver for the infant while the mother continues her schooling and teenage activities; the father has contact with the child. In this setting, the unwed teenager is more likely to receive the loving support so needed at this critical time.

The teenage couple sometimes decides to marry when pregnancy occurs. Food, clothing, shelter, and health care then become primary concerns. Because of their age and lack of educational preparation and job experience, it may be impossible to obtain employment adequate to sustain them. Consequently, they may have to live with his or her parents. The success of this arrangement depends largely on the previous relationship between the parents and the couple and their feelings toward the pregnancy. Stress and conflict may develop in the couple if they are not permitted to participate in decisions which concern their own welfare and the pregnancy. They may also be made to feel guilty for adding to the financial burdens of the family by allowing the pregnancy to occur and for disappointing the parents' hopes for their futures. As a result, the parents and couple may become estranged. The couple may feel trapped by the pregnancy and may develop negative feelings toward it. These negative feelings may eventually be passed on to the child after birth. The couple may however be drawn closer to each other and may become more protective of the pregnancy and the child as they defend a situation that has occurred because of their love for one another. On the other hand, if the parents can overcome their initial shock and disappointment and can work together with the couple to achieve the best possible outcome for this situation, the family bonds are strengthened, everyone grows, and positive feelings toward the pregnancy and child are encouraged.

In the past, maternal–child health professionals have largely ignored the teenage father when caring for the teenage mother. Because the father is a vital part of the support system for the mother and because of the influence he will have on the child, he needs to be included in the decision making and in the care. He can be more effective in his role as support person if his own coping needs are recognized and he is helped to resolve them. Furthermore, his attitude toward the pregnancy and the expected child is more likely to be positive if he is recognized as a valuable member of the triad. The teenage father may need counseling and help regarding preparation for fatherhood, contraception and responsible sexuality, job training, and caretaking decisions. Whether or not the couple marry, he may have an important influence both in training the child and, if it is a son, as a role model.

SINGLE PARENTS

Today's society has a fast growing segment composed of single parents. A single parent may be either an unmarried person who adopts a child or gives birth to a child and keeps it, or a parent who was married but has lost a partner through death, divorce, or desertion. Forced separation of a spouse due to imprisonment or military service can create a situation simulating single parenthood.

Although some single parents receive some financial assistance for child support from their former spouse, social security, or aid to dependent children, many assume full responsibility for the support of themselves and their child or children. In many instances the single parent must work outside the home. This may be a problem if there is a lack of suitable employment or if she has inadequate educational preparation and no job experience. Finding competent, dependable child care while she works may also be a problem unless she has family or friends who are able and willing to provide it.

The self-supporting woman who becomes pregnant may experience the same feelings and effects of pregnancy as the married woman, but her adjustments and responsibilities may be greater since they are not shared with a spouse. She may also have to modify her life-style in preparation for the child. For example, if she lives in an apartment complex that does not accept children, she must make other living arrangements. She may have spent much of her income on clothes or entertainment before becoming pregnant; now she may spend less on these in order to buy the items needed for the baby.

Parenting requires that the parent and child spend time together getting to know each other. Providing financial security for the family also requires time. In assuming the parenting responsibilities usually provided by both parents, the single parent may find that her dual roles of mother and provider may sometimes conflict with performance of one actually jeopardizing the other. Such might be the case when she loses time from work because of a sick child or when she fails to spend time with the child because of the demands of her job.

The self-supporting single woman has responsibilities to herself as well as to her child. If she spends all of her time parenting and earning a living, she may soon feel so "tied down" that she is unable to cope with her situation. She needs to have time away from the child when she can participate in adult social functions and pursue interests that promote her personal growth. Finding the time and opportunity for these may be a problem. In some communities, single parents have formed organizations where they can meet for social activities and discussion of parenting problems. Groups of parents have arranged among themselves for weekend baby-sitting on a rotating basis so that, within a particular period of time, each parent has a weekend free of children. No expense is involved since each parent takes her turn baby-sitting for the others.

PLANNING FOR THE NEW BABY

Although the parent(s) must initiate and direct the planning for the new baby, all members of the family can be involved. Children will be cooperative instead of resentful of changes affecting them if they are included in the planning. The parent(s) will need to decide whether to obtain everything at once or only those items needed immediately, with others to be added as the need arises.

The most important immediate needs of the baby include food, clothing, and nursery supplies. The nutritional requirements of the infant can be met either by breast-feeding or by formula-feeding. In deciding which method to use, the woman will usually be influenced by her own personal feelings and preferences; her husband's feelings and wishes; her doctor's advice; her health; whether or not she plans to continue employment; her financial status; and social pressures. If she decides to breast-feed, she should realize that this is an emotionally satisfying practice. She should also understand the importance of a proper diet and adequate rest to the quality and quantity of her milk supply. If she chooses to formula-feed, she should know that the infant's nutritional needs can be met satisfactorily by this method, as can the emotional needs, if the infant is held while being fed. She should know that she can prepare formula inexpensively by using evaporated milk, water, and some form of carbohydrate, or that she can buy formula that is already prepared but is more expensive (see Chap. 15).

The entire family can be involved in the selection of the layette and nursery supplies (Fig. 2-1). To be comfortable the clothing should be soft, have smooth seams, be warm for winter and cool for summer, should not have frills around the neck, and should not be constricting. To be practical the clothing should be of material that can take repeated washings, be made so that it will not come apart after being worn a few times, and be not so small that the baby will soon outgrow it.

The type and amount of clothing included in the layette depends on the family's budget and personal preferences, their laundry facilities, and the time of year the infant is due to be born. The number of diapers included

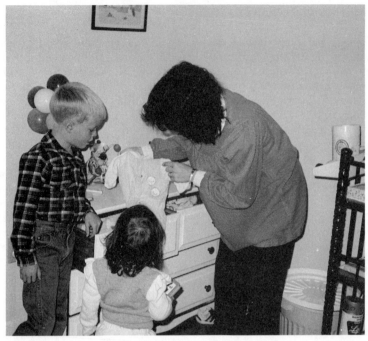

FIG. 2-1. *Children who are included in the planning for the new baby are more likely to anticipate the event with joy.*

in the layette depends on whether the mother plans to use disposable diapers, a diaper service, or launder them herself.

The following list of clothing and nursery supplies is suggested for immediate use by the newborn:

CLOTHING	NURSERY SUPPLIES
o 3 to 6 shirts	o Bassinet or crib
o 4 to 6 gowns or kimonos	o Mattress
o 2 to 3 receiving blankets	o Bathtub
o 3 to 5 dozen diapers	o Diaper pail
o 2 pairs waterproof pants	o Crib sheets
o 2 waterproof pads	o Quilted pads
o 2 blankets	o Bathtowels and washcloths
	o Crib-size blankets
	o Soap and soap dish
	o Safety pins
	o Cotton balls

PLANNING FOR FAMILY CARE

During the latter part of pregnancy the woman must make arrangements for family members to be cared for during her hospitalization. If they are new to the community or if there are no friends or relatives who can help, other arrangements are necessary. If the budget permits, a housekeeper can be employed, but if the family cannot afford one, the services of a social worker may be needed to study the total home situation and assist in obtaining a "homemaker" or a "home-aid." The family pays for the services of this individual according to their financial ability.

The woman will also want to plan for the care of the family and the new baby and herself for the first week or so after she and the baby come home from the hospital. These plans may be a continuation of the arrangements made for the family while she is in the hospital. In planning for her hospital stay the woman will want to pack a suitcase with items she will need and those needed for bringing the baby home. Suggested items to take to the hospital are:

FOR MOTHER	FOR BABY
o Toiletries	o Shirt
o Bras	o Diaper and pins
o Gowns	o Gown, suit, or dress
o Robe	o Receiving blanket
o Slippers	o Blanket
o Clothing to wear home	o Booties, bonnet, or cap as desired

This planning will promote the expectant mother's peace of mind and make her hospital stay more enjoyable, because she will know that her family will be cared for in her absence and also that she will have the personal items necessary to her comfort. In addition it will save time, minimize confusion, and provide a smoother transition from hospital to home on the day she is dismissed from the hospital.

CLINICAL REVIEW

ASSESSMENT: On August 2, Mrs. R., who had given birth to a 7 lb 6 oz (3345 g) baby on August 1, was standing at the nursery window looking at her baby. A nurse asked: Do you have a favorite in there?

Mrs. R.: Yes, I surely do. This is my fourth. We just knew it was going to be a girl; but are we ever glad it's a boy!

Nurse: Are your other children girls?

Mrs. R.: No, I have a son, nine. My daughters are 11 years old and 5 years old. But this is our last!

Nurse: Oh?

Mrs. R.: We didn't expect to have this one. When I first suspected I was pregnant, I told my husband if I were I'd kill him! He's been real tickled all
along about it; but I was a bear. It was purely an accident! I've been
president of the Fruitdale PTA this year and I kept saying I thought I
was pregnant, but the girls said, "Oh, Betty, maybe it's just nerves, with
you being so busy and all!" and I said, "Well, maybe." But I knew I never
skipped a period before without being pregnant. And then when my
stomach got upset, I knew it had to be. But I fought it every step of
the way. I kept saying to my husband, "If I am I'm gonna kill you!" And
he kept saying "I'm sorry!" But he was as happy as could be. And now,
well, it was worth it. We're all as proud as can be.

Nurse: How did the children feel about it?

Mrs. R.: My son hoped it would be a boy. And I said, "Well, son, it may be a
girl." Well, he made a face and was really unhappy for a while, but then
finally decided a girl would be all right—said he would "beat up" on
her. When I called him after the baby was born and told him we had
a boy he couldn't believe it. He is so happy! Now he keeps wanting to
know if the baby can talk yet and what he's like. He wants to know if
he can play with him.

Nurse: He's eager to have you bring him home?

Mrs. R.: Yes! And my 11-year-old daughter told me on the phone today that
she has cleaned the house and washed and everything is done. I had
told her the doctor said I couldn't do anything when I came home. So
now she's got everything done so I can come home.

Nurse: How do you think your 5-year-old will feel about the baby? Will she be
jealous since she's been the baby for so long? Or is she old enough not
to resent your attention to the baby?

Mrs. R.: Oh, I'm afraid she'll be jealous, especially when her daddy holds the baby.
She's her daddy's girl. My husband's family had 11 boys and he's been
real partial to his girls. That's another reason I'm glad it's a boy—for my
son's sake. I asked my little girl if her daddy could hold the baby when
it came and she hesitated a bit, then said, "Yes, after I go to bed."

At this point Mrs. R.'s doctor arrived and she went to her room.

1. From the above conversation, which members of this family seemed to
   make the fastest adjustment to this pregnancy? Support your answer.

2. Do you think Mr. R. helped his wife adjust to the pregnancy? Give reasons
   for your answer.

3. How did her friends seek to reassure Mrs. R.? Do you think they helped
   or hindered her in adjusting to the pregnancy? Or did they not influence
   her adjustment?

4. Which of the children do you think will be affected most by the new
   baby? Give reasons for your answer.

5. Why do you think Mrs. R. told her son the baby might be a girl? Why do
   you think he reacted the way he did at first to this? Why did he react
   the way he did after he had thought about it for a while?

6. What do you think of the 11-year-old's reactions?

7. What was the 5-year-old saying when she said her father could hold the baby after she went to bed? What do you think could have been done to help her adjust to the baby before it was born? What can be done now to keep her from resenting her father's attentions to the new baby?

BIBLIOGRAPHY

Brown MA: Marital support during pregnancy. J Obstet Gynecol Neonatal Nurs 15:475, 1986

Dresen S: The young adult adjusting to single parenting. Am J Nurs 76:1286, 1976

Earls F, Siegel B: Precocious fathers. Am J Orthopsychiatr 50:469, 1980

Fischman SH: Delivery or abortion in inner city adolescents. Am J Orthopsychiatr 47:127, 1977

Griffith S: Pregnancy as an event with crisis potential for marital partners: A study of interpersonal needs. J Obstet Gynecol Neonatal Nurs 5:35, 1976

Helton A: Battering during pregnancy. Am J Nurs 86:910, 1986

Hott JR: The crisis of expectant fatherhood. Am J Nurs 76:1436, 1976

Jensen MD, Bobak IM: Maternity Care: The Nurse & The Family, 3rd ed, pp 65–95, 195–205, 293–307. St. Louis, CV Mosby, 1985

Obrzut LAJ: Expectant fathers' perception of fathering. Am J Nurs 76:1440, 1976

Reeder SR, Martin LL: Maternity Nursing, 16th ed., pp 57–68, 126–133, 299–310. Philadelphia, JB Lippincott, 1987

Wuerger MK: The young adult stepping into parenthood. Am J Nurs 76:1283, 1976

Nursing and Maternity 2
Care

the past and present in 3 maternity care

BEHAVIORAL When the goals of this chapter are reached, the student will
OBJECTIVES be able to:

○ *Explain the similar origins of obstetrics and midwifery.*

○ *Explain how the term cesarean section probably came into use.*

○ *Tell what each of the following contributed to obstetrics: Palfyne, Raynaldes, Johan Peter Frank, Oliver Wendell Holmes, Ignaz Philipp Semmelweis, Louis Pasteur, Hendrik van Deventer.*

○ *Name the man who first used anesthesia in obstetrics, tell what the anesthetic was, and tell when and where it was used.*

○ *Tell what contribution Queen Victoria made to obstetrics.*

○ *List three or four advances that have been made in obstetrics in the 20th century.*

○ *Discuss the choices available to expectant couples as to types of services and facilities and how these became available.*

OBSTETRICS AND MIDWIFERY

The word "obstetrics" is believed to be derived from the Latin word *obstetrix*, which means midwife, or the Latin verb *obstare*, which means to stand by or in front of. In England, as well as in the United States until the latter part of the 19th century, obstetrics was synonymous with midwifery. A midwife in the original sense was one who stood by or in front of the woman giving birth. The definition of the term indicates the rather passive attitude that existed toward the woman in childbirth. In normal cases mothers and babies survived probably because there was no intervention, while in problem cases they usually died for lack of intervention.

For many years a midwife was a female attendant at childbirth. In time, male physicians began to perform this function. A physician attendant at childbirth was known as a midman or man-midwife. Later, the more acceptable term "accoucheur" (one who practices obstetrics) was used. The physician who undertook the practice of midwifery was limited by prejudices and was even more limited in his approach. As late as 1857 the American Medical Association decreed that any physician who could not conduct labor by touch alone should not undertake midwifery.

OPERATIVE OBSTETRICS

CESAREAN SECTION

Among the ancient Egyptians, cesarean section was performed on dead mothers. However, it is generally agreed that the first cesarean section on a live patient was performed by Trautmann of Wittenberg in 1610.

After this time many cesarean sections were done on live patients. The death rate, however, was high due to hemorrhage and infection, because the wound was not sutured and aseptic technique was not employed.

The origin of the term "cesarean section" has long been a question. Some say it originated with Julius Caesar, who supposedly was delivered by this method. This is doubtful, since his mother lived for several years after his birth. A more logical explanation is that the term was derived from the law *Lex Regis* (later called *Lex Caesaris* under the Caesars), which required that this operation be performed on a pregnant woman who died, so that mother and baby could be buried separately.

OBSTETRIC FORCEPS

The Egyptians were also known to have used obstetric forceps; however, for many years there were none. Then, about 1580 *Peter Chamberlen* is supposed to have invented them. He did not make his invention known or available to the medical profession, preferring to keep it a family secret.

Therefore, official credit for the invention of obstetric forceps is given to *Palfyne*, who in 1770 designed a pair and presented a copy to the Academy of Medicine in Paris. Later in the same century William Smellie improved the forceps by adding a steel lock and curved blades.

EARLY OBSTETRIC PUBLICATIONS

One of the earliest manuals on obstetrics was *Ta Sheng P'Ien*, a Chinese publication the author of which was convinced that it was the final word on the subject and needed no additions or deletions. The first English textbook on obstetrics, *Byrthe of Mankynd* by Raynaldes, and its German counterpart by Roesslin were published during the Renaissance. Johan Peter Frank in Germany wrote about obstetrics between 1779 and 1817. Through his writings, entitled *System einer vollstandigen medicinischen Polezey*, his ideas spread beyond Germany and were widely accepted. He believed that all childbirths should be attended by trained persons and that the midwife who was to attend the birth should be contacted before the expected date of confinement. Frank also proposed legislation providing state aid to the newly delivered mother, if necessary, so that she could have a period of rest following the birth and could give the necessary attention to her infant.

PUERPERAL SEPSIS

During the 17th, 18th, and 19th centuries, most births occurred at home. This was perhaps fortunate, for hospital conditions left much to be desired. Long hair and long beards were the style, and the germ theory and aseptic technique were unknown. Physicians customarily wore their street clothes while attending patients, performing operations, and delivering babies. Handwashing and wearing gloves were not a part of the practice. After treating a patient with a contagious disease or performing an autopsy on a patient who had died of puerperal fever, the physician would proceed to the bedside of a patient in labor and examine her vaginally and deliver the baby. No wonder it is estimated that as many as one of every ten women who delivered in hospitals died from puerperal infection. That is a conservative estimate; in some places the rate was twice that number. And this was in the best clinics of Paris and Vienna.

To compound the tragedy, only an occasional physician seemed concerned about the high death toll, and little attention was given to finding out the cause and correcting the situation. One of those in the United States who was appalled at the maternal mortality from puerperal sepsis was *Oliver Wendell Holmes*, of Harvard University. After studying puerperal infection and obstetrics as it was practiced, in 1843 he accurately described the nature of puerperal sepsis and established guidelines which, if followed, would prevent the disease. He was the first in the United States to do so. However, his findings and recommendations were scorned and rejected by the physicians of his day.

About the same time that Oliver Wendell Holmes was presenting his views on the contagiousness of puerperal fever in this country, *Ignaz Philipp Semmelweis* of Vienna was studying the same problem in the Viennese clinics. He observed that in Clinic II, where patients were commonly attended during labor and delivery by midwives, the death rate from puerperal infection was much lower than in Clinic I, where physicians were in attendance. To reduce the death rate in Clinic I, Semmelweis tried to follow the practice of Clinic II, but without the desired results. Then one day his friend and colleague, Kalletschka, cut his finger while performing an autopsy on a woman who had died of puerperal fever. Kalletschka died, and the autopsy findings were identical with those of puerperal sepsis. From this dramatic and tragic event, Semmelweis concluded that physicians were carrying the disease from the autopsies to the women in labor. He therefore demanded that all physicians wash their hands in chloride of lime following autopsies and before attending women in labor. He had finally found the key to reducing the maternal mortality in Clinic I. Later, he discovered that puerperal fever could be transmitted from an infected patient to a noninfected patient by contact with contaminated materials and by attendants, as well as being transmitted from the autopsy room. In 1861 he published his findings under the title, *The Cause, Concept and Prophylaxis of Puerperal Fever.*

Although Semmelweis proved without question the nature of the source and transmission of puerperal sepsis, many of his colleagues distorted, criticized, and wholly rejected his findings. After relentless persecution he died in 1865. His work, however, has withstood the test of time, and he is recognized today as having made a great contribution to obstetrics.

The findings of Semmelweis received support when in 1879 *Louis Pasteur* demonstrated the organism that caused puerperal infection in a drop of blood taken from an infected patient. Pasteur recommended controlling the spread of the organism by the use of aseptic technique.

FATHER OF MODERN OBSTETRICS

Although many have made contributions to the knowledge of obstetrics, *Hendrik van Deventer* of Holland (1651–1724) is honored as the father of modern obstetrics. He is credited with making the first accurate description of the pelvis, its deformities, and their effect on childbearing. He was also one of the first to describe the mechanism of labor.

OBSTETRIC ANESTHESIA

Just as the other advances in obstetrics received much opposition, so also did the early attempts at lessening or relieving pain in childbirth. This opposition, mostly from the male population, particularly the clergy, was based on the belief that women were *supposed* to suffer during childbirth, because the Bible says "in sorrow thou shalt bring forth children" (Genesis 3:16). So strong were the protests and so powerful the protestors that not until 1847 was the first anesthetic used in obstetrics. The anesthetic was ether, which had been discovered in America but was first used in obstetrics by *Sir James Y. Simpson* in Great Britain. Later, when chloroform became available, he used it instead of ether. *Queen Victoria* helped to silence some of the opposition to anesthesia in childbirth when she accepted chloroform for delivery in 1853.

TECHNOLOGIC ADVANCES

In the 20th century much progress has been made in the area of analgesia and anesthesia for childbirth. In addition, advances have been made in antepartal care, diet and nutrition during pregnancy, antibiotic therapy and chemotherapy in the prevention and treatment of infection, and in measures to prevent, control, and treat hemorrhage. These advances, combined with the knowledge passed down from earlier generations, have resulted in the lowest maternal mortality rates in history.

Advances have also been made in technology to diagnose and treat fetal conditions before birth, and in the genetic screening of newborns after birth. For example, intrauterine transfusions can now be given to the fetus with erythroblastosis fetalis, and a ventriculoamniotic shunt can be placed under ultrasound guidance in the fetus with hydrocephalus. Furthermore, advances in neonatology and perinatology have dramatically changed the outlook for infants born with problems. Owing to these technologic advances and to the highly skilled care available in neonatal intensive care units (NICUs), infants weighing only 1000 g at birth now have a good chance of survival. Where the technology and NIICUs are available, even infants weighing 600 g to 700 g at birth may survive; these infants, however, may be severely impaired.

The ability to save the lives of very small infants has given rise to many legal, moral, and ethical questions. Doubtless it would be better to prevent the preterm birth than to try to save the life of the very small infant who may be severely and permanently impaired. However, little progress has been made in preventing preterm birth in the past quarter century. Largely because of the high incidence of preterm births, the United States ranks 16th among developed countries in perinatal mortality.

The signs of preterm labor are often difficult to detect, and the diagnosis may not be made until labor is advanced or the membranes have ruptured. The contractions in preterm labor may be painless, or the woman, not expecting contractions at this time, may confuse them with intestinal cramps or fetal movement. One method being tried to prevent preterm birth is monitoring women who are at high risk for preterm labor. The woman wears a tocodynamometer on a belt around her abdomen about 2 cm below the umbilicus; a small recorder-transmitter is carried in a pocket. Any increase in uterine activity is detected and appropriate measures can be taken to prevent preterm labor. The tocodynamometer can be worn while the woman is at home or at work. Great strides have also been made in the technology devoted to helping infertile couples. These include in vitro fertilization and embryo transplants (see Chap. 5).

ALTERNATIVE BIRTHING CENTERS

Interesting developments are taking place in maternity care as well, in response to consumer demands for a voice in the type of services and care provided. A few years ago there was a trend to home delivery because some couples thought that health-care providers were not responsive to their needs in maternity care. As a result, in some areas alternative birthing centers (ABCs) were established so that couples could have a choice as to the place of birth, plan of care, and persons present at the birth. ABCs, located in hospitals or as free-standing clinics associated with hospitals, provide an alternative to home delivery. A homelike atmosphere is maintained and active participation by family and friends in the birth is possible; in addition, qualified personnel and equipment are available to deal with emergencies. Thus, ABCs are more humane than some hospital maternity departments and safer than home delivery.

Only women who have been screened and found to be low risk and who, with their mates, have been prepared by attending expectant parents' classes, are accepted to give birth in ABCs. The practice of pubic shaving, medication, and electronic monitoring and the use of stirrups, episiotomy, and forceps may be minimized or eliminated completely in this setting. The mother has a choice of position, lighting, persons present, and their participation during labor and birth. Many women go home with their infants the day of delivery, although certain medical criteria must first be met. In some areas, a follow-up visit by a nurse-midwife or nursing specialist within 24 hours after discharge is arranged so that the conditions of mother and infant can be assessed.

Other choices available in the type of setting for childbirth include the traditional setting, birthing rooms, and single-unit care facilities. In the traditional setting, the mother labors in one room, delivers in a second, recovers in a third, and spends her postpartum stay in a fourth. The husband can usually be present for the birth. The infant usually stays in the nursery most of the time.

In *birthing rooms* the mother labors, gives birth, and recovers in the

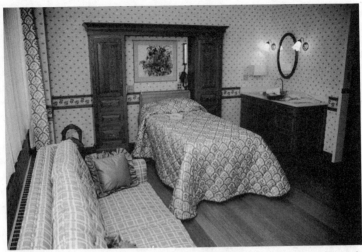

FIG. 3-1. *A single room where the woman labors, gives birth, and spends her postpartum hospital stay. The couch opens into a queen-sized bed where the husband and children can sleep.* (Photo courtesy Porter Memorial Hospital, Denver, Colorado.)

same room. Then she is transferred to the postpartum unit for the remainder of her stay. The couple can have family or friends present for the birth. The infant can be with the mother as much as she likes.

In the *single-unit* or *single-room facility*, the mother is admitted to a comfortably furnished room where she labors, gives birth, recovers, and stays during the postpartum hospitalization (Fig. 3-1). The bed, which provides several options for positioning, allows the mother to select the position most comfortable for giving birth. There is a couch that opens into a bed for her husband and other children, and a lounge where the children can play, usually under the supervision of a hospital volunteer. Anyone the couple wishes to have can be present at the birth. The same nurse usually takes care of the mother and infant throughout their hospital stay. The infant can stay in the room with the mother at all times or can be taken to a nearby nursery or holding room when the mother wishes to rest or be alone.

As more and more health-care providers have listened to what consumers say they want in maternity care, other choices are becoming available. These include classes for couples anticipating cesarean birth or normal birth, classes for grandparents, and classes for siblings; the choice of medicated or "natural" childbirth; jacuzzis in the labor room; unrestricted sibling visitation; participation by family or friends in the birth; and the presence of the husband during cesarean birth. The couple also have a choice regarding length of hospital stay. Many, because of financial or other considerations, choose early discharge. Even some preterm infants are being discharged much earlier than previously. As a result of this trend, hospital nurses in some areas are doing telephone or home visit follow-up.

BIBLIOGRAPHY

Brooten D et al: A randomized clinical trial of early hospital discharge and home follow-up of very low birth-weight infants. N Engl J Med 315:934–939, 1986

Gill PJ, Katz M: Early detection of preterm labor: Ambulatory home monitoring of uterine activity. J Obstet Gynecol Neonatal Nurs 15:439–442, 1986

Groeneveld M: Sending infants home on low-flow oxygen. J Obstet Gynecol Neonatal Nurs 15:237–241, 1986

Jansson P: Early postpartum discharge. Am J Nursing 85:547–550, 1985

Jensen MD, Bobak IM: Maternity Care: The Nurse and The Family, 3rd ed, pp 6–10, 49–68, 1076–1104. St. Louis, CV Mosby, 1985

Reeder SR, Martin LL: Maternity Nursing, 16th ed, pp 561–578. Philadelphia, JB Lippincott, 1987

Waryas FS, Luebbers MB: A cluster system for maternity care. Am J Maternal Child Nurs 11:98–100, 1986

the nursing process in 4 maternity care

BEHAVIORAL OBJECTIVES When the goals of this chapter are reached, the student will be able to:

o *Define: obstetrics, maternity nursing, birth rate, marriage rate, neonatal death rate, neonatal death, fetal death, stillbirth, infant mortality rate, perinatal mortality rate, maternal mortality rate.*

o *Discuss the aim of maternity care.*

o *Describe the following and tell what care each provides in the maternity cycle: family practice physician, obstetrician, pediatrician, midwife, nurse-midwife.*

o *Name three or four other health personnel who may be involved in providing maternity care.*

o *Discuss the services provided by each of the following facilities in relation to maternity care: doctors' offices, hospitals, birthing centers, public health departments, private agencies, adoption agencies, Planned Parenthood, U.S. Children's Bureau, National Office of Vital Statistics.*

o *List three things the birth certificate proves.*

o *List three or four factors that influence the number of women who become pregnant.*

o *Discuss the effects of socioeconomic status on maternity care in relation to: where care is sought, number of prenatal visits, and time at which care is sought.*

o *Discuss how parity, education, and race affect the number of prenatal visits.*

o *Name four or five developments that have contributed to improved maternity care in recent years.*

o *Name and discuss two or three current problems in maternity care.*

o *Define the nursing process and describe the five steps involved in it.*

o Discuss the nursing diagnosis and explain how it differs from the medical diagnosis.

o List four or five types of forms used for charting. Which form reflects the nursing process?

o Explain the nurse's responsibility in relation to the Standards of Care.

o Explain why charting is important.

o Explain why it is important for the nurse to understand a patient's culture and tell how the nurse can become acquainted with the patient's ethnicity.

Obstetrics is the branch of medicine devoted to the care of women during the entire period of pregnancy, labor, birth, and for at least 6 weeks following birth. It is based on a body of scientific knowledge that covers both normal and abnormal conditions during this time, and it recognizes the effects that other health and life conditions have on pregnancy and childbirth, as well as the effects that pregnancy and childbirth have on the health and life of the mother and her child. Recently, because of its broader meaning of the care of the mother and her offspring throughout the reproductive experience, the term "maternity care" has come into use. Because of the interdependence of obstetrics and maternity nursing, a definition of obstetrics would not be complete without a definition also of maternity nursing.

Maternity nursing is care rendered by the nurse to the expectant woman during pregnancy and to her and her child during labor, birth, and the puerperium. It also includes assisting the physician in the care rendered during this time. Maternity nursing involves establishing relationships of trust and understanding with individuals and families, recognition of needs and problems, and action based on knowledge, judgment, and available means and resources to meet the needs or solve the problems.

AIM OF MATERNITY CARE

It is the aim of maternity care to assist every mother to go through pregnancy, labor, and birth with minimal discomfort and optimal health and well-being, and to maintain the unborn child in the highest possible state of health throughout pregnancy, labor, and birth (Fig. 4-1). It has also become the aim of many maternity care providers to satisfy the wishes of the expectant parents regarding the type of environment and emotional atmosphere present at the time of birth. This has led to modifications of the hospital setting for labor and delivery and the establishment of alternative birthing centers. Thus, the aim of maternity care has broadened to include not only the physical health of mother and baby but also the emotional and spiritual well-being of those involved.

In a broad sense, maternity care begins with the health and education of potential parents. It is concerned not only with their physical health and well-being but also with the development of wholesome attitudes toward family relationships. The educational goals include knowledge of the responsibilities of parenthood and the development of judgment and abilities that will enable parents to meet these responsibilities in a confident and satisfying manner.

PROVISION OF MATERNITY CARE

If the broad aims of maternity care are to be achieved, care must be begun by the parents in the home, continued by the religious group and

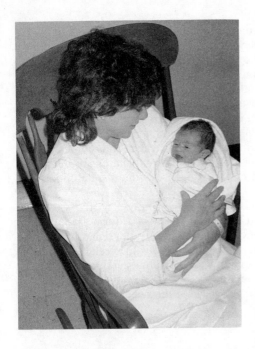

FIG. 4-1. *The aim of maternity care is a healthy mother and infant.*

the school, and completed by the community health team and all the facilities dedicated to this purpose.

Maternity care may be provided by many different types of health-care workers (see the box Providers of Maternity Care on p. 42). Similarly, many types of health care facilities are involved in providing maternity care (see the box Facilities for Providing Maternity Care on pp. 43–44).

STATISTICS

It is a legal requirement in all 50 states and the District of Columbia that a birth certificate be filled out on every birth and sent to the local registrar (Fig. 4-2). After the birth is registered locally, a complete report is sent to the *National Office of Vital Statistics* in Washington, D.C. Parents who want a certified copy of the child's birth certificate can obtain it from the local registrar for a small fee.

The birth certificate is legal proof of age, citizenship, and family relationships. In addition, the information on these records forms the basis for numerous statistical studies essential to those agencies concerned with human reproduction. These studies are compiled by the National Office of Vital Statistics and deal with such topics as:

The birth rate. The number of births per 1000 population.

The marriage rate. The number of marriages per 1000 population.

H105.142 Rev. 5 78

TYPE OR PRINT IN PERMANENT INK

COMMONWEALTH OF PENNSYLVANIA
DEPARTMENT OF HEALTH
VITAL STATISTICS
CERTIFICATE OF LIVE BIRTH

PRIMARY DIST. NO. _____

STATE FILE NO. _____

CHILD—NAME
1. FIRST | MIDDLE | LAST | SEX 2. | DATE OF BIRTH (Mo. Day Year) 3a. | HOUR 3b. ___ AM / PM

HOSPITAL NAME (If not in Hospital, Give Street and Number) 4a. | City, Boro, or Twp. of Birth 4b. | COUNTY OF BIRTH 4c.

I CERTIFY THAT THE STATED INFORMATION CONCERNING THIS CHILD IS TRUE TO THE BEST OF MY KNOWLEDGE AND BELIEF
5a. (Signature) ▲ | DATE SIGNED (Mo. Day, Year) 5b. | CERTIFIER—NAME AND TITLE (Type or Print) 5c.

Name and Title of Attendant at Birth if other than Certifier (Type or Print) 5d. | CERTIFIER'S MAILING ADDRESS (Street or R.F.D. No. City or Town, State, Zip) 5e.

MOTHER—MAIDEN NAME
6a. FIRST | MIDDLE | LAST | AGE (At time of this Birth) 6b. | STATE OF BIRTH (If not in U.S.A., Name Country) 6c.

MAILING ADDRESS 7. STREET AND NUMBER | CITY AND STATE | ZIP CODE

WHERE DOES MOTHER ACTUALLY LIVE? 8. STATE | COUNTY | CITY, BORO, TWP. (Specify)

FATHER—NAME
9a. FIRST | MIDDLE | LAST | AGE (At time of this Birth) 9b. | STATE OF BIRTH (If not in U.S.A., Name Country) 9c.

INFORMANT 10a. | Relation to Child 10b. | REGISTRAR'S SIGNATURE AND DATE RECEIVED 11. ▲

A. _____
B. _____
C. _____
D. _____
E. _____
F. _____
G. _____
H. _____
I. _____

CONFIDENTIAL INFORMATION FOR MEDICAL AND HEALTH USE ONLY

RACE—MOTHER (e.g., White, Black, American Indian, etc. — Specify) 12. | RACE—FATHER (e.g. White, Black, American Indian, etc. — Specify) 13. | EDUCATION—MOTHER (Specify only highest grade completed) ELEMENTARY OR SECONDARY (0-12) 14. / COLLEGE (1-4 or 5+) | EDUCATION—FATHER (Specify only highest grade completed) ELEMENTARY OR SECONDARY (0-12) 15. / COLLEGE (1-4 or 5+) | IS MOTHER MARRIED TO FATHER? 16. ☐ Yes ☐ No

PREGNANCY HISTORY (Complete each section)
LIVE BIRTHS (Do not include this child) 17a. Now living Number / None ☐ | 17b. Now dead Number / None ☐ | OTHER TERMINATIONS (Spontaneous and induced) 17d. Before 16 wks. Number / None ☐ | 17e. After 16 wks. Number / None ☐ | Date Last Normal Menses Began (Mo. Day, Year) 18. | Month of Pregnancy Pre Natal Care Began (1st, 2nd, etc.) (Specify) 19a. | Pre Natal Visits – Total (If none, so state) 19b. | Length of Pregnancy in weeks. 20.

17c. Date of Last Live Birth (Mo. Year) | 17f. Date of Last Other Termination (Mo. Year) | BIRTH WEIGHT 21. | THIS BIRTH—Single, Twin, Triplet, etc. (Specify) 22a. | If NOT Single Birth – Born First, Second, Third etc. (Specify) 22b. | APGAR SCORE 1 Min. 23a. / 5 Min. 23b.

Method of Delivery 24. | COMPLICATIONS OF PREGNANCY (Describe or write "none") 25.

CONCURRENT ILLNESSES OR CONDITIONS AFFECTING THE PREGNANCY (Describe or write "none") 26. | COMPLICATIONS OF LABOR AND/OR DELIVERY (Describe or write "none") 27.

BIRTH INJURIES OF CHILD (Describe or write "none") 28. | CONGENITAL MALFORMATIONS OR ANOMALIES OF CHILD (Describe or write "none") 29.

Death Under One Year Of Age–
Number of Death Certificate For This Child
Multiple Births Enter State File Number for Mate(s)
Live Birth(s)
Fetal Death(s)

FIG. 4-2. *Certificate of live birth used by Pennsylvania Department of Health. Similar forms are used by other cities and states.*

⚹**The fertility rate.** The number of births per 1000 women between the ages of 15 and 44 years.

⚹**The neonatal death rate.** The number of neonatal deaths per 1000 live births. A *neonatal death* is death of an infant during the first 4 weeks following birth. A *fetal death* or *stillbirth* is death of the fetus in the uterus after 20 or more weeks' gestation.

⚹**The infant mortality rate.** The number of infant deaths before the first birthday per 1000 live births.

⚹**The perinatal mortality rate.** The total number of deaths of fetuses and infants weighing 1000 g or more that occur between 28 weeks' gestation and 4 weeks of age.

⚹**The maternal mortality rate.** The number of maternal deaths per 100,000 live births. Death of a woman from any cause during pregnancy or within 42 days after the pregnancy has terminated, regardless of the duration or location of the pregnancy, is a maternal death. The leading causes of maternal mortality in this country are hemorrhage, infection, and pregnancy-induced hypertension. (P I H)

PROVIDERS OF MATERNITY CARE

PHYSICIANS

Family practice physician: Specializes in care of all family members; refers problems of pregnant woman to *obstetrician;* refers problems of newborn to *pediatrician*

Obstetrician: Specializes in care of women during pregnancy, childbirth, and post partum; usually a *gynecologist* as well (specialist in diseases of women)

Pediatrician: Specializes in care of infants and children

Resident: Physician who is preparing to specialize in a particular branch of medicine, such as obstetrics

MIDWIVES

Lay midwife: Provides care under supervision of physician but physician not present unless problem exists; education limited; practices in areas where few physicians are available

Nurse-midwife: Registered, professional nurse with additional special preparation in an accredited midwifery program; provides total care to expectant mother throughout pregnancy and labor, and to mother and baby after birth; responsible to and practices under supervision of physician but he is not present unless problem arises; practices wherever state laws permit

NURSES

RN: Assists physicians in providing continuous and complete care to mother and infant throughout maternity cycle

LPN or LVN: Assists RN and physician in providing total care

OB-Gyn nurse practitioner: RN with additional preparation in obstetrics and gynecology; provides total care during prenatal and postnatal period to mother and infant and assists physician during labor

OTHERS

Laboratory technicians, social workers, nutritionists, geneticists, mental hygienists, radiologists, dentists

FACILITIES FOR PROVIDING MATERNITY CARE

DOCTORS' OFFICES

Provide antepartum care and postpartum follow-up care to the mother
Provide prenatal and neonatal care to the infant
Source of information and guidance in healthful living and family planning

HOSPITALS

General—Outpatient facilities for prenatal care and postpartum follow-up
 Maternity department with labor-delivery suite, newborn nursery, postpartum unit
 Facility for expectant parent classes
Special—Children's hospitals: Specially equipped to care for premature and other high-risk infants
 Homes for retarded children: Provide for children who need special, prolonged care
 Homes and hospitals for unwed mothers: Operated by Salvation Army, Florence Crittendon Homes, etc.; may provide counseling services, employment, opportunity for continuing education, and shelter and medical care

ALTERNATIVE BIRTHING CENTERS

Free-standing facility separate from hospitals
Provide alternative to home or hospital as place for childbirth
More freedom for couple to choose who is present at birth; humanistic aspect of birth stressed
Safer than home delivery
Qualified personnel and emergency equipment available

PUBLIC HEALTH DEPARTMENTS

Set standards of care
Do case finding
Provide follow-up care through referrals from doctors and hospitals
Conduct antepartum, postpartum, well-baby, and family planning clinics

GENETIC COUNSELING CENTERS

Provide genetic diagnostic studies and counseling regarding risk of producing defective children

ADOPTION AGENCIES

Resource to woman who relinquishes her child and to couples who wish to adopt
Operated by Welfare Departments and some religious organizations

U.S. CHILDREN'S BUREAU

Federal agency, part of the Department of Health and Human Services
Established in 1912 during administration of President Theodore Roosevelt

(continued)

Concerned with everything that pertains to health and well-being of children

Co-operates in international program for maternal-child care and in state programs

Staff composed of specially prepared doctors, nurses, social workers, nutritionists

Guides in setting of standards of care at state and local levels

Furnishes expert advice to state and local departments

Prepares and prints pamphlets and booklets on infant and child care

Finances certain maternal and child health clinics and family planning programs

HOMEMAKER SERVICES

Offer services of "home care helpers" or "home health aides"

Provide care for family on 24-hour basis while mother is in hospital and for as long as needed afterward

PLANNED PARENTHOOD ASSOCIATION

Offers services and information to individuals and couples who wish to limit the size of their families and to space their pregnancies

RECIPIENTS OF MATERNITY CARE

NUMBER OF RECIPIENTS

Generally, the recipients of maternity care are women between the ages of 15 and 44. Several factors that influence the number of women who become pregnant and therefore recipients of maternity care are listed below.

The marriage rate. This rate is the number of marriages per 1000 population. In recent years there has been a decline in the number of married couples who elect to have children and an increase in the number of children born to couples not in traditional marriages (for example, social contract and other nonlegal unions). Therefore, the marriage rate is not as significant a factor in predicting the number of women who will become pregnant as it once was.

The number of women in their 20s. Although all women between the ages of 15 and 44 are considered potential recipients of maternity care, the highest number of actual recipients are women in their 20s.

The desire of a woman to bear a child. There are many reasons why a woman may desire to have children. She may wish to have children because society expects her to, or she may wish to prove her femininity or to fulfill her desire for achievement if she failed to do so in a career. She may desire to bear children because she is eager for the relationship she expects to have with them, or she may feel her home is incomplete without them.

The availability of acceptable methods of birth control. Within the past few years safe, effective, easy-to-use contraceptive measures have become available (see Chap. 15). Consequently, many couples have been able to postpone the time of beginning their families, to limit the size of their families, and to space their children. To a greater extent than ever before children are being conceived because they are wanted, and not solely as a result of the sexual drive.

CHARACTERISTICS OF RECIPIENTS

Some characteristics of recipients of maternity care in relation to socioeconomic status are:

1. Most women in the lower socioeconomic group visit medical facilities (clinics, hospitals) for care, while women in the middle and upper socioeconomic groups visit physicians.

2. Women in the middle and upper socioeconomic groups make more prenatal visits than those in the lower group.

3. Women in the lower socioeconomic group seek care later in pregnancy than those in the middle and upper groups.

4. Women in the lower socioeconomic group have higher rates of illegitimacy than those in the middle and upper groups.

Other characteristics, based on parity (*parity* denotes the number of viable pregnancies a woman has had), education, and race in relation to the number of prenatal visits and the time care is sought are: (1) women having their first baby make more prenatal visits than women who have had other children; (2) women who have completed more grades in school make more prenatal visits; and (3) white mothers seek care earlier than nonwhite mothers.

HEALTH CARE AND CULTURE

Health workers too often assume that patients have the same attitude toward health care as they do. And too often they are mistaken, particularly when they are providing care to persons with an ethnic background different from their own. To avoid this error, and to make the care more acceptable and therefore more effective, the health-care provider must become acquainted with the culture of the population she serves.

Culture has to do with a way of life. It is expressed in the feelings, beliefs, attitudes, and practices of individuals in relation to diet, language, religion, art, history, family values, social patterns, childbearing and childrearing, healing, and health.

When a nurse or other health-care provider is confronted with cultures different from her own, she should be careful not to be judgmental and not to stereotype individuals just because they are members of a particular ethnic group. No two people are alike, even though they may be of the same ethnicity. Instead, the nurse should do all that she can to learn as much as possible about the individual and her culture and try to adapt the health care so that it will be more acceptable. If there is a language barrier, the nurse should try to find an interpreter among health workers with the same ethnicity. If this is not possible, then an interpreter may be found among the patient's relatives. Because it is often difficult for the lay person to translate scientific terms, the nurse should keep her language simple. She should also keep in mind that the lay interpreter may include her own ideas in the information given to the patient and may even delete information with which she does not agree.

The patient is frequently the best source of information about her own culture. A good way to obtain this information is to visit the patient's home, a privilege that may not be possible unless one is a public health nurse. If a home visit is not possible, the nurse should listen very carefully to what the patient has to say and glean as much information as she can from contacts with her. Reading the literature on a patient's ethnic group is also helpful. Being well informed on scientifically sound health practices is essential and necessary for the nurse, but her knowledge will not be helpful unless the patient accepts it, and it will not be accepted if it conflicts with the patient's beliefs.

Those trying new life-styles attach great significance to the emotional and spiritual aspects of childbearing. Therefore, in selecting antepartal services and in planning for the birth, they are likely to choose those that permit participation by the father and their significant others. If they have access to a medical facility with birthing rooms or alternative birth centers, they may utilize them because of the homelike atmosphere and because their significant others can participate in the birth. If these facilities are not available, they may elect to give birth at home rather than in a maternity unit with rigid rules that restrict visitors and deny participation by the father and significant others.

The health worker dealing with this segment of society is more likely to be successful if she realizes that members of communes are often well educated and may tend to be of a philosophical nature. Some members may be skeptical of traditional organized medicine, and the health-care worker should anticipate that they will ask questions and be prepared to document her answers with rational explanations and practical experiences. She should expect that they may reject some of her advice, but she should treat this decision with respect. As with all couples, she should show genuine concern and courtesy in her relationships with them.

CURRENT PROBLEMS IN MATERNITY CARE

Many outstanding developments have been made in maternity care in recent years. These include preparation of better qualified personnel; establishment of a wide variety of well-equipped facilities; improved diagnostic methods; spread of antepartal care; advances in obstetric anesthesia and analgesia; availability of antibiotics and chemotherapy in the prevention and treatment of infection; advances in the prevention, control, and treatment of hemorrhage; and more family-centered approaches. However, despite these developments, some problems are still apparent in present-day maternity care.

Infant mortality.   One of the biggest problems in maternity care today is infant mortality. In recent years there has been a decline in infant mortality in the United States, perhaps due in part to such factors as a falling fertility rate, better contraceptive practices, increasing availability of safe abortion, and a higher standard of living in the general population. However, this decline has not been as apparent among those in the lower socioeconomic group. Much attention is being directed toward ways of reducing infant mortality in this group. Measures that have been successful include community maternal-infant care programs that provide prenatal and infant care for high-risk mothers and infants through the first year of life, and the development of newborn intensive care units in hospitals.

The main causes of death during the first 4 weeks of life are preterm birth and low birth weight. Other important causes are respiratory distress syndrome, asphyxia and atelectasis, congenital malformations, and birth injuries.

Distribution of care.   Another major problem is the distribution of care. Expectant mothers in some communities may have access to several facilities or agencies, while those in other areas may have no facilities to serve them. To compound the problem, some women choose not to take advantage of the care that is available. These include women from low-income families who are not used to seeking medical care for nonemergency conditions and do not recognize pregnancy as a condition requiring care. Or some women may have gone for one visit but became discouraged because of the impersonal manner of those providing the care, because of the long waiting required, or for other reasons. Also included in this group are some unwed mothers who may not seek care because they are ignorant of the need or the availability of facilities, or fear being condemned. The number of pregnant women who are addicted to drugs is increasing rapidly. The main concern of these women is obtaining money to support their habit; they are not concerned with prenatal care. They may resort to prostitution to obtain funds.

Another group of women who often do not seek care are those living in communes. Often this group consists of young unmarried girls who may have used controlled drugs before and after becoming pregnant. In addition to not seeking antepartal care, they may choose to give birth in the commune unattended by medical or nursing personnel.

Quality of care.   Women in the middle or upper income brackets usually have a good education and realize the value of the basic essentials to a healthy outcome of pregnancy and seek to obtain them. Therefore, they usually have good nutrition and the best available medical care throughout pregnancy, labor, birth, and the puerperium. Women in the lower income bracket, on the other hand, who probably do not have an adequate diet at any time, and who usually have more pregnancies and a higher chance of having problems during pregnancy, usually receive less medical care or poorer quality care than the women in the other levels.

Abortion. The controversy over voluntary abortion continues in spite of the 1973 U.S. Supreme Court decision. Prior to that decision, each state had its own laws governing abortion. Some had very strict laws that made it impossible for abortion to be performed legally unless the woman's life or health was jeopardized by continuation of the pregnancy. During this era, women who wished to have an abortion for nonmedical reasons had to resort to illegal means to obtain it. As concern for control of population growth mounted and as a result of pressure from various groups for women's rights, some states relaxed their abortion laws. This made it possible for women living in these states to obtain abortions more easily if they could afford them. Women living outside the states with liberal abortion laws often had to travel great distances and spend considerable money to obtain abortions.

The decision by the Supreme Court defines the extent to which the states can regulate abortion. In effect, the Court ruled that during the first trimester the decision for abortion rests with the woman and her physician, and the state cannot interfere. During the second trimester the state "may, if it chooses, regulate the abortion procedure in ways that are reasonably related to maternal health . . ." (Hall, p. 3). This means the state can require that persons performing abortions have certain qualifications and that the facilities where abortions are done meet certain standards and be equipped to provide aftercare and to cope with emergencies that may arise.

During the third trimester the state has more authority: "For the stage subsequent to viability the State, in promoting its interest in the potentiality of human life, may, if it chooses, regulate, and even proscribe, abortion except where it is necessary, in appropriate medical judgment, for the preservation of life or health of the mother" (Hall, p. 3).

The Supreme Court decision on abortion was based on the woman's right of privacy as set forth in the Fourteenth Amendment. Those who are opposed to voluntary abortion for moral or religious reasons contend that life begins at conception rather than at the age of viability (stage of gestation at which the fetus has a chance of survival if it is born). According to this view, the unborn conceptus is a person from the time of conception, and therefore is entitled to the right to live. The "right to life" movement is seeking to pressure legislators into passing an amendment to the Constitution that would guarantee the right to life of the unborn. One week after the Supreme Court handed down its decision, such a resolution was introduced into the House of Representatives. Although the "right to life" movement has received considerable support, it has not been able to negate the Supreme Court decision through such an amendment.

 THE SUPREME COURT DECISION ON ABORTION

o Did not decide the issue of *when* life begins.

o Did define viability as that point of development when the fetus can survive outside the uterus at about 22 to 23 weeks' gestational age.

o Did imply that the fetus is not a person, for purposes of protection under the Fourteenth Amendment.

o Did deny the woman's spouse or father of the fetus the right to prevent abortion.

o Did not provide for abortion on demand. (The physician still has the right and obligation to exercise professional judgment.)

o Did not mention pregnant minors. (In most states minors can obtain abortion without parental consent.)

In December 1978 Congress passed the Hyde Amendment, which states that Medicaid funds can be used for abortion only if (1) the woman's life is endangered by carrying the fetus to term; (2) two physicians determine that the woman would suffer severe and long-lasting physical damage as a result of the pregnancy; or (3) the pregnancy was the result of rape or incest and was reported promptly to a law enforcement or public health agency. In July 1980, in a class action suit, the U.S. Supreme Court upheld the constitutionality of the Hyde Amendment.

The reasons a woman may seek abortion are numerous. The pregnancy may be (1) a threat to her health or life, (2) the result of rape or incest, or (3) likely to produce a defective child because of a disease, such as German measles, contracted by the mother during pregnancy; or the pregnancy may be unwanted because of (4) economic reasons, (5) large size of family, (6) disaffection for father of the child, (7) lack of desire for children, or (8) unmarried state of the mother.

The Roman Catholic Church opposes abortion on religious grounds. Protestants generally oppose it as a birth control measure; otherwise, they hold varying opinions.

Availability and utilization of qualified personnel. There are not enough qualified personnel to administer high-quality care to all maternity patients. Furthermore, some of the better qualified are not being used to best advantage. For example, nurse-midwives who are qualified to render total and continuous care throughout pregnancy, labor, birth, and the postpartum period are limited in their function by legal restrictions in some areas and by prejudice in other areas.

Another problem area of utilization is that of the clinic for low-income patients. Here there is a tremendous need for care by experienced nurses, obstetricians, and pediatricians with the best qualifications.

THE NURSING PROCESS AND FAMILY-CENTERED CARE

The *nursing process* is a way of identifying and solving patient health problems within the scope of nursing practice. It consists of five overlapping steps, or stages, that are based on the scientific method of reaching conclusions through logical, rational analysis of data that are systematically collected.

The steps, or stages, are
1. Assessment
2. Analysis
3. Planning
4. Implementation
5. Evaluation

Assessment is the collection of subjective and objective data on the patient and her health problem. Subjective data are provided by the patient and reflect her understanding of her present health needs as well as her medical and reproductive history. Objective data are obtained by the nurse through observation of the patient, from health care records, from laboratory test results, from family or friends, or from physicians, nurses, and other members of the health care team. Subjective data and much objective data are obtained in the dialogue between patient and nurse. The initial assessment by the nurse becomes the *data base*, and this is updated and changed as more information is obtained.

Analysis is interpretation of the data. Analysis involves judgment and decision-making. What does the information mean? How does it compare with or differ from what is considered normal? What is the nursing problem as seen by the nurse? What is the problem from the patient's viewpoint? From analysis of the data the *nursing diagnosis* is formulated. The nursing diagnosis is a statement in which the analyzed data are summarized to indicate the nature and extent of the patient's health problem. It must be within the limits of nursing practice as presented in the local nurse practice act. A patient may have more than one nursing diagnosis. The nursing diagnosis should be stated in as few words as possible and should be as specific as the data allow. It must be a patient problem that the nurse can treat.

Planning of care involves defining desired or expected goals or outcomes of care and then organizing them according to importance (setting priorities). It also involves choosing appropriate actions to attain the desired outcome. When possible the patient, and perhaps family members, should be involved in the setting of goals. The patient's culture and life-style should also be considered. This is essential to willing participation by the patient in her own health care, which is necessary for a successful outcome. The goals are stated in patient-centered terms.

Setting priorities is influenced by whether or not the health problem is life-threatening. If it is not life-threatening, then the patient's or nurse's preference can be considered.

This step in the nursing process results in the development of a *nursing-care plan*. The care plan can be an effective tool in communicating the needs of the patient and how they can be met. In addition, it aids in providing continuity of care.

Implementation consists of the actions or interventions taken by the nurse to achieve the desired goals or outcomes. These actions are of different kinds. They may be observations to obtain information about the problem. They may be measures to bring about healing or to promote comfort. They may be explanations or instructions designed to detect, correct, or prevent health problems and to promote positive health.

Evaluation involves determining the progress the patient has made toward the desired goals, and changing the care plan if that is found to be necessary. For evaluation to be meaningful, goals must be stated so that they are measurable; they must be specific and realistic. Depending on the nature of the health problem, evaluation may take place within minutes, and the care plan changed immediately, or it may take place over a period of time. Evaluation not only reveals how well a goal has been reached, it may also indicate the need for changing the goal or the nursing actions, or for collecting more data.

To use the nursing process skillfully, the nurse must have a broad base of general nursing knowledge and skills. In addition, she must have specific knowledge in specialty areas, such as maternal–newborn nursing, as well as adequate clinical experience in these areas.

FAMILY-CENTERED CARE

Sensitivity is an important attribute that each nurse must develop if she does not already possess it. In order to bring the family-centered approach into the nursing process, the care-giver must be sensitive to and demonstrate respect for the individual's and the family's feelings, beginning with the first contact and continuing throughout their relationship.

During the first interview the nurse should seek to put the patient at ease by being sensitive to her need for privacy. The interview should be conducted in a quiet area apart from others or in a private room. The patient should be assured that the information she gives will be kept confidential. This may mean excluding family members from the interview if the patient so desires. The nurse can ask the patient if she wants a family member or friend with her during the interview, but this should be done when the nurse is alone with the patient. Patients may withhold information or give incorrect information in the presence of someone they do not want to have the information.

During the physical assessment, exposure of the "private" parts of the body may be embarrassing to the patient. The sensitive nurse can anticipate this and take measures to reduce the patient's anxiety. These include explaining beforehand what will be done, staying with the patient during the doctor's examination, keeping the patient's body covered as much as possible during the examination, and making sure that the examination is done in private with the door or curtain to the exam area closed.

The nurse must also be sensitive to the husband's feelings and his need to be involved in the pregnancy. The nurse who is sensitive to the family members' needs for each other in sharing the experience of pregnancy and childbirth and who encourages involvement by them in the care will find that implementing her plan of care will be easier and more successful than if she had not considered their needs.

CHARTING

Many types of forms are used for recording information on the patient and the nursing process. These may be short forms for quick reference, or long forms for detailed recording. Some of the more common types are the data base record, nursing-care plan, nurse's notes, progress notes, graphs, flow sheets, Kardex, and discharge summary.

The **data base record** contains the information obtained when the patient is admitted or first seen. It includes the patient's vital signs, subjective and objective symptoms and reason for admission, present and past medical history, family history, obstetric history, laboratory findings, and a brief statement regarding life-style. The data base is updated with each patient visit.

The nursing process is reflected in the **nursing-care plan.** Standard care plans can be developed that apply to all patients with the same or similar conditions or problems. These plans can then be modified to fit the individual patient's problems. Care plans are continually updated to include new data as they become available and to delete problems as they are resolved. Care plans can be effective as a communication tool when they are available to everyone involved in the care of the patient. They can also be helpful in providing continuity and consistency of care.

Nurse's notes are records by the nurse of nursing information. Each hospital or clinic has a preferred style of charting in the nurse's notes. It may simply be a narrative statement regarding nursing assessments and actions and the patient's response, or any other information relevant to the patient or her condition; or it may be in the format of a problem-oriented record (POR) using the SOAP format described below. In this method, the patient's problems are listed on a separate problem sheet and numbered. The SOAP format is then used in recording the plan for each problem:

S—subjective; problem as seen by the patient

O—objective; observations and findings by examiner and laboratory test results

A—assessment; conclusion reached after analyzing subjective and objective data

P—plan; detailed course of action to be taken regarding problem

Another style of recording in the nurse's notes consists of documenting variances—positive or negative changes—as they occur. In this system, assessment of the patient is recorded every shift, and more often as necessary as changes occur.

Regardless of the style of charting, the information should be pertinent and stated clearly and concisely.

Progress notes may be used in addition to or instead of nurse's notes. When they are used, all members of the health team contribute to them.

The **graphic** is a type of short form on which the vital signs are recorded and graphed. Other concise information, such as fluid intake and output, can also be recorded on the graphic. This form is valuable as a quick reference to determine trends in the direction the temperature is taking, the ratio of fluid intake to output, and other responses to treatment.

The **flow sheet** is a short form that can be used for frequent recordings of a patient's vital signs and other aspects of her condition, such as height and tone of fundus, amount of lochia, and the like, in the immediate postpartum period. By a quick glance at the flow sheet used during recovery following delivery, the nurse can readily detect fluctuations in blood pressure and other changes in the patient's condition. The flow sheet is a convenient tool for recording daily postpartum and newborn assessments.

The **Kardex** is a short form on which pertinent information, including the nursing-care plan, can be recorded and easily updated. It is available to all care-givers.

The **discharge summary** usually contains a brief description of the patient's condition, a short review of specific instructions, and a statement regarding the patient's understanding of teaching regarding her condition or self-care. Any follow-up care is stated in detail. The discharge summary is useful in providing continuity of care and as a general evaluation of the patient's response to care.

LEGAL ACCOUNTABILITY

Each health care facility usually has *Standards of Care* that act as guidelines for the nurse in the performance of her duties. These may be spelled out by the specific institution in its policy and procedure manual or by an accrediting agency such as the Joint Commission on Accreditation of Hospitals (JCAH), or they may be recognized as the accepted practices and policies of a community. It is the responsibility of the nurse to acquaint herself with the standards of care in the area of her practice, for she is legally accountable for performing her nursing duties in harmony with them.

The nurse is also legally responsible for performing her duties within the scope of nursing function as defined by the nurse practice act in her state and according to her level of skill and training. A nurse who fails to meet the standards of care or who does not stay within the legally established boundaries of care for her level of expertise may jeopardize her patient's safety and may, as a result, cause legal action to be brought against herself and her employer.

Another area of legal significance is the recording, or charting, by the nurse. Her observations of her patient's condition, the nursing actions or interventions she performed in response to her observations, and the results of her nursing care should be carefully charted. Entries should be made frequently throughout the shift and a summary statement entered at the end of the shift. Because a written record of specific actions recorded at the time they occurred is more reliable than memory when legal actions are taken, the importance of accurate, pertinent charting is obvious.

BIBLIOGRAPHY

Bryn RM: The new jurisprudence. JAMA 236:359, 1976

Cates W Jr et al: Legal abortion mortality in the United States: Epidemiologic surveillance, 1972–1974. JAMA 237:452, 1977

Chol ESC, Hamilton RK: The effects of culture on mother-infant interaction. J Obstet Gynecol Neonatal Nurs 15:256, 1986

Hall RE: The Supreme Court decision on abortion. Am J Obstet Gynecol 116:1, 1973

Jensen MD, Bobak IM: Maternity Care: The Nurse & The Family, 3rd ed, pp 3–43. St. Louis, CV Mosby, 1985

Ladewig PA, London ML, Olds SB: Essentials of Maternal-Newborn Nursing, pp 2–13. Menlo Park, Addison-Wesley, 1986

Little DE, Carnevali DL: Nursing Care Planning, 2nd ed. Philadelphia, JB Lippincott, 1976

Reeder SR, Martin LL: Maternity Nursing, 16th ed, pp 4–5, 58–68. Philadelphia, JB Lippincott, 1987

Sullivan E. et al: Legal abortions in the United States, 1975–1976. Fam Plann Perspect 9:22, 1977

Weinstock E, et al: Legal abortions in the United States since the 1973 Supreme Court decision. Fam Plann Perspect 7:23, 1975

Human
Sexuality 3
and
Reproduction

the
reproductive 5
system

BEHAVIORAL When the goals of this chapter are reached, the student will
OBJECTIVES be able to:

○ *Identify the female external reproductive organs.*

○ *Tell the functions of the acini, sinuses, and tubercles of Montgomery.*

○ *Describe the vagina and list three of its functions.*

○ *Describe the size and location of the uterus and explain how it is held in place.*

○ *Name the three parts and three layers of the uterus.*

○ *Define: ovaries, primordial follicle, graafian follicle, ovulation, corpus luteum.*

○ *Trace the pathway of the ovum from the ovary to the outside of the body.*

○ *Diagram and explain the hormonal control of the menstrual cycle.*

○ *Name and describe the four bones comprising the pelvis.*

○ *Name and describe the three parts of the true pelvis, and explain why pelvic size is important in childbirth.*

○ *Explain how the bladder and rectum may affect and be affected by pregnancy.*

○ *Name the male external organs of reproduction.*

○ *Describe the testes and tell where the sperm are produced.*

○ *Name the components of the spermatic cord.*

○ *Tell which of the following are ducts or passageways for the sperm and which are glands providing fluid for transport of the sperm: epididymis, vas deferens, seminal vesicles, prostate, bulbourethral glands.*

○ *Compare ova and sperm as to appearance, size, and number produced.*

o *Trace the pathway of the sperm from the testis to the outside of the body.*

o *Describe the methods of contraception and evaluate the effectiveness of each method.*

o *List three causes of male infertility and three causes of female infertility.*

o *Discuss recent developments that may help some infertile couples have children.*

o *Prepare a sample nursing care plan for an infertile couple, including assessments, nursing diagnosis, goals, interventions, and evaluation.*

FEMALE REPRODUCTIVE SYSTEM

EXTERNAL REPRODUCTIVE ORGANS

Vulva. The external female organs of reproduction are located from the lower border of the abdomen downward to the anus (Fig. 5-1). They have protective as well as sexual functions.

The uppermost of these structures is the *mons pubis*, situated at the lower border of the abdomen. The name is derived from its shape (*mons* = mountain) and its location (over the pubis). This mound of fatty tissue, which is covered with hair at puberty, protects the delicate tissue it surrounds from trauma. Extending downward and backward from the mons are two folds of fatty tissue that also protect the underlying tissue from trauma. These are the *labia majora* (large lips), containing the sebaceous Bartholin's glands that provide moisture for the entrance to the vagina. At puberty, the labia majora become covered with hair. Within and parallel to the labia majora are two flat, delicate folds of skin that are highly sensitive to manipulation and trauma. These are the *labia minora* (lesser lips).

Important to sexual activity is the *clitoris*, a small, cylindrical, erectile organ located at the upper end of the labia. The clitoris is an extremely sensitive body comparable to the penis in the male. The folds of tissue covering the clitoris create a dimple which, during catheterization, may be mistaken for the opening to the urethra.

The urethra, vagina, Bartholin's glands, and Skene's glands open into a small triangular area enclosed by the labia minora called the *vestibule.*

FIG. 5-1. *Female external reproductive organs.*

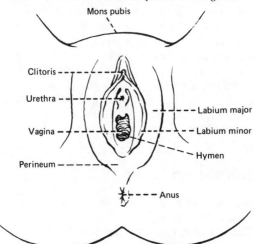

The vaginal opening is surrounded by a fold of mucous membrane called the *hymen*. The hymen is usually lacerated during the first sexual intercourse, with further lacerations occurring during childbirth. An intact hymen was once considered evidence of virginity, while a torn hymen indicated a lack of virginity. Today the condition of the hymen is considered of little significance in determining virginity, since it may be torn or stretched in childhood accidents, in active sports, or by tampons.

Bartholin's glands are two small glands situated one on either side of the vagina. These glands secrete a yellowish mucus that acts as a lubricant during sexual activity.

Skene's glands are two small glands situated just inside the urethra. In acute gonorrhea these glands are almost always infected.

Collectively, these external female organs of reproduction are called the *vulva* or *pudendum.*

Perineum.   The *perineum* is the area extending from the lower border of the vaginal opening downward to the anus. Because of its location, it plays an important part in the birth process. It is made up of the levator ani muscles and fascia, the deep transverse perineal muscles and fascia, and the muscles of the external genitalia. These muscles support the pelvic organs. The pudendal arteries and nerves supply the muscles, fascia, and skin of the perineum. At the time of delivery, an anesthetic agent may be injected into the pudendal nerve so that an incision can be made into the perineum to prevent lacerations of the area.

Breasts.   The breasts are classified with the organs of reproduction because of their functional relationship, that is, to secrete milk for the infant. The two breasts, or mammary glands, are situated on the anterior wall of the chest. Each breast consists of 15 to 20 lobes, and each lobe contains many lobules. The lobules contain many tiny cells called *acini* or *alveoli.* Leading from the lobules are ducts that extend to the surface of the nipple. Near the surface of the breasts, just before reaching the nipples, each duct widens to make a sinus, then narrows again. The acini secrete the milk, which is carried along the ducts to the sinuses near the nipple. The sinuses act as reservoirs to collect the milk until the baby suckles. The pigmented area surrounding the nipples is called the *areola.* Within the areola are sebaceous glands called *tubercles of Montgomery,* which secrete oil that lubricates the nipples, protecting them when the baby suckles (Fig. 5-2). The size of the breasts depends on the amount of fatty tissue deposited between the lobes and does not indicate the amount of milk the breasts will produce.

INTERNAL REPRODUCTIVE ORGANS

The female internal reproductive organs include the vagina, uterus, fallopian tubes, and ovaries (Fig. 5-3).

Vagina.   The vagina is located in the pelvic cavity and is a 3-to 4-inch (7.5- to 10-cm) long curved tube leading from the uterus to the external

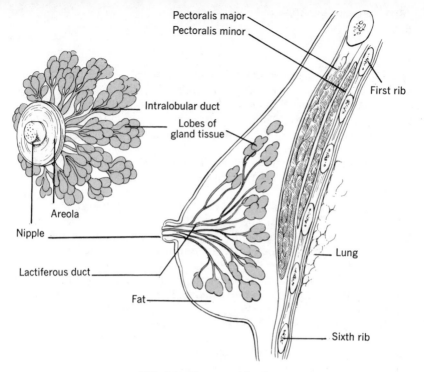

FIG. 5-2. *Mammary gland.*

FIG. 5-3. *Schematic drawing of female reproductive organs, showing path of oocyte from ovary into uterine tube; path of sperm is also shown, as is the usual site of fertilization.*

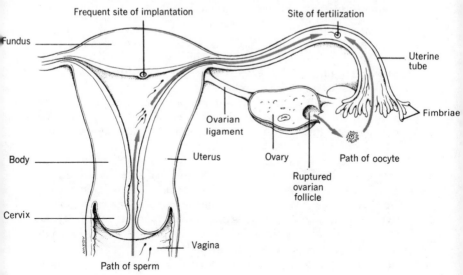

opening in the vestibule, with the urinary bladder in front and the rectum behind. It extends beyond and surrounds the part of the cervix (the *fornix*) of the uterus that protrudes into it. It consists of muscle and connective tissue and is lined with mucous membrane, which contains many folds called *rugae*. The rugae permit considerable stretching of the vagina without tearing.

During sexual intercourse the vagina receives the penis; during menstruation uterine discharges pass through it; and during delivery it is part of the birth canal.

Uterus. The uterus is a hollow, pear-shaped, muscular organ, approximately 1 inch (2.5 cm) thick, 2 inches (5 cm) wide, and 3 inches (7.5 cm) long in a nonpregnant woman. It is situated in the middle of the pelvic cavity between the bladder and the rectum. The uterus is held in place by ligaments that allow its upper portion to be freely movable. The most important of these are the round ligaments and the broad ligaments. During pregnancy the ligaments become pulled and stretched, frequently causing backache.

The uterus has three parts. The upper triangular part is called the *corpus*, or body. On each of its upper corners the corpus is joined to the fallopian tubes. The area of the corpus between the fallopian tubes is called the *fundus*. The lower cylindrical part of the uterus is called the *cervix*. Part of the cervix protrudes into the vagina. The abundant blood supply of the uterus is provided by the uterine and ovarian arteries.

The uterus is composed of three layers:

The *perimetrium*, the outer serous layer that is continuous with the peritoneum

The *myometrium*, the thick, middle muscular layer

The *endometrium*, the inner mucous membrane layer

The myometrium is the largest of the three layers and contains a network of muscle fibers that run in all directions. These muscles are capable of great growth and stretching. The myometrium is thickest in the fundus and thinnest in the cervix. This is significant during labor, since the fundus must contract more forcibly than the lower part of the uterine wall and the cervix must stretch and dilate to permit birth. Interwoven among the muscle fibers are many blood vessels. As the uterus contracts following delivery, these muscle fibers control bleeding by tightening around the blood vessels.

The endometrium is the inner mucous membrane lining of the uterus. It is made up of three layers: (1) a compact surface layer (stratum compactum), (2) a spongy layer of connective tissue (stratum spongiosum), and (3) a dense inner layer (stratum basale) that attaches to the underlying myometrium. Within the spongy layer are branched tubular glands that extend to the myometrium. The blood supply to the endometrium consists of straight arteries to the dense inner layer and spiral arteries to the compact and spongy layers. During menstruation and following birth of a baby, the compact and spongy layers of the endometrium slough off. This is accompanied by bleeding from the torn vessels.

The endometrium lines the cavity of the uterus. This cavity is triangular, with an opening at each point of the triangle. The upper openings join with the fallopian tubes; the lower opening joins the narrow cavity in the cervix called the *cervical canal.* The cervical canal has an opening at each end. The upper opening, the *internal os,* joins with the cavity of the uterus; the lower opening, the *external os,* opens into the vagina.

The uterus is the organ in which the fetus develops and grows and from which it is expelled when mature. The lining of the uterus, the endometrium, sloughs off and is discharged during menstruation.

Fallopian tubes. The two fallopian tubes are approximately 4 inches (10 cm) long. They are joined to the upper corners of the uterus, one on each side. Each tube extends laterally from the uterus to the ovary on the same side. The end of the fallopian tube nearest the ovary is spread out and contains fingerlike projections known as *fimbriae.* These fimbriated ends of the tubes receive the ovum as it is expelled from the ovary. Within each fallopian tube is a tiny canal extending the length of the tube; the mucous membrane lining of the canals contain *cilia.* The wavelike movements of the cilia, along with the peristaltic action of the tube, propel the ovum along the tube toward the uterus. The mucosa of the tubes is continuous with that of the uterus and vagina and therefore often becomes infected by gonococci or other organisms introduced into the vagina. Because it is also continuous with the peritoneum, inflammation of the tubes (salpingitis) may readily spread to become inflammation of the peritoneum (peritonitis), a serious condition. In the male there is no such direct connection by which microorganisms can reach the peritoneum from the exterior.

FUNCTIONS OF THE UTERUS

o Menstruation—sloughing of the compact and spongy layers of the endometrium with bleeding from torn vessels.

o Pregnancy—houses and supports fetus.

o Labor—contractions of muscular wall and dilation of cervix force fetus down and out of uterus.

The *ovum* is the egg cell produced by the female. It is about 0.2 mm in diameter and relatively immobile. It contains a nucleus and much cytoplasm. The nucleus of the ovum is a small spherical body within the cytoplasm enclosed in a nuclear membrane. Within the nucleus are the chromosomes containing the genes, which determine the hereditary characteristics of the individual. The cytoplasm is enclosed in a cell membrane and contains a store of food (yolk and other granules of varying sizes, weights, and chemical compositions) that is readily available should the ovum be fertilized.

Ovaries. The ovaries are two small, almond-shaped glands located on either side of the uterus. The ovaries are the female sex glands and are connected to the uterus by the *ovarian ligaments.* At birth the ovaries contain hundreds of thousands of immature follicles called *primordial,* or *primary, follicles.* One of these follicles ripens or matures each month from puberty until menopause. The mature follicle, known as the *graafian follicle,* contains the ovum. Once a month a graafian follicle ruptures and the mature ovum is expelled; this process is called *ovulation.* Ovulation usually occurs 14 days before the beginning of the next menstrual period.

In addition to producing, maturing, and expelling ova, the ovaries also produce the hormones estrogen and progesterone. *Estrogen* is the female sex hormone responsible for the development of the distinctive female characteristics, such as the breasts. *Progesterone* is necessary for reproduction, since it prepares the endometrium for pregnancy and maintains it during pregnancy. It also suppresses ovulation during pregnancy. Both estrogen and progesterone are active in breast development: estrogen stimulates growth of the ducts of the mammary glands and progesterone stimulates development of the alveoli, the cells that actually secrete milk.

MENSTRUAL CYCLE

The menstrual cycle is controlled by interaction among hormones produced by several glands. The anterior lobe of the *pituitary gland* secretes two hormones that influence ovarian activity. These are the follicle-stimulating hormone (FSH) and the luteinizing hormone (LH). The *hypothalamus* secretes FSH- and LH-releasing hormones that stimulate the anterior lobe of the pituitary gland to produce FSH and LH. The hypothalamus is a part of the brain that is located just above the pituitary gland and is connected to it by blood vessels; it is connected to the central nervous system by neurons. The two hormones (estrogen and progesterone) produced by the *ovaries,* in turn, not only bring about changes in the endometrium of the uterus but also influence the production of FSH and LH.

Beginning on the first day of the menstrual cycle, the anterior lobe of the pituitary gland secretes FSH. FSH stimulates the primordial follicle in the ovary to grow and develop into a mature, or graafian, follicle. As the follicle grows it produces estrogen in increasing amounts. The estrogen stimulates the endometrium of the uterus to thicken and its glandular activity to increase. By about the 10th day of the menstrual cycle the follicle is mature and the estrogen level is high. As the estrogen increases, FSH decreases and LH increases. On about the 14th day of the menstrual cycle the graafian follicle, under the influence of LH, ruptures, expelling the mature ovum. The follicle, still under the influence of LH, becomes a yellowish body called the *corpus luteum.*

The corpus luteum secretes progesterone and some estrogen. For pregnancy to occur, the ovum must be fertilized within 48 hours after ovula-

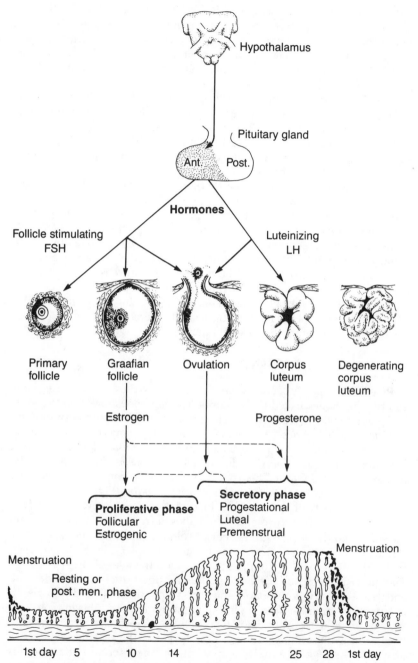

FIG. 5-4. *Hormonal control of the normal menstrual cycle.*

tion. When fertilization does occur, it takes about 6 to 8 days for the fertilized ovum to become embedded in the endometrium prepared for it. The corpus luteum then continues to produce progesterone and estrogen to maintain the thickened endometrium until the placenta produces these hormones in sufficient quantity to maintain the endometrium throughout pregnancy.

If pregnancy does not occur, the corpus luteum is maintained for about 8 days and then begins to regress, eventually disappearing completely. This regression brings about a reduction in the amount of progesterone and estrogen produced. As these hormones decrease, the endometrium sloughs off, and another menstrual cycle begins (Fig. 5-4). The unfertilized ovum is cast out with the menstrual flow.

A woman who plans to use the rhythm method to space her pregnancies needs to know when she ovulates each month. To find out when ovulation probably occurs, she can take her temperature, either rectally or orally, immediately on awakening and before getting out of bed each morning. An accurate recording of the temperature is graphed (Fig. 5-5). Usually, a drop in temperature immediately precedes ovulation; a rise in temperature follows ovulation. The rise in temperature is believed due to the high progesterone levels following ovulation. If pregnancy is desired, intercourse should take place the same day or evening following the drop in temperature. If pregnancy is not desired, intercourse should not take place for 5 days before and 3 days after ovulation.

PELVIS AND PELVIC ORGANS

Pelvis. The pelvis is composed of four bones: the *coccyx*, the *sacrum*, and two hip bones called the *os coxae*. The hip bones make up the sides and front of the pelvis. In the back, the sacrum is situated between and adjoining the hip bones. The coccyx is below, adjoining the sacrum. Each hip bone is made up of three bones fused: the *ilium*, the *ischium*, and the *pubis*. The upper flaring side of each hip bone is the ilium, and the underpart is the ischium. The front part of each hip bone is the pubis. The two pubes join in front to form the *symphysis pubis* (Fig. 5-6).

The upper part of the pelvis, formed by the ilia, is known as the *false pelvis*. The lower part, formed by the pubes in front, the ilia and ischia on the sides, and the sacrum and coccyx behind, is known as the *true pelvis*. The true pelvis has an *inlet*, a *cavity*, and an *outlet* (Fig. 5-7). The brim that separates the false from the true pelvis is the inlet of the true pelvis. The outlet is the space between the ischial tuberosities on the sides, the end of the coccyx in the back, and the symphysis pubis and pubic arch in front. The *cavity* is the area between the symphysis pubis in front and the sacrum and coccyx in back. The cavity is shaped like a curved canal because it is three times as long in the region of the sacrum and coccyx as it is in the region of the symphysis pubis. The internal female organs of reproduction, the urinary bladder, and the rectum are located within the cavity of the true pelvis (Fig. 5-8).

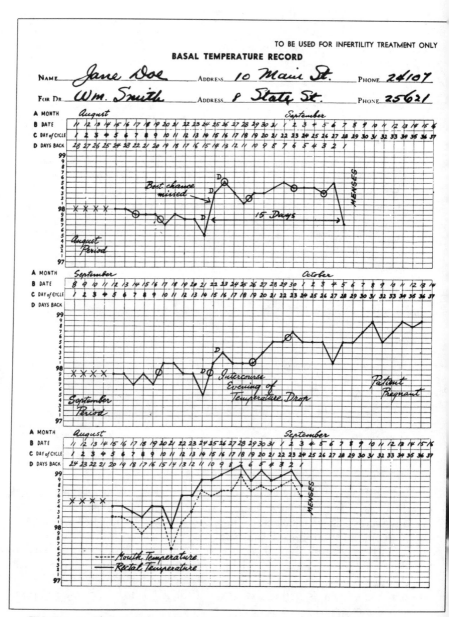

FIG. 5-5. *Basal temperature record is kept to show times of ovulation. (From Margaret Sanger Research Bureau)*

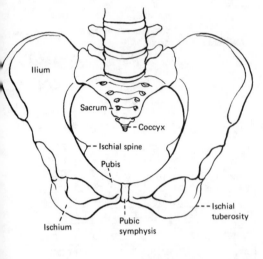

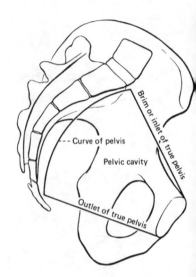

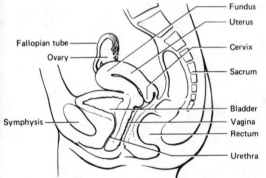

FIG. 5-6 (upper left). *The pelvis.*

FIG. 5-7 (upper right). *Lateral view of the pelvis, showing inlet, outlet, cavity, and curvature.*

FIG. 5-8 (lower left). *Sagittal section of the female pelvis, showing anatomic relationships of the organs.*

The false pelvis supports the growing uterus during pregnancy and directs the fetus into the true pelvis near the end of gestation. Some physicians believe that determining the size of the false pelvis is helpful in estimating the size of the true pelvis. The size of the true pelvis is important because the baby must pass through it in order to be born. If the inlet, the cavity, or the outlet is small, the baby may be unable to pass through it or labor may be prolonged and harder. Measurement of the pelvis is known as *pelvimetry;* x-ray of the pelvis to determine its size is called x-ray pelvimetry (see Chap. 8).

There are important differences between the female pelvis and the male pelvis. The female pelvis is adapted to permit the function of child-bearing. The inlet, the cavity, and the outlet of the true pelvis are larger than in the male. In addition, the arch formed by the pubes is wider and the coccyx is more movable than in the male pelvis (Fig. 5-9).

FEMALE   MALE

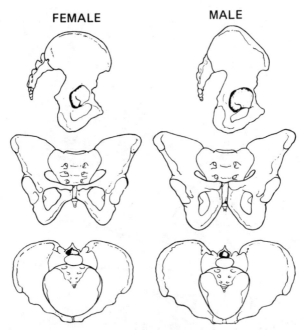

FIG. 5-9. *Contrast in female and male pelvis. (Top) Lateral view. (Middle) Front view. (Bottom) Inlet view.*

Bladder and rectum. The urinary bladder is a musculomembranous organ situated in the pelvic cavity in front of the uterus and vagina. The rectum, the lower end of the alimentary tract, lies behind the uterus and vagina. The bladder and the rectum may influence the position of the uterus and they, in turn, may be influenced by the uterus. As the uterus enlarges during pregnancy, pressure is placed on the bladder, causing frequent urination. Pressure from a full bladder or rectum can affect the position of the uterus.

The external opening of the rectum, the *anus*, has an abundant blood supply. During pregnancy, pressure from the uterus may cause the veins in the anus to become overdistended and form painful masses called hemorrhoids.

MALE REPRODUCTIVE SYSTEM

EXTERNAL REPRODUCTIVE ORGANS

The male external reproductive organs consist of the penis and scrotum (Fig. 5-10).

Penis. The penis is made up of three cylinders of erectile tissue covered by skin. Two of these, the *cavernous bodies*, contain blood spaces

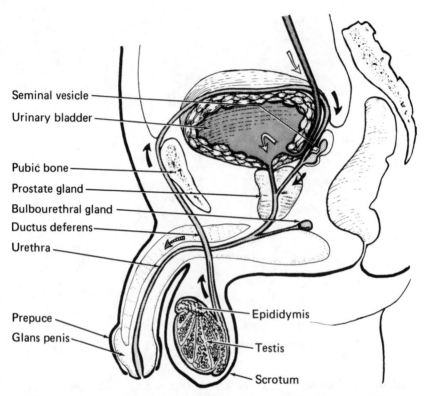

Seminal vesicle
Urinary bladder

Pubic bone
Prostate gland
Bulbourethral gland
Ductus deferens
Urethra

Prepuce
Glans penis

Epididymis

Testis

Scrotum

FIG. 5-10. *Male reproductive system. Dark arrows indicate the direction the sperm travel from the testicle to the exterior. Light arrows show the urinary path from the ureters and bladder.*

that, when empty, cause the penis to be flaccid (limp). When psychic or mechanical sexual stimulation occurs, these spaces fill with blood and the penis becomes swollen, elongated, and stiff. The third cylinder of erectile tissue, the *spongy body*, lies beneath the cavernous bodies. Through it passes the urethra from the bladder. The penis is the male organ of copulation and also part of the urinary system.

The head of the penis is composed of an enlarged portion of the spongy body called the *glans penis*. The glans is covered loosely by a fold of skin known as the *prepuce* or *foreskin*. Circumcision consists of removal of the foreskin for health, religious, or cultural reasons.

Scrotum.   Lying beneath the penis and outside the abdominal cavity is the scrotum, a sac or bag that contains the testes and related structures. The scrotum is divided into two compartments by a wall down the middle. Each compartment contains a testis (testicle), an epididymis, and a portion of the spermatic cord. The temperature of the scrotum is a few degrees cooler than body temperature. This is important, because sperm require a slightly lower temperature for development and maintenance. The optimum temperature for the sperm is promoted by the response to temperature changes of the muscles that hold the scrotum in place. When the internal body temperature increases, these muscles relax so that the scrotum is suspended farther away from the body; when the internal temperature decreases they contract, drawing the scrotum closer to the body.

During early fetal life, the testes are located in the abdominal cavity, but they descend through the inguinal canals into the scrotum about 2 months before birth. Rarely, an infant is born with undescended testicles (a condition known as *cryptorchidism*). This condition can be detected quickly and easily by simple palpation of the scrotum. To prevent permanent sterility caused by exposure of sperm to the higher temperature inside the abdominal cavity, the testes must be brought down into the scrotum surgically.

INTERNAL REPRODUCTIVE ORGANS

The male internal reproductive structures are the testes, epididymis, vas deferens (ductus deferens), seminal vesicles, prostate gland, and bulbourethral glands (Cowper's glands) (see Fig. 5-10).

Testes. The two testes are oval shaped and about 1½ to 2 inches (3.7 to 5 cm) long and 1 inch (2.5 cm) wide. Each testis is divided into about 250 tiny compartments or lobules. Each lobule contains one to three twisted and coiled *seminiferous tubules* in which the spermatozoa are produced. Between the seminiferous tubules are located the cells of Leydig (interstitial cells), which produce testosterone, the male sex hormone.

The internal spermatic arteries supply blood to the testes. These arteries and veins as well as the lymphatic vessels, nerves, and the vas deferens make up the spermatic cord.

Epididymis. The epididymis is a small, firm, oblong body situated behind the testis. It consists of a coiled tube or canal approximately 20 feet (600 cm or 6 m) long when stretched out. The upper end of the epididymis is enlarged to form a head; the lower end is less enlarged to form a tail. The spermatozoa enter the epididymis from the testis and pass through it to the vas deferens.

Vas deferens. The vas deferens, a duct about 18 inches (45 cm) long, is a continuation of the canal of the epididymis. It passes from the epididymis upward through the spermatic cord into the pelvis to the posterior side of the bladder to the point where it joins the duct of the seminal vesicle to form the *ejaculatory duct*. The vas deferens provides a passageway for the spermatozoa from the epididymis to the ejaculatory duct. The ejaculatory duct opens into the portion of the urethra surrounded by the prostate gland.

Seminal vesicles.   The seminal vesicles are two saclike structures located at the base and rear of the bladder. Each vesicle is made up of a 4- to 5-inch (10- to 12.5-cm) thin coiled tube enclosed in a capsule. This tube tapers into a short duct that joins the vas deferens to form the ejaculatory duct. The seminal vesicles produce a secretion that contributes a large portion of the seminal fluid in which the spermatozoa are transported at ejaculation.

Prostate gland.   The prostate gland completely surrounds the urethra just below the bladder. It is composed of glandular tissue enclosed in the fibrous capsule. About 20 to 30 ducts enter the urethra from this gland. Prostate secretions are thin and alkaline; they make up the largest part of the seminal fluid. This alkalinity is important to sperm motility, which is greatest in neutral or slightly alkaline media. (Acid depresses or, if strong enough, kills sperm.) The ejaculatory ducts pass through the upper part of the prostate and open into the urethra.

Bulbourethral glands.   The bulbourethral glands are two small glands about the size of a pea that are situated one on each side of the prostate gland. The ducts of these glands open into the urethra just as it enters the penis. They product a mucoid secretion that also forms part of the seminal fluid.

The *spermatozoa* are produced in the testes and accumulate in the epididymis. From the epididymis they pass through the vas deferens to the ejaculatory duct and into the urethra in the penis. At intercourse they are deposited by the penis in the vagina. The seminal vesicles, prostate gland, and bulbourethral glands provide secretions that create a fluid medium in which the spermatozoa are sustained and transported.

Spermatozoa are much smaller than ova and resemble tadpoles with oval heads and long tails (Fig. 5-11). They are produced in tremendous

Ovum

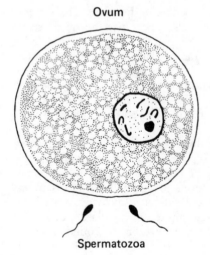

Spermatozoa

FIG. 5-11. *Relative size of ovum and spermatozoa.*

numbers. At each ejaculation about 300 million spermatozoa are deposited in the vagina. Many of these enter the cervix, uterus, and fallopian tubes of the female, but only one penetrates and thereby fertilizes the ovum, if an ovum is available. Once the sperm enters the female reproductive tract it may retain its potential for fertilization for hours or even days.

HUMAN SEXUAL DEVELOPMENT

PUBERTY

Puberty is the transitional period from childhood to adulthood. During this time certain changes occur that signal the approach of sexual and therefore reproductive maturity.

In boys, the changes that occur during puberty include the growth of hair on the face and chest, under the axilla, and on the pubes; voice changes; growth of the testes and penis; an increase in body growth; and muscular development. Puberty generally begins later in boys than in girls and covers a period of 2 to 3 years.

The changes that occur in girls during puberty include growth of axillary and pubic hair; an increase in the size of the external genitalia; growth and maturing of the breasts;.a sudden increase in body growth; and the onset of menstruation. The physical changes that characterize sexual maturity are accompanied by emotional growth and maturing. Puberty in girls covers a period of 4 or 5 years.

MENSTRUATION

Menstruation is the periodic discharge of blood, mucus, and epithelial cells from the uterine mucosa. The first menstrual period is called the *menarche*. The onset of the menstrual cycle usually occurs simultaneously with the onset of the ovarian ovulatory cycle. Therefore, with the onset of menstruation, the individual is considered capable of reproduction. Once established, menstrual periods continue to occur at more or less regular intervals from puberty to the menopause, except during pregnancy and early lactation.

The age at which menstruation begins varies considerably, influenced by factors such as race, climate, heredity, nutrition, and environment. In the United States the onset is usually between the ages of 12 and 16, with the average being 12 or 13.

Most commonly menstruation occurs at 26- to 31-day intervals and lasts 3 to 7 days. The total amount of blood lost by a healthy woman during a normal menstrual period is 25 to 60 ml. However, there is wide variation in the intervals between periods, the duration of the period, and the amount of flow.

There should be no pain associated with a normal menstrual period. However, just prior to their periods, some women experience a feeling of fullness in the pelvis and breasts that may be accompanied by slight nausea, headache, and, occasionally, by skin eruptions on the face. Painful menstruation is called *dysmenorrhea* and may be caused by psychological or physical factors.

Personal hygiene is important at any time and becomes even more so during the menstrual period. Although there are considerable differences between individuals regarding the frequency of menstrual periods, as well as their duration and the amount of flow, usually each person develops a pattern that is fairly consistent for her. She can therefore be alert to her particular pattern and be prepared to cope with its appearance in a healthful manner. There are numerous commercial products on the market for both external and internal use in coping with the flow. One should decide which type best meets her needs and keep a supply on hand. Frequent baths or showers, as well as frequent changes of pad or tampon, are essential to cleanliness and a sense of well-being during the menstrual period.

The purpose of menstruation has often been questioned. Probably the most logical explanation is that it is the casting out of the "nest" which the body prepares each month in anticipation of the fertilized egg. When the egg is not fertilized, the nest is not needed and is subsequently discarded. Normal menstruation is not an illness, and under normal circumstances the healthy individual need not curtail her usual activities during her period.

MENOPAUSE

The female reproductive potential persists from puberty until the menopause, an average time of about 35 years. The *menopause* is the permanent cessation of the menstrual periods. The age at which the menopause occurs varies, with about one half of women experiencing it between the ages of 45 and 50, one fourth before the age of 45, and one fourth after the age of 50. The menstrual periods may stop abruptly, or the flow may gradually decrease in amount until it ceases altogether, or the periods may be spaced farther apart until they stop completely.

The critical period in a woman's life when menstruation ceases and the ovaries stop producing estrogen is known as the *climacteric*. Lay people call it "the change of life." The climacteric may last from 1 to 4 or 5 years. As with any aspect of life, women react differently to this time in their lives. Some women go through the climacteric experiencing few or none of the annoyances it causes others.

As a result of the diminishing supply of estrogen during the climacteric, some women periodically experience a sudden surge of heat flooding the body from feet to head. The woman has no control over this excessive production of heat, which may occur at any time or place regardless of the temperature of the environment. The term "hot flash" has been used to describe this condition, which comes on suddenly and lasts from 30 to 60 seconds. As the hot flash occurs, the face becomes flushed and, as the heat reaches its peak, the face and body become covered with perspiration. Because the facial flushing and perspiration are quite visible for anyone to see, this may be a source of embarrassment to the woman, who may already be extremely uncomfortable from the wave of heat. In severe hot flashes the woman may become nauseated and feel as if she were suffocating.

Other symptoms that may occur during the climacteric include growth of hair on the chin or lip, severe mood changes with excessive irritability, pain and weakness in the shoulders and thighs, and swelling of the joints.

Careful medical checkups, good nutrition, rest, exercise, appropriate clothing, and good personal hygiene are important to the well-being of the woman during the climacteric.

FAMILY PLANNING

The rapid increase in the population during this century has been cause for concern. This concern is based on the knowledge that when the population exceeds the resources available to sustain it, suffering and deprivation result. Overpopulation can result in malnutrition or starvation, overcrowded schools, inadequate housing, spreading ghettos, diminished employment opportunities, traffic congestion and inadequate transportation, decrease in open space and land for recreation, and a shortage of medical personnel and facilities to adequately care for the sick.

Two outstanding reasons are apparent for suggesting population control to the individual family. First, there is the high cost of providing for the needs of a family. Second, in the urban and suburban areas, where most of the population tends to congregate, there is limited space for family dwellings.

Couples who wish to limit the size of their families have access to several safe and effective methods of contraception (Fig. 5-12). The method chosen by a couple should be psychologically acceptable as well as physically suitable to their needs.

Oral contraceptive. The "pill" is an oral contraceptive composed of synthetic estrogenlike or progesteronelike compounds, or both. It acts by building up a high blood concentration of these substances and thereby preventing the development of a follicle and its ovum each month. Since there is no mature ovum to be expelled, ovulation does not occur, and consequently pregnancy cannot occur.

Originally, the pill was taken every day for 20 days, beginning on the fifth day of the menstrual cycle. Three or four days after the pill was stopped, menstruation occurred. Beginning on the fifth day of the cycle, the pill was taken again for 20 days, and so forth. The pill can still be

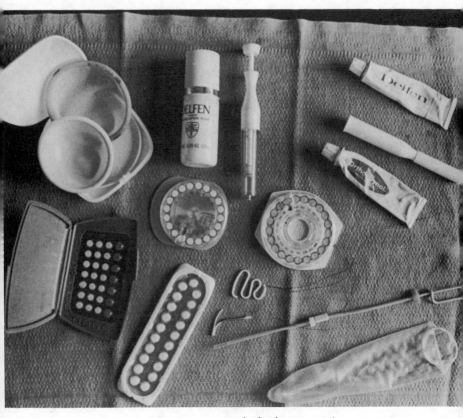

FIG. 5-12. *Common methods of contraception.*

taken this way, and in most instances it probably is. However, there are also other ways to take it. It can be taken for 3 weeks and then stopped for one week. A woman who takes it this way can control when her menstrual periods occur by starting and stopping the pill on the same day each month. It is also possible to get the pill in packages of 28 so that a pill is taken every day. By taking a pill every day there is less chance of forgetting to take it. The last seven pills for each cycle are not birth control pills but rather are placebos.

The pills come in calendar packs, dial packs, and punch packs, among others, which specify the day or date that each pill is to be taken. This helps the woman remember to take them; it is also helpful if she places them near something that she uses each day, such as her toothbrush or alarm clock. Taking them at the same time each day establishes a habit and reduces the chance of forgetting.

While she is on the pill, the woman may notice that her menstrual flow is decreased and that she does not have cramps. The advantages of the pill, when taken as directed, are that it is one of the most effective contraceptives; also, it is convenient, inexpensive, and aesthetically acceptable in that its use is separate from the sex act.

The use of oral contraceptives is not without risks, some of which are so serious that the Food and Drug Administration (FDA) requires that a patient information sheet, explaining the risks, be included with each packet of pills sold. Women who take oral contraceptives are more likely than nonusers to develop venous and arterial thromboembolism, thrombotic and hemorrhagic stroke, myocardial infarction, visual disorders, hepatic tumors, gallbladder disease, and hypertension. If a woman becomes pregnant while on the pill or soon after discontinuing it, there is an increased risk of fetal abnormalities. Estrogen, a component of oral contraceptives, may increase the risk of uterine cancer when given for periods of more than 1 year to women after the menopause. Although studies have not confirmed that oral contraceptives cause cancer in humans, when certain animals are given estrogen continuously for long periods, cancers may develop in the breasts, cervix, vagina, and liver.

The risks associated with use of oral contraceptives increase with age, so that women who are over 40 years old probably should not use this method of contraception. In addition, the risks are so great to women who are heavy smokers and to women who presently have, or who have a history of hypertension, diabetes, pregnancy-induced hypertension, or hyperlipoproteinemia, that they probably should not use oral contraceptives at any age. Women who now have, or who have had in the past, such conditions as heart or kidney disease, hepatic disease or jaundice, thrombophlebitis, stroke, migraine headaches, fibroid tumors or cancer of the uterus, breast nodules or abnormal mammograms, or gallbladder disease probably should use some other method of contraception.

Adverse reactions that may be experienced with the use of oral contraceptives include nausea, vomiting, abdominal cramps, spotting, edema, amenorrhea, chloasma, tenderness and enlargement of the breasts, breast secretions, jaundice, migraine headaches, allergic rash, elevated blood pressure, alopecia, and mental depression.

A woman who uses oral contraceptives should have periodic checkups by her physician. When she wants to become pregnant she should discontinue the pill and use another contraceptive method for at least 3 months before becoming pregnant. This is to decrease the risk of fetal abnormalities caused by the pill.

Intrauterine device. An intrauterine device (IUD) is a small, flexible appliance in the form of a spiral, loop, or ring that is made of plastic tubing, nylon thread, or stainless steel (Fig. 5-13). This device is inserted into the uterine cavity by a physician, a specially trained nurse, or a midwife. Many of these devices have a nylon string attached that rests in the vagina after the device is in place. The woman can reassure herself that the device is in place by locating the string, which also makes removal of the device easy.

The exact way IUDs prevent pregnancy is not known. They are effec-

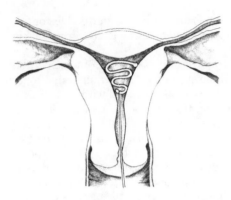

FIG. 5-13. *Intrauterine device positioned in the uterine cavity.*

tive in 97% of cases when they are retained for 6 to 9 months. Until it is retained for that long, the woman should check prior to intercourse to make sure that it is in place. The advantages of this method are that it has fewer side effects than the pill; it is second only to the pill in effectiveness; it is inexpensive; it can be easily removed when children are desired; and the woman need not worry about contraception except to check occasionally to make sure that it is in place. There are disadvantages to IUDs. About 10% to 30% of women cannot tolerate them either because of the cramps and bleeding they cause or because they are expelled spontaneously. It is believed by some authorities that there is an increase in the incidence of pelvic inflammatory disease with use of IUDs, but others disagree. In rare instances, IUDs have caused perforation of the uterus.

Diaphragm.   The diaphragm is a shallow rubber cup that may vary in size from 7 to 10 cm. It is filled with a sperm-killing cream or jelly and before intercourse is inserted into the vagina to cover the cervix (Fig. 5-14). The purpose of the diaphragm is to hold the sperm-killing preparation against the opening of the cervix during and for at least 6 hours after intercourse. The advantages of the diaphragm are that it is inexpensive and free from side effects (except in rare cases of allergy to the spermicides or to rubber), and when used properly, it is effective. The disadvantages are that it is messy; it requires planning, which detracts from the spontaneity of sex; after one or more pregnancies some women cannot be fitted with a diaphragm; and the vaginal manipulation necessary to insert the arc flex diaphragm is objectionable to some women. However, this latter disadvantage can be overcome by the use of the flat or coil spring diaphragm, which has an inserter.

Condom.   The condom is a thin sheath made of rubber or fine material that is used to cover the penis and collect semen during intercourse. The advantages of the condom are that it is cheap, easily available, can be used without medical advice, and, when put on before any penetration, it is safe. The disadvantage to this method is that it lessens sexual pleasure.

Rhythm. The rhythm method of contraception requires knowing when ovulation occurs. The woman who has regular menstrual cycles may have no difficulty finding out when she ovulates, since ovulation occurs approximately 14 days before the onset of menstruation. However, even in regular menstrual cycles, menstruation may occur 1 or 2 days early or 1 or 2 days late. When this happens ovulation will also vary.

The woman who has irregular menstrual cycles may, theoretically, determine the time of ovulation by taking her temperature every morning and recording it (see Fig. 5-5). When there is a rise in her temperature that is sustained for 3 days, she can assume that ovulation has occurred and that she will not become pregnant if she has intercourse.

Whether her periods are regular or irregular, the woman using this method should know that, although the ovum is capable of being fertilized for only 48 hours after ovulation, the sperm may survive and be able to fertilize the ovum for as long as 5 days after ejaculation. This means that if the rhythm method is to be effective, there should be no intercourse for at least 5 days before ovulation, on the day of ovulation, and for 2 days following ovulation. In addition, allowance must be made for variations of a day or two in the menstrual cycle.

This method is effective for some couples and is the only contraceptive method approved by the Roman Catholic church. The disadvantages are that it requires self-control, necessitates the keeping of accurate records of daily body temperatures if the menstrual cycle is irregular, and is the least effective of the methods.

Coitus interruptus. This method involves withdrawal of the penis from the vagina before sperm are deposited. The disadvantages to this method are that it requires concentration and willpower on the part of the man and may lead to frustration and conflicts in the husband-wife relationship. Also, it is unreliable because some sperm usually escape prior to orgasm.

Jellies, creams, and suppositories. The use of spermicidal creams, jellies, and suppositories is usually ineffective because the woman cannot be sure that they are properly placed and that they stay in place. The advantages are that they are cheap and available without a prescription from a physician.

Foam. Used alone, foam is probably no more effective than jellies, creams, or suppositories. Used in combination with a condom, its effectiveness nearly equals that of oral contraceptives, without the risks associated with them. When foam is used with a condom, both partners are involved in the contraceptive effort. When a woman discontinues the pill because she wants to become pregnant, foam with the condom can be used effectively for a few months until her hormonal balance is restored and her menstrual cycle is reestablished. Like jellies, creams, and suppositories, foam is inexpensive and available without a physician's prescription. It should be inserted in the vagina no more than one-half hour before intercourse, and it should be used with each intercourse. The woman

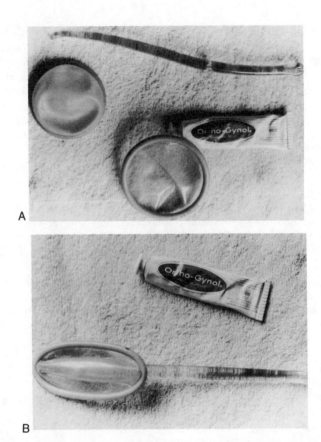

FIG. 5-14. *(A) Diaphragms, spermicidal jelly, and inserter. (B) Diaphragm in position on inserter. (C) Diaphragm with spermicidal cream applied. (D) Diaphragm compressed ready for manual insertion.*

should not douche for at least 8 hours after intercourse when foam is used for contraception.

Lactation. As a contraceptive method lactation is very unreliable. Although menstruation usually does not occur during lactation, ovulation may. The nursing mother should understand that ovulation will occur before she has her first menstrual period.

Sterilization. For those couples who do not want more children, sterilization, a permanent fertility control measure, can be performed. In the woman, sterilization is usually accomplished by tubal ligation or tubal cauterization; it may also be accomplished by removal of the uterus (hysterectomy). Removal of both of the ovaries (oophorectomy) or removal of both of the fallopian tubes (salpingectomy) also results in sterilization, although these procedures are not usually performed for that purpose.

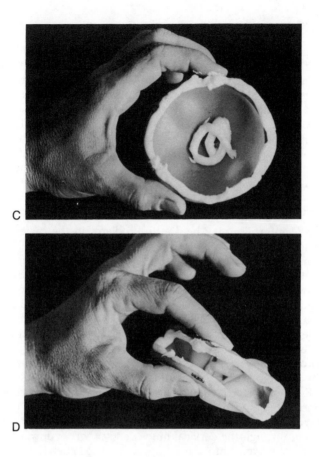

When a tubal ligation is done, each fallopian tube is ligated (tied) in two places about an inch apart. Then a segment of the tube between the ties is cut and removed, thus preventing the sperm and ovum from meeting. This procedure is accomplished through an abdominal incision or through the vagina. Cauterization of the tubes is usually accomplished by laparoscopy. The laparoscope is inserted through a small incision in the umbilicus after the abdomen has been distended with carbon dioxide. The tubes and ovaries are visualized and then the tubes are grasped with a coagulating instrument, cauterized, and severed.

Sterilization can be accomplished in the man by vasectomy. In this procedure an incision is made into the upper part of the scrotum and the sperm-carrying tube, the vas deferens, is severed.

The failure rate in tubal ligation and vasectomy is about 1%. Neither procedure affects the capacity for or the pleasure of sexual relations.

INFERTILITY

Infertility is the inability to produce offspring. For a couple to produce offspring, the man must have an intact nervous system so that erection and ejaculation can occur, and he must be capable of producing healthy, motile sperm in sufficient quantity and quality. The woman must be able to produce a healthy ovum and must have healthy, open fallopian tubes through which the ovum and sperm can travel and meet. The sperm must be able to travel to the ovum and unite with it at the optimal time for conception. The fertilized ovum must have proper and adequate nourishment and a protected environment in which to thrive and develop. Failure in any aspect of these requirements may result in infertility.

MALE INFERTILITY

The cause of infertility may be due to problems in the male or in the female. The most common causes of infertility in the male relate to the production, motility, transportation, or deposition of the sperm.

Production. A normal ejaculate consists of 2 to 5 ml of semen containing more than 20 million sperm per milliliter. These sperm must be of good quality and highly motile. Any of the following may so affect the production of sperm as to decrease their number to levels that are incompatible with fertility: (1) high fever, (2) orchitis following mumps, (3) excessive exposure to radiation, (4) varicocele or undescended testicle, (5) malformation or atrophy of the testicles, (6) serious trauma or castration, or (7) prolonged or continuous temperature elevation within the testicles. Emotional stress, extreme fatigue, or ingestion of certain drugs may temporarily decrease sperm production.

Motility. The motility of sperm is vital to fertility since sperm must be able to swim through the cervical mucus and progress upward through the uterine cavity and into the fallopian tube to meet the ovum. The motility of sperm may be hampered by (1) a decrease in the amount of secretions from the prostate gland as a result of chronic prostatitis or by an absence of secretions following removal of the prostate gland, (2) immunologic reactions in which a man produces antibodies against his own sperm, (3) hormonal factors, (4) an excessively high sperm count, or (5) very infrequent sexual relations.

Transportation. Stricture or blockage of the passageway through which sperm must travel from their origin to the exterior may prevent transportation of sperm. Most commonly this blockage is related to (1) scarring and adhesions caused by infections such as venereal disease, (2) trauma to the vas deferens during surgical repair of inguinal hernia, or (3) vasectomy, which is the severing of the vas deferens for the purpose of sterilization.

Deposition. Premature ejaculation, impotence, congenital malformations of the penis such as hypospadias or epispadias, improper sexual technique, or problems such as spinal cord injury may prevent the sperm from being deposited properly within the vagina.

FEMALE INFERTILITY

Common causes of infertility in the female include (1) mechanical barriers to union of ovum and sperm, (2) endocrine problems, and (3) structural defects.

Mechanical barriers. Any blockage of the passageway in the female reproductive tract that prevents the sperm and ovum from meeting results in infertility. Scarring and adhesions in the cervix, uterus, fallopian tubes, or around the ovaries may cause blockage. Blockage may result from infections such as gonorrhea or peritonitis following a ruptured appendix. Endometriosis, a condition in which endometrial tissue grows in abnormal places such as the tubes, ovaries, or peritoneal cavity and bleeds during menstruation, also causes scarring and adhesions that may result in infertility.

Endocrine problems. Ovulation is essential to fertility. Ovulation does not occur in congenital absence of the ovaries and following surgical removal of the ovaries. When any of the endocrine glands that regulate the menstrual cycle fail to function properly, a hormonal imbalance may occur and ovulation may cease or may occur infrequently. Hormonal imbalance with a decrease in estrogen secretion may cause the cervical mucus to become hostile rather than receptive to the sperm. Decreases in progesterone secretion may prevent the normal buildup of the endometrium necessary for the maintenance of the fertilized ovum.

Structural problems. Infertility in the female may be caused by such structural problems as congenital absence or surgical removal of the uterus, ovaries, or tubes; multiple fibroid tumors; congenital malformation of the uterus; or extreme malposition of the uterus.

DIAGNOSIS OF INFERTILITY

When a couple decides to seek help in finding the cause of their inability to have children, both partners should be evaluated. In the cases where the cause of infertility can be determined, approximately 35% of the problems are due to the male and approximately 35% to the female. About 30% are due to combined male–female problems. In about 10% of all cases of infertility, no definite cause can be found.

Medical history. Early in the workup, a thorough medical history of each partner should be obtained. Such disclosures as past venereal disease in either or both, or surgical procedures such as inguinal hernia repair or vasectomy in the man or hysterectomy, oophorectomy, salpingectomy, or dilation and curettage in the woman may be extremely helpful to the investigation. The menstrual cycle pattern and the frequency and technique of sexual relations should also be ascertained. Information relating to the occupation and habits of each partner may reveal excessive exposure to radiation or the use of certain drugs that affect fertility.

Physical examination. A complete physical examination of each partner, including a thorough pelvic examination of the woman, should be done. Structural defects or other obvious health problems that can cause infertility may be detected during the examination, making further testing unnecessary. If the history and physical examination reveal no apparent reason for the couple's inability to have children, they must then decide whether to continue to search for the cause. They should understand that further testing may take considerable time to complete, may be expensive and painful, and involves the risks of not finding the cause or of finding a cause that is not correctable. If the couple chooses to submit to further testing, it should be started with the man because it is easier, less expensive, and less painful to test him.

Tests. An infertility study may include semen analysis, postcoital testing, tubal insufflation, hysterosalpingography, laparoscopy or culdoscopy, and endometrial biopsy. A *semen sample* is evaluated for volume, sperm density, percentage of motile forms, quality of the motility of the sperm, and the percentage of abnormal sperm. The *postcoital test* is done on a sample of mucus taken from the cervix within 12 hours after intercourse. The couple is instructed to have intercourse a day or two before ovulation is expected. At this time, because of high estrogen levels, the cervical mucus is normally clear and abundant and most receptive to sperm. This test provides information regarding the proper deposition of sperm, as well as the quality of the cervical secretions and their ability to support the life of the sperm. When more than 20 sperm per high-power field are present in areas of clear, abundant mucus, the test result is considered normal.

Tubal insufflation and hysterosalpingography are tests to determine the patency of the fallopian tubes. In *tubal insufflation* (the Rubin test), carbon dioxide is blown under controlled pressure into the uterus and tubes. When there is no obstruction present, the carbon dioxide flows through the uterus and tubes out into the peritoneal cavity. Pain in the shoulder is then experienced by most women when they sit up. If an obstruction is present, additional pressure is exerted, within safe limits, until no more carbon dioxide can be inserted. Occasionally, the pressure from the gas will remove small adhesions, and the patency of tubes will be restored.

Hysterosalpingography is performed in the radiology department. A radiopaque material is placed into the uterus and fallopian tubes. Fluoroscopy is used to observe the path of the material as it travels through the uterus and, if no interference is encountered, through the tubes and out into the peritoneal cavity. X-rays are taken as the material moves along so that a permanent record is available for study.

This test is scheduled during the first half of the menstrual cycle (2 to 6 days after cessation of the menstrual flow), in order to avoid irradiation of a conceptus, in case the woman should be pregnant and not be aware of it. If an oil-based dye is used, hysterosalpingography may actually correct an infertility problem due to blockage of tubes caused by adhesions or mucous plugs, or due to sluggish tubal activity. In such instances, the dye acts like a hydrostatic wedge to separate adhesions, dislodge mucous plugs, and stimulate tubal cilia.

Direct visualization of the ovaries and tubes is accomplished by inserting an endoscope through the cul-de-sac (*culdoscopy*) or through the umbilicus (*laparoscopy*). While the examiner is looking through the endoscope, the patency of the tubes can be determined by injecting dye into the uterus and observing the ends of the tubes for spillage. The presence of endometriosis and adhesions can also be detected through culdoscopy or laparoscopy.

Because ovulation is vital to fertility, it is important early in the infertility workup to find out if and when the woman ovulates. Some women have no difficulty knowing when they ovulate because of the discomfort they experience at this time. This discomfort is referred to as "mittelschmerz" because it occurs midway between menstrual periods. Others experience no discomfort and have no way of knowing when ovulation occurs. Methods used to find out when ovulation occurs include obtaining a history of the menstrual periods, using the basal body temperature graph (see Fig. 5-5), and examining a sample of the cervical mucus for the characteristic changes that occur in it during ovulation. In addition, *biopsy of the endometrium* can be performed during the latter part of the menstrual cycle. Endometrial biopsy can also provide information as to the quality of the lining in preparation for the implantation and maintenance of the fertilized ovum. Late in the menstrual cycle, blood samples may be taken to determine the plasma progesterone levels.

TREATMENT OF INFERTILITY

Treatment of infertility consists of correcting the cause if one is found and is correctable. Temporary use of hormone therapy in the man may be beneficial to improve the quantity and quality of sperm if normal sperm-producing tissue is present. He can be advised to avoid prolonged use of athletic supports, frequent hot showers, saunas, or other things that can cause temperature elevation in the testicles. Surgery can be performed to correct varicocele or undescended testicles. Antibiotics can be prescribed in cases of chronic prostatitis to improve sperm motility. Steroid therapy may also be helpful in improving sperm motility. The couple may be encouraged to have sexual relations more frequently during the woman's fertile time of the month, since it appears that sperm motility improves with frequent sexual activity. Correction of blockage of the vas deferens may be impossible, although occasionally surgery is successful. Sexual counseling may be helpful to the couple whose problem is the improper deposition of sperm.

The woman who does not ovulate or who ovulates infrequently may be treated with drug therapy. Among the more common drugs used to stimulate ovulation are clomiphene citrate (Clomid) and human menopausal gonadotropin (hMG). The use of these drugs, particularly hMG, may overstimulate the ovaries so that more than one ovum is released in a cycle. Multiple pregnancies may then occur.

When endometriosis is the cause, treatment consists of surgical removal or cautery of all visible areas of endometrial tissue and surgical removal of adhesions. This may be followed by administration of estrogen and progesterone in amounts sufficient to suppress menstruation. These levels are comparable to those attained during a normal pregnancy and, in effect, create a "pseudopregnancy." This appears to be effective in treating endometriosis because the increased hormone levels cause degeneration and death of the endometrial tissue found outside the uterus.

Antibiotics can be prescribed for infections that are causing infertility. In some instances surgery may be helpful in removing adhesions or scarring in the uterus or in correcting certain congenital problems such as a bicornuate uterus. Surgical removal of fibroid tumors of the uterus may be effective treatment for these problems. Correction of mechanical barriers, such as blockage of the fallopian tubes, may be difficult or impossible.

HELP FOR INFERTILE COUPLES

Until recently, a couple with an infertility problem of unknown or uncorrectable etiology had little hope of having a family. They could choose to remain childless, try artificial insemination of the wife with donor semen, or adopt children. With advances in technology, however, other possibilities are now available. Among these are surrogate embryo transfer, *in vitro* fertilization and embryo transfer, and gamete intrafallopian transfer.

In surrogate embryo transfer, a fertile woman is artificially inseminated with sperm from the husband of the infertile couple. About 5 days after fertilization, the uterus is washed out and the embryo is recovered from the washings and transferred to the uterus of the infertile woman. This procedure is technically complex and problems can arise at any stage. In some instances, the surrogate mother is paid by the infertile couple to carry the pregnancy to term. When the baby is delivered it is given to the infertile couple. There are legal and ethical aspects to be considered in both of these situations.

In *in vitro* fertilization and embryo transfer, the infertile woman's ovaries are stimulated by intramuscular doses of hormones to produce and mature follicles. When the egg is mature, laparoscopy is performed and one or more eggs are removed from her ovary. The eggs are fertilized in a laboratory dish with sperm from the husband, cultured to the four- to eight-cell stage, and transferred into the woman's uterus.

In gamete intrafallopian transfer, large doses of hormones are given intramuscularly at precise times to the infertile woman to stimulate follicular development. Pelvic ultrasound or serum estradiol levels are used to determine when the follicles have reached maturity. Then one or more eggs are aspirated from the ovary by laparoscopy and fertilized with sperm from the husband. The fertilized egg is loaded into a catheter. The catheter is inserted through a laparoscope and its contents are deposited into the fallopian tube of the wife through the fimbriated end of the tube. Usually the procedure is repeated for the other fallopian tube.

Although these procedures may result in a much-desired child for the infertile couple, the failure rate is high. Whether the outcome is successful or not, the emotional and financial costs may be tremendous. In addition, some religions disapprove of these methods, and the legal and ethical considerations are yet to be resolved.

THE NURSING PROCESS AND THE INFERTILE COUPLE

To fulfill her role appropriately, the nurse who cares for the infertile couple must be familiar with the diagnostic procedures used and the physiological basis for the tests and treatments performed. This will enable her to supplement and reinforce the doctor's explanations to the couple when necessary. She also must be aware of the emotional impact of childlessness on the couple that wants to conceive. Often they experience frustration, anger, resentment, isolation, guilt, depression, and low self-esteem.

Assessments by the nurse are made through interviewing the couple, reviewing their records, and observing their behavior. The nurse should ascertain the couple's knowledge of the reproductive process, their sexual behavior and techniques, their usual coping behavior (supporting each other, sharing responsibility, or blaming each other), their feelings about their inability to conceive, their understanding of the tests that may be performed, and their understanding of the potential for success or failure.

After *analysis* of the assessment data, the *nursing diagnoses* may include knowledge deficits regarding reproductive anatomy and physiology, foreplay and sexual techniques, and available support groups (such as Resolve, Inc.), which are available in many cities throughout the United States. Other nursing diagnoses may be anxiety, feelings of inadequacy, low self-esteem because of the couple's inability to conceive, and embarrassment and pain due to the procedures and tests performed.

In *planning* the nursing care for the infertile couple, the *goals* would include assisting the couple to obtain the information they need; reducing anxiety, fear, pain, and embarrassment; and helping them to cope.

Implementation of nursing actions or interventions is directed toward resolving the nursing diagnoses and reaching the goals. In infertility cases, the interventions by the nurse might include providing accurate information, allowing time and opportunity for the couple to express their feelings and to ask questions in an accepting atmosphere, explaining procedures and tests before they are done, providing privacy, suggesting ways to reduce the discomfort caused by tests and procedures, and being warm and friendly during each contact with the couple.

Evaluation of the effectiveness of the nursing interventions is done by *listening* to see if the couple verbalize accurate information, and by *observing* a decrease in their anxiety and fear, a display of support for each other, and a positive attitude about themselves.

CLINICAL REVIEW

ASSESSMENT. While you are working in the clinic you become acquainted with Judy, a 17-year-old high school dropout, who is in her sixth month of pregnancy. She is a warm, friendly person and you quickly establish rapport with her. She talks freely to you about herself, her pregnancy, her husband Mike, and their plans for the future. You learn that 18-year-old Mike is also a high school dropout and has had difficulty getting a job. Recently, though, he has been able to get a "good job," as Judy puts it, as a carpenter's helper. They are both happily anticipating the coming of the baby, but Judy admits that she sometimes feels frightened when she thinks about the responsibilities of being a mother.

Judy is 5 feet tall, and before she became pregnant, weighed about 110 lb (50 kg). She has one younger sister and no brothers. This is her first pregnancy. Her menstrual periods started when she was 11 years old, arrive regularly every 28 days, and last 4 days. She has never had any health problems. Mike is 6 feet tall and weighs 165 lb (75 kg). He has two older brothers and one younger sister. Both Judy and Mike are Catholics.

Mike accompanies Judy to the clinic one day when he can't work because of bad weather. He is pleased about the pregnancy, although he confesses that they have a lot to learn because they are "new at this." He expresses amazement that the baby is actually growing inside Judy and wonders how it will ever get out. They confide to you that they have decided that Judy should breast-feed the baby but they wonder if she will be able to since her breasts are small. They also reveal that, although they would love to have a large family, they hope they don't have any more children until they are better able to care for them (Table 5-1).

TABLE 5-1 CLINICAL REVIEW: NURSING CARE PLAN FOR JUDY AND MIKE

NURSING DIAGNOSES	INTERVENTIONS	EXPECTED OUTCOME
Knowledge deficit related to anatomy and physiology of reproduction	Use pictures, charts, etc. to explain anatomy and physiology of reproduction	Couple verbalizes understanding of anatomy and physiology of reproduction
Anxiety related to responsibilities of parenting	Allow time for couple to verbalize their feelings; encourage them to ask questions; answer questions in language they can understand; encourage them to use their parents as resources when they have questions; listen to their concerns and help them deal with them; encourage them to take one day at a time	Anxiety decreased
Fear related to Judy's ability to breast-feed	Discuss physiology of breast-feeding and explain that size of breasts is not important	Fear reduced or eliminated
Anxiety related to controlling size of family	Explain birth control options	Anxiety decreased

1. In considering the nursing care plan for Judy and Mike, what other information might be helpful to you in preparing a more complete care plan for them?
2. What other nursing diagnoses and interventions might be included, using the data available?
3. From the data available, what would you expect would *not* be a problem with this new family?

BIBLIOGRAPHY

Anthony CP, Thibodeau GA: Textbook of Anatomy and Physiology, 10th ed, pp 606–647. St. Louis, CV Mosby, 1979

Chaffee EE, Lytle IM: Basic Physiology and Anatomy, 4th ed, pp 545–547. Philadelphia, JB Lippincott, 1980

Coskey RJ: Eruptions due to oral contraceptives. Arch Dermatol 113:333, 1977.

Dennison CF: Oral contraceptives: Another look at the risks of the pill. Patient Care 10:147, 1976

Hawkins JW, Higgins LP: Maternity and Gynecological Nursing, pp 51–98. Philadelphia, JB Lippincott, 1981

Huxall LK: Today's pill and the individual woman. Am J Maternal-Child Nurs 2:359, 1977

Kane FJ Jr: Evaluation of emotional reactions to oral contraceptive use. Am J Obstet Gynecol 126:968, 1976

Kistner RW, Seigler AM, Behrman SJ: Suggested classification for endometriosis: Relationship to infertility. Fertil Steril 28:1008, 1977

Menning BE: Infertility: Facts and Feelings, 2nd ed. Belmont, MA, Resolve Inc, 1975

Mishell DR Jr: Current status of oral contraceptive steroids. Clin Obstet Gynecol 19:743, 1976

Ortho Patient Information Sheet. Raritan, NJ, Ortho Pharmaceutical Corp., 1978

Reeder SR, Martin LL: Maternity Nursing, 16th ed, pp 146–168, 235–252. Philadelphia, JB Lippincott, 1987

Zeitz AN: Oral contraceptives: Women's rights, nurses' responsibilities. J Obstet Gynecol Neonatal Nurs 5:54, 1976

description and effects 6 of pregnancy

BEHAVIORAL OBJECTIVES When the goals of this chapter are reached, the student will be able to:

○ *Define: conception, parturition, pregnancy, gestation, gravida, para, viable, lunar month, trimester, embryo, fetus.*

○ *Determine a pregnant women's estimated date of confinement using Naegele's rule.*

○ *State the usual length of pregnancy in days, weeks, lunar months, and calendar months.*

○ *Explain why pregnancies vary in duration.*

○ *Give the gestation period in weeks for each of the following: preterm, term, postterm.*

○ *Name the presumptive signs of pregnancy and explain why each is not a reliable indication of pregnancy.*

○ *Name and describe the probable signs of pregnancy.*

○ *Explain the basis for pregnancy tests.*

○ *List the advantages of the immunologic tests for pregnancy.*

○ *Explain why positive pregnancy tests are not considered positive signs of pregnancy.*

○ *Name the positive signs of pregnancy.*

○ *Describe the possible psychological effects of pregnancy and tell how they can be influenced by whether the pregnancy is planned or unplanned.*

○ *Describe how pregnancy affects the uterus with regard to weight, blood supply, muscle fibers, and lymphatic and nerve tissue.*

o *Describe the changes that occur in the cervix during pregnancy.*

o *Explain the purpose of the mucus plug.*

o *Explain the effects pregnancy has on the fallopian tubes, ovaries, and ovulation.*

o *Describe the changes that occur in the vagina and perineum during pregnancy and state the purpose of these changes.*

o *Discuss how the mammary glands and nipples are affected by pregnancy.*

o *Describe the changes that occur in the pelvis during pregnancy, and explain the physiological basis for the backache experienced by some women late in pregnancy.*

o *Explain how pregnancy affects blood volume, blood pressure, respiration, gastrointestinal peristalsis, metabolism, and endocrine activity.*

o *Describe the effects of pregnancy on the pelvic veins, the gums, the bladder and ureters, and the skin.*

o *Define: lactation, colostrum, striae gravidarum, linea nigra, chloasma, diastasis recti.*

TERMINOLOGY

The beginning of a new human life occurs when a mature sex cell from the male unites with a mature sex cell from the female. This union of the two sex cells is called _conception_ or _fertilization._ The fertilized cell develops into a fetus that grows inside the uterus (womb) of the mother until it is mature enough to survive outside her body, at which time it is expelled by the process known as birth or _parturition._ _Pregnancy_ is that period of time between conception and birth during which the baby is developing within the uterus; it is also spoken of as the _gestation_ period.

Gravida is the medical term for a pregnant woman. A woman who is pregnant for the first time is a gravida I, or a _primigravida._ During subsequent pregnancies she is a gravida II, a gravida III, a gravida IV, and so forth, or a _multigravida._

Para is the term for a woman who has carried a _viable_ fetus—that is, capable of surviving outside the uterus—regardless of whether the child was born alive or dead. Therefore, a pregnancy that ended in abortion or miscarriage of a nonviable fetus is not counted in the para, while a pregnancy that terminated in a live birth or a stillborn infant (born dead) is counted.

Para is often interpreted to mean the number of _children_ a woman has given birth to. However, it actually refers to _pregnancies,_ not _children._ Thus, a pregnancy that terminates with the birth of twins or triplets is counted as one _para._

A woman who is pregnant for the first time is a primigravida and a _nullipara_ (_null_ = none), or she is said to be a gravida I, para 0.

After giving birth to her first child (thus terminating her first pregnancy after the age of viability), she is a _primipara._ After she has had more than one pregnancy that terminated after the age of viability she is a _multipara._

One method commonly used in maternity centers to indicate not only the number of pregnancies a woman has had but also the outcomes utilizes five digits separated by dashes. The first digit denotes all pregnancies she has had, including the present one; the second is the total number of deliveries; the third is the number of premature births; the fourth is the number of abortions; and the fifth is the number of children living at this time. Using this system, a pregnant woman who has five living children, all single births, and who has had no premature births and no abortions would be a gravida 6-5-0-0-5 (Fig. 6-1).

DURATION OF PREGNANCY

The duration of pregnancy is commonly determined by counting from the first day of the last normal menstrual period (LMP). When a diagnosis of pregnancy is established, the physician tells the expectant mother an approximate date on which her baby may be born. This estimated date of

Total of all pregnancies	Total number of deliveries	Number of premature births	Number of abortions	Number of living children
6 -	5 -	0 -	0 -	5

FIG. 6-1. *System of five digits used by some maternity centers to denote the number of pregnancies and their outcomes.*

confinement (EDC) or estimated date of delivery (EDD) is determined by adding 7 days to the first day of the LMP and counting back 3 months. This method of arriving at the EDC is known as *Naegele's rule.* Using Naegele's rule, the EDC of a woman whose last menstrual period began August 12 would be May 19. It should be remembered that this is an *estimated* date and that birth may not occur on this date. Only a small percentage of births do occur on the estimated date, most occurring a week or so before or after.

The duration of pregnancy is approximately 280 days. This period of time is measured in 28-day months called *lunar* months. There are approximately 10 lunar months (40 weeks, 280 days) in a full-term pregnancy (Fig. 6-2). This is approximately the same as 9 calendar months. Because of the variation in ovulation time among women and because fetuses seem to mature at different rates, some pregnancies may last only 240 days while others continue for 300 days with perfectly normal outcomes.

For convenience the 9 months of pregnancy are divided into 3-month periods called *trimesters.* Thus, there are three trimesters in a pregnancy.

During the first 5 weeks of pregnancy, the developing organism is called an *embryo;* thereafter, until birth it is called a *fetus.*

Not all pregnancies continue to term. A pregnancy that terminates before the fetus is viable is called an *abortion.* A pregnancy that terminates after the age of viability but before full term is classified as premature or preterm labor.

Until recently the criteria for viability were a gestational age of at least 28 weeks and a fetal weight of more than 1000 g. As a result of the progress made in maternal and newborn care in the past few years, some authorities now recommend that the criteria for viability be a gestational age of at least 26 weeks and a birth weight of 601 g or more (Jensen and Bobak, p. 264).

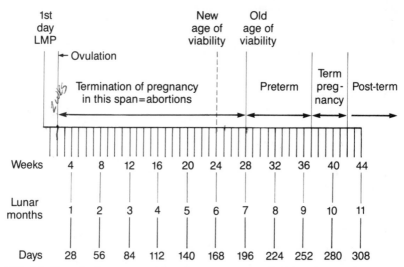

FIG. 6-2. *Length of pregnancy. Note that some experts feel that the age of viability should be reduced from 28 weeks' gestational age to 24 weeks because of advances in maternal and newborn care.*

SIGNS AND SYMPTOMS

Pregnancy produces many physical changes in the woman. Some of these changes are slight and may not be easily detected; others are marked and may be not only obvious but also annoying. Many of the changes, or symptoms, may also be present in conditions other than pregnancy.

The signs and symptoms commonly seen during pregnancy are classified as *presumptive signs, probable signs,* and *positive signs.* The presumptive signs appear very early but are not reliable evidence of pregnancy. Probable signs also make their appearance during the early months of pregnancy and are more likely to be detected by the physician. These are more reliable indicators of pregnancy, especially when two or more are present. Until the advent of ultrasound scanning and the Doppler probe, the positive signs of pregnancy were not detectable until the pregnancy had reached the halfway mark. With these devices, pregnancy can be confirmed at a much earlier date. Their use is discussed in Chapter 9.

PRESUMPTIVE SIGNS

The presumptive signs that may make a woman suspect that she is pregnant are *amenorrhea* (cessation of menstruation), *nausea and vomiting, breast changes, pigmentation, frequent urination,* and *quickening.*

√ **Amenorrhea** is one of the first and most important signs of pregnancy.

SIGNS AND SYMPTOMS OF PREGNANCY

PRESUMPTIVE

- Amenorrhea
- Nausea
- Breast changes
- Pigmentation
- Frequency of urination
- Quickening

PROBABLE

- Enlargement of the abdomen
- Chadwick's sign
- Goodell's sign
- Hegar's sign
- Ballottement
- Braxton Hicks contractions
- Pregnancy tests
- Fetal outline on palpation

POSITIVE

- Fetal heartbeat heard
- Fetal movements felt by examiner
- Bony outline of fetus on x-ray
- Detection of products of conception by ultrasound

It is particularly significant if the woman's menstrual cycle is usually regular and if the expected period is overdue by 10 days or more. But since amenorrhea may also be caused by emotional disturbances, disease conditions, fatigue, and other factors, it can only be a presumptive sign of pregnancy. In addition, it is possible for pregnancy to occur in the absence of menstruation, as in the case of a woman who becomes pregnant again shortly after giving birth and before menstruation has been reestablished.

Nausea, with or without vomiting, is present in about half of all pregnancies during the 4th to the 12th weeks. Since it occurs most often in the morning hours it is called "morning sickness." Usually the nausea disappears in a few hours, only to reappear again the following morning. Frequently, the woman can obtain relief by eating a dry cracker before getting out of bed in the morning.

One theory attributes morning sickness to psychological factors. As such it is considered a manifestation of the expectant woman's subconscious rejection of her pregnancy. In some instances this may be true;

however, in cases where a woman experiences morning sickness before she is aware that she is pregnant, other factors doubtless are involved. Another theory attributes the nausea and vomiting of pregnancy to physiological changes, such as changes in carbohydrate metabolism and an increase in hormones. Should the nausea and vomiting persist, they may become a serious complication of pregnancy.

Breast changes that may be noticed during the early weeks of pregnancy include enlargement, heaviness, tingling, and increased sensitivity of the breasts and nipples. However, these same breast changes are experienced by many women just before their menstrual periods begin, and therefore are not necessarily indications of pregnancy. Another change involving the breasts is increased pigmentation (darkening) of the nipples and areolar tissue surrounding the nipples.

Pigmentation is also increased in the abdomen and face (see Fig. 6-10). The pigmentation of the abdomen appears as a dark line running from the umbilicus to the symphysis and is called *linea nigra.* The face may have irregular areas of pigmentation, called *chloasma,* which give the appearance of a blotchy, suntanned mask. Although the increased pigmentation usually disappears following pregnancy, it may remain from one pregnancy to the next. Chloasma is not unusual in women taking birth control pills, because of the hormones in them. This chloasma may not fade after the contraceptive is discontinued.

Frequency of urination, present in certain diseases of the urinary system, often occurs early in pregnancy as the growing uterus puts pressure on the bladder, thereby decreasing its capacity.

Quickening is the term for the first movements of the baby felt by the expectant mother. Since these first movements are light and fluttery, it is possible for a woman who thinks she is pregnant to mistake the movement of gas within her bowel for movements of the baby. This presumptive sign usually appears between the 18th and 20th weeks of pregnancy. Knowing the time that quickening occurred may be helpful to the physician in estimating the date of delivery in instances where a woman's menstrual periods are irregular or if she has had no period since the birth of a previous child.

PROBABLE SIGNS

When one or more of the presumptive signs of pregnancy are experienced, the woman should visit her doctor to confirm her suspicions. In his examination, the doctor looks for the probable signs of pregnancy, such as enlargement of the abdomen, Chadwick's sign, Goodell's sign, Hegar's sign, ballottement, Braxton Hicks contractions, fetal outline, and positive pregnancy tests.

Enlargement of the abdomen in pregnancy is due to the growth of the uterus. In nonpregnant conditions, as when a tumor is present, the abdomen may also become enlarged.

✓**Chadwick's sign** is a bluish or purplish discoloration of the vulva and vagina that is caused by an increased blood supply. It is seen after the fourth week of pregnancy.

✓**Goodell's sign** consists of the characteristic softening of the cervix that accompanies the increased blood supply and increased hormone production associated with pregnancy. It occurs about the time of the second missed menstrual period.

✓**Hegar's sign,** which is perceptible about the sixth week of pregnancy, is the softening of the lower uterine segment. This softening can be felt by the physician as he places the fingers of one hand behind the cervix through the vagina and feels with the fingers of the other hand above the cervix through the abdominal wall (Fig. 6-3).

✓**Ballottement** is the rebounding of the fetus against the physician's fingers after he has made it move by giving it a push through the vagina or the abdomen. The fetus can then be felt rebounding against his fingers (Fig. 6-4). This sign appears during the fourth or fifth month when the fetus is small in comparison to the amount of fluid surrounding it.

FIG. 6-3. *Hegar's sign.*

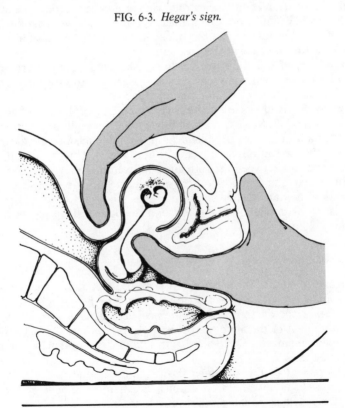

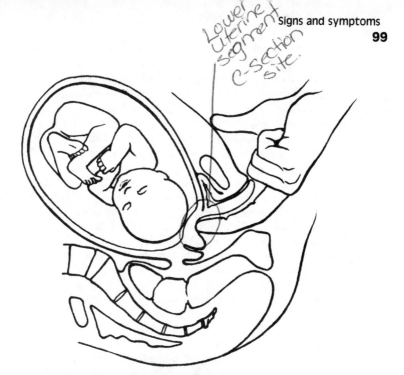

Lower uterine segment + c-section site.

FIG. 6-4. *Ballottement.*

√ **Braxton Hicks contractions** are painless uterine contractions that occur at 5- to 10-minute intervals throughout pregnancy and may be observed by the physician in the later months. These contractions are usually not noticed by the expectant woman until near the end of her pregnancy.

√ **A fetal outline** may be determined by the doctor by *palpation*. However, because it is possible for a tumor to have irregular parts and thereby be confused with a fetus, this is not a definite sign of pregnancy.

√ **Pregnancy tests,** when properly done, are accurate in 90% to 98% of cases and therefore are quite reliable indications of pregnancy. Most pregnancy tests are based on the presence of human chorionic gonadotropin (hCG), a hormone produced by the chorionic villi of the placenta and present in the blood and urine of pregnant women by about the 15th day of pregnancy. Since this hormone is present early in pregnancy, tests can be very helpful in making a probable diagnosis of pregnancy. However, the pregnancy tests that depend on hCG also may be positive in the presence of hydatidiform moles and choriocarcinoma (see Chap. 16) and therefore are not positive signs of pregnancy.

Biologic and immunologic tests may be used to detect pregnancy. Biologic tests commonly used in the past were the Ascheim-Zondek (immature female mice), the Friedman (immature female rabbits), and the male frog tests. These have been largely replaced by the immunologic tests, which are available in kits yield results within a few minutes or a few hours. Other advantages of the immunologic tests are that they can detect pregnancy within 10 days after a missed period; they are more accurate than the biologic tests; animals are not used, eliminating the necessity for obtaining and maintaining them; and the urine specimen can be collected at any time during the day, thus eliminating the inconvenience of withholding fluids, collecting the first specimen in the morning, and refrigerating it. However, since serum cannot be used in these tests, it is important that the urine specimen not contain blood. If the woman is bleeding, the specimen must be obtained by catheterization. In the tests, which also depend on the presence of hCG in the urine, an antiserum is added to the urine specimen. Then an antigen is added to the urine-antiserum mixture. In a negative test, agglutination occurs; in a positive test, no agglutination occurs. The Gravindex test, the UCG-Slide test, and the Pregnosticon Accuspheres test are examples of pregnancy tests based on the immunologic principle.

One of the most sensitive and accurate tests for pregnancy has recently been developed. This is a *radioimmunoassay* capable of detecting hCG in maternal serum from about the eighth day after fertilization, thus making diagnosis of pregnancy possible before a menstrual period is missed. This test is expensive and is not readily available.

Just as the presumptive signs of pregnancy may be present in conditions other than pregnancy, so also may the probable signs. However, when two or more probable signs are present, it is fairly safe to assume that the woman is pregnant.

POSITIVE SIGNS

The presence of the following positive signs ensures a definite and unquestionable diagnosis of pregnancy.

✓**The heartbeat of the fetus can be heard.** At first the fetal heartbeat is a faint, distant sound and may be difficult to detect. As pregnancy progresses it becomes more audible. The fetal heart tones (FHT) are very rapid, normally ranging from 110 to 160 beats per minute. While one is listening to the fetal heart tones, the pulsation in the aorta of the mother may be mistaken for the heartbeat of the baby. To avoid this error, the radial pulse of the mother should be felt at the same time the fetal heart tones are auscultated; the mother's pulse is considerably slower than the baby's heartbeat. To make listening easier, all extraneous noise should be minimized.

The sound produced by touching the stethoscope while counting the fetal heart tones may interfere with hearing and an incorrect count may result. To avoid this problem, a *fetoscope* or a Leffscope, instruments designed especially for this purpose, may be used to listen to the heart tones. The fetoscope has a band that fits over the head of the listener, making handling of the instrument unnecessary while the heart tones are counted (Fig. 6-5). The metal band also aids in bone conduction of sound so that the heart tones are more easily heard. The Leffscope has a weighted end

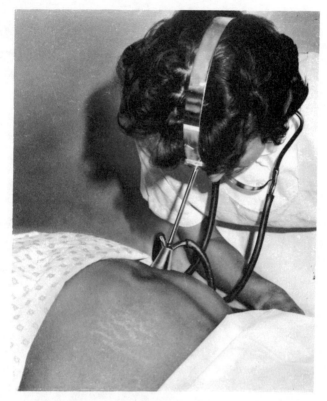

FIG. 6-5. *The band of the fetoscope fits over the head of the nurse making handling of the instrument unnecessary while counting the heart tones. Note striae gravidarum and linea nigra on the abdomen.*

which, when placed on the mother's abdomen, makes holding it in place unnecessary. The Doppler probe, a low-energy ultrasound flow probe, can also be used to detect fetal heart activity very early in pregnancy. It is a small, compact instrument that some physicians use exclusively for auscultation of fetal heartbeat in their offices (Fig. 6-6).

Other sounds one may hear while listening to the fetal heartbeat are the funic souffle and the uterine souffle. The *funic souffle* is a soft, swishing sound made by the blood as it is propelled through the umbilical cord. The rate of the funic souffle is the same as the fetal heart rate, since the blood is forced through the cord by the fetal heart. The *uterine souffle* is a soft, swishing sound made by maternal blood as it rushes through the large vessels of the uterus. The rate of the uterine souffle is the same as the maternal pulse rate, because this blood is propelled by the maternal heart.

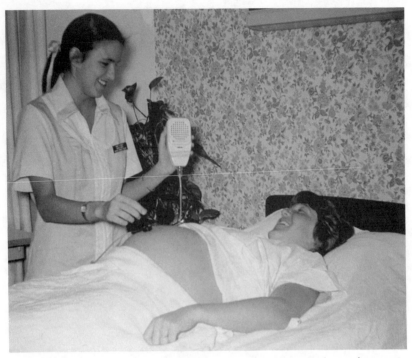

FIG. 6-6. *Listening to fetal heart tones with a Doppler probe. Mother and nurse can hear the fetal heart at the same time.*

√ **Fetal movements can be felt by the examiner.** After the fifth month of gestation fetal movements can be felt by placing a hand on the mother's abdomen while she is in the supine position. The movements are made by the baby as it kicks, stretches, and changes position. At first the movements are light and concentration is required to detect them. As the fetus grows, its movements become stronger, causing the mother to complain about its kicking, especially when she is trying to rest or sleep.

√ **The bony outline of the fetus can be seen on x-ray.** After the fourth to fifth month of pregnancy, an x-ray film offers undeniable proof of pregnancy. However, if pregnancy is suspected, radiography is not recommended unless a justifiable condition warrants its use, because exposure to radiation can cause developmental defects in the fetus, especially in early pregnancy. Ultrasound scanning is a useful means of diagnosing pregnancy early. And, unlike radiography at the present time there are no known harmful effects on the fetus (see Chap. 11). Using ultrasound scanning, it is sometimes possible to identify the embryo as early as the fourth week of gestation. This method is very accurate after the third month of pregnancy.

PSYCHOLOGICAL EFFECTS

When a pregnancy is confirmed, the initial response by those involved usually is either strongly positive—joy, elation, happiness; or strongly negative—anger, resentment, dismay, disappointment. Seldom is a casual reaction toward pregnancy recorded initially. Pregnancy affects every aspect of a woman's life, and it affects, in some way and to some degree, every member of the household involved. Although the initial reaction to an unplanned pregnancy may be one of shock, disappointment, resentment, and anger, it is of utmost importance to the health and well-being of the mother, the expected child, and the other family members that these negative attitudes be replaced by positive attitudes as soon as possible. This is accomplished gradually as adjustments are made and the pregnancy is accepted. Continued rejection of a pregnancy is destructive and damaging to the mental and emotional health of the mother and thus undermines her physical health. At the same time the health and future of the expected child are placed in jeopardy.

The background and circumstances of individuals are important factors in determining the psychological effects a pregnancy will have on them. Other factors include their physical health and well-being, age, emotional maturity and stability, financial status, housing, marital status, partner's feelings about pregnancy and children, number of children already in the family, plans for the future, how family members feel they will be affected by the pregnancy, and timing (see Chap. 2).

To the physically healthy, emotionally mature woman who desires a family and who has the security of her husband's love, respect, and understanding and to whom finances are no major problem, pregnancy may be seen as a welcome and happy experience that promotes the fulfillment of her role as a woman, a wife, and a mother. On the other hand, an unwed woman who is solely responsible for her own support, who knows there is no possibility of marrying the father of the expected child, and who realizes that her church, her parents, and her peers frown upon pregnancy out of wedlock may see pregnancy as a disaster of major proportions.

A woman sometimes wants children so much that she becomes obsessed with the idea of being pregnant. She thinks about it so much that she convinces herself that she is pregnant. Then she convinces her husband, if she is married, and her family and friends. Her abdomen may become enlarged and her menstrual periods may stop. This condition is known as pseudocyesis, or false pregnancy.

CHANGES IN THE REPRODUCTIVE SYSTEM

UTERUS AND CERVIX

In order for the developing fetus to have room for growth, the cavity of the uterus must expand. To allow this, the walls of the uterus distend, stretch, and become very thin. The muscle fibers in the walls grow to about 5 to 10 times their original size. However, this expansion in itself is not quite sufficient to accommodate the growing fetus; therefore, new muscle cells develop within the uterine wall. To add to the strength and elasticity of the walls, an additional supply of connective and elastic tissue develops, forming a network around the muscle bundles.

The blood supply to the uterus must be increased to provide nutrients for the developing fetus and for the growing uterus; therefore, the blood vessels become larger. In addition, there is an increase in the size of the lymphatic and nervous tissue.

As a result of these changes, the uterus grows from an organ approximately 3 inches long, 2 inches wide, and 1 inch deep (7.5 cm × 5 cm × 2.5 cm) to one approximately 12 to 14 inches long, 8 to 10 inches wide and 8 to 9 inches deep (30 to 35 cm × 20 to 25 cm × 20 to 22.5 cm). Its weight increases from approximately 2 oz (56.7 g) to about 2 lb (907 g), and its capacity increases to more than 500 times what it was before pregnancy. During the first 3 months of gestation, the growth of the uterus is stimulated by hormones; during subsequent months, pressure of the growing fetus against the uterine wall plays an important part in stimulating its growth. The growth of the uterus is greatest in the region of the fundus and at the placental site.

The cervix of the uterus becomes shorter and softer during pregnancy. These changes prepare the cervix for the thinning (*effacement*) and enlargement (*dilatation*) of its os, which are necessary to permit the infant to pass from the uterus at birth. The softening of the cervix (Goodell's sign) is one of the first observable signs of pregnancy, occurring as early as a month after conception; it is the most outstanding change in the cervix during pregnancy.

The softening is due to the increased blood supply, an increase in the number of the glands of the cervix, and edema. The secretions from the cervical glands form a mucus plug in the cervical canal that acts as a barrier preventing vaginal bacteria from entering the uterus (Fig. 6-7). Just before or during labor, this mucus plug, along with a small amount of blood, is discharged as the "show."

The connective tissue in the cervix becomes looser during pregnancy. Unlike what happens in the uterus, the number of muscle cells in the cervix decreases, but those that remain increase in size.

FALLOPIAN TUBES AND OVARIES

The blood supply to the ovaries and tubes increases during gestation. As a result of this excellent blood supply, the corpus luteum becomes quite large, but new follicles do not mature and ovulation does not occur.

The position of the ovaries and tubes changes from horizontal to almost vertical. This is brought about as the enlarging uterus, to which they are attached, rises upward into the abdominal cavity.

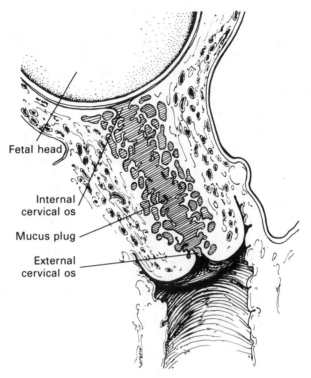

FIG. 6-7. *Cervix with mucus plug.*

Fetal head

Internal
cervical os

Mucus plug

External
cervical os

VAGINA AND PERINEUM

The changes that occur in the vagina and perineum prepare these structures for the tremendous stretching they must undergo as the baby is born. The greatest change in the vagina is an increase in its blood supply. The congestion resulting from the increased blood supply causes the vagina to become a bluish or purplish color, one of the signs of pregnancy (Chadwick's sign). Other changes that promote distention of the vagina are thickening of the mucosa, loosening of the connective tissue, and hypertrophy of the muscle cells, which results in a lengthening of the vaginal walls. During pregnancy there may be an increased amount of vaginal secretions.

The changes in the perineum are very similar to those in the vagina. There is an increased blood supply, hypertrophy of the skin and muscles, and loosening of the connective tissue.

BREASTS

The changes that occur in the breasts prepare them for secreting milk for the infant (Fig. 6-8). They are believed to occur as a result of hormonal stimulation. The production of milk is called *lactation*. Before pregnancy, the glands that secrete milk are undeveloped. During the early weeks of gestation, as these glands begin to develop, the pregnant woman may experience tenseness and a tingling sensation in her breasts. After about the second month, she may notice that her breasts are becoming larger. Later, the superficial veins may be seen through the thin skin. Thin, red streaks, called *striae gravidarum,* may appear on the breasts of some pregnant women.

The nipples also prepare for suckling by the infant. They become larger and more erectile and, along with the areola, more deeply pigmented. There seems to be a correlation between the degree of pigmentation and the complexion of the individual, since brunettes become more deeply pigmented than blondes. The sebaceous glands in the areola, the tubercles of Montgomery, increase in size in preparation for lubricating the nipple during lactation. After the early months of gestation, a think, yellowish fluid called *colostrum* may be expressed from the nipples. Colostrum is present until it is replaced by the milk about the third or fourth day following delivery.

FIG. 6-8. *Comparison of the mammary glands at the nonpregnant, pregnant, and lactating stages. (Adapted from Ross Nursing Education Aids, No. 10. Ross Laboratories, Columbus, Ohio)*

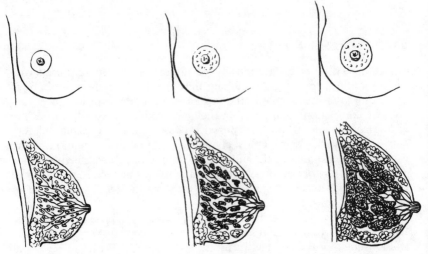

CHANGES IN OTHER BODY SYSTEMS

MUSCULOSKELETAL SYSTEM

Hormonal changes occurring during pregnancy and the increased blood supply to the pelvis are believed responsible for relaxation and increased mobility of the sacroiliac, sacrococcygeal, and pubic joints. Because of this relaxation, some of the weight of the heavy uterus moves to the surrounding muscles and ligaments. As the uterus enlarges, it causes the abdomen to extend forward. The woman's posture is affected, and lordosis develops as the center of gravity shifts back over the lower extremities. Changes in posture and mobility of the joints may be partially responsible for some of the discomforts (such as backache) experienced by the woman late in pregnancy and also for the waddling gait of many pregnant women.

Sometimes the enlarged uterus stretches the abdominal wall so much that the rectus muscles separate. This separation is termed *diastasis recti*, and may be slight or extensive. When diastasis recti is present, it is often possible to feel the parts of the fetus very easily through the thin wall of the uterus.

CIRCULATORY SYSTEM

For the blood supply to the reproductive organs to increase during pregnancy without depleting the blood supply to the rest of the body, there must be an increase in the total amount of blood in the circulatory system. During pregnancy, the blood volume increases approximately 30% due primarily to an increase in plasma content, although there is some increase in the erythrocyte volume as well. Because of these changes, there may be a slight dilution of the hemoglobin content of the blood. However, it is believed that the woman who has an adequate storage of iron when she becomes pregnant or whose daily diet contains an adequate amount of iron will manifest very little, if any, drop in hemoglobin or hematocrit levels during pregnancy. A hemoglobin of at least 12 g/dl and a hematocrit of at least 35% should be maintained throughout pregnancy to meet the iron needs of the mother and fetus.

The additional blood volume increases the work load of the heart. For the healthy heart this creates no problems; the patient with a diseased heart may require careful medical supervision during pregnancy.

In normal pregnancy there is no increase in the blood pressure. There may even be a slight lowering of the blood pressure, but it usually returns to nonpregnant levels during the last month of pregnancy.

In the latter months of pregnancy, the enlarged uterus places considerable pressure on the pelvic veins, thus slowing down the return flow of blood from the legs. As the blood accumulates, the pressure in the veins builds up and some fluid escapes through the vessel walls into the

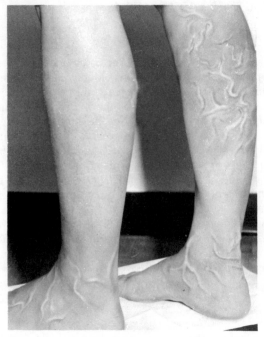

FIG. 6-9. *Varicose veins.*

tissues of the feet and ankles, causing edema in these areas. The distention of the veins with blood causes varicose veins to develop in women who have weak vessel walls (Fig. 6-9). The occasional formation of hemorrhoids during pregnancy was noted earlier.

RESPIRATORY SYSTEM

It has been estimated that about three fourths of all pregnant women experience some reddening and swelling in the larynx, which causes the voice to sound hoarse. Some women have difficulty breathing because of nasal congestion due to the increased blood supply. Nosebleeds are not uncommon during pregnancy, and may be due to the increased blood supply and hormonal activity.

In the later months of pregnancy, the diaphragm is pushed upward by the large uterus. This may cause some pregnant women to experience shortness of breath, especially when lying down. The pressure from the uterus makes the height of the chest shorter, but the chest widens so that there is just as much breathing space as before. In fact, studies have shown that there is an actual increase in the amount of air inspired during pregnancy.

GASTROINTESTINAL SYSTEM

Some pregnant women complain that their gums bleed when they brush their teeth or when other slight irritations occur. The bleeding is due to softening of the gums from large amounts of estrogen present in the body.

Some women also complain of excessive salivation, called ptyalism. In its severe form, increased salivation may cause maceration of the skin around the mouth.

There is a slowing down of peristaltic action of the stomach and the bowel. Heartburn, flatulence, and vomiting, which frequently accompany pregnancy, have been attributed to this decreased gastric motility. The stomach and the bowel lose some of their tone, and the stomach is pushed upward into a more or less horizontal position. The loss of tone of the gastrointestinal tract is believed responsible, in part at least, for the constipation suffered by at least one half of all pregnant women.

URINARY SYSTEM

Early in pregnancy the growing uterus places pressure on the bladder, causing a decrease in the amount of urine the bladder can hold. Consequently, the pregnant woman has frequency of urination. Later, as the pelvis becomes too small to accommodate the enlarging uterus, the bladder is brought along with the rising uterus into the abdominal cavity. Then, near the end of pregnancy, as the presenting part settles into the pelvic cavity, pressure is again exerted on the bladder, with frequency of urination returning.

During pregnancy the ureters become dilated and their peristaltic action, which is necessary to propel the urine from the kidneys to the bladder, decreases. The urine is not carried as rapidly as usual from the kidneys to the bladder so that some of it accumulates in the kidneys, contributing to infections in the urinary system during pregnancy. The dilatation of the ureters and their decreased motility are believed to be due to hormonal activity.

WEIGHT AND METABOLISM

The desirable weight gain for the average, healthy woman during pregnancy is about 25 to 30 lb (11–13 kg). However, it is generally recognized that weight gain should be individualized, with special consideration given to those who are under or over average weight at the beginning of pregnancy. Emphasis should be on a good, balanced diet rather than on weight gain. Only about 2 to 4 lb (1 to 2 kg) are gained during the first trimester, with the remainder being gained during the last two trimesters. Much of the weight gain due to the products of conception, fluid retention, and increased blood volume may be lost at delivery or shortly thereafter; weight gained as fat deposits is usually more difficult to lose.

DISTRIBUTION OF WEIGHT GAINED DURING PREGNANCY

- infant—6 to 8 lb (2722 to 3629 g)
- Placenta—1 to 1½ lb (454 to 680 g)
- Amniotic fluid—1 to 1½ lb (454 to 680 g)
- Breasts—2 to 3 lb (907 to 1361 g)
- Uterus—2 to 3 lb (907 to 1361 g)
- Increased blood and fluids—8½ lb (3855 g)

In the latter half of pregnancy, the basal metabolism increases by 5% to 25%. This is believed to be due to the fetus rather than to an increase in the basal metabolism rate of the maternal tissues.

ENDOCRINE SYSTEM

The major endocrine gland during pregnancy is the *placenta*. Soon after implantation of the fertilized ovum occurs, the chorionic villi begin to produce hCG, which causes the corpus luteum to continue to survive and to produce the estrogen and progesterone essential to the growth and maintenance of the pregnancy. After the first 2 months of pregnancy, the placenta becomes the major source of estrogen and progesterone. The chorionic villi of the placenta also produce human placental lactogen (chorionic somatomammotropin). This hormone is important to the somatic cell growth of the fetus and aids in the preparation of the breasts for lactation. Ovulation ceases and the ovaries become relatively inactive during pregnancy.

The *pituitary gland* enlarges during pregnancy, but it is not essential to the maintenance of pregnancy. Estrogen and progesterone levels during normal pregnancy are sufficient to inhibit release of gonadotropins by the anterior lobe of the pituitary. Oxytocin, a hormone that has a strong stimulating effect on the uterine muscle, is produced by the posterior lobe of the pituitary. Oxytocin is used to prevent or treat hemorrhage after delivery and to stimulate or induce labor. As a nasal spray, oxytocin is effective in promoting milk let-down in mothers who breast-feed their infants. Synthetic oxytocin is marketed under the brand names of Pitocin and Syntocinon.

The *thyroid gland* enlarges during pregnancy but its activity does not increase.

Probably the most significant change in the *adrenals* during pregnancy is an increase in the secretion of aldosterone. Since this hormone is responsible for retention of sodium by the kidneys, an uncontrolled intake of salt by the pregnant woman can result in excessive fluid retention.

SKIN

The noticeable changes that may occur in the skin of the pregnant woman include the appearance of *striae gravidarum* and the increased pigmen-

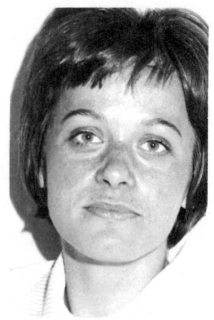

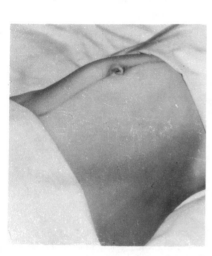

A   B

FIG. 6-10. *(A) Note the pigmented line, linea nigra, on the abdomen and (B) the patchy pigmentation, chloasma of the face.*

tation of certain areas. Striae may develop on the skin of the breasts, abdomen, thighs, or buttocks due to stretching. After delivery, the striae lose their redness and become silvery in appearance.

In addition to the pigmentation of the nipples and areola, there is a darkening of the line in the center of the abdomen that extends from the symphysis pubis upward to, and sometimes above, the umbilicus. This pigmented line is referred to as the *linea nigra.* An irregular, patchy pigmentation, known as *chloasma* or "mask of pregnancy," appears on the face of some pregnant women (Fig. 6-10). The cause of this pigmentation is not definitely known, but it is believed to be due to hormonal activity. Usually the pigmented areas become lighter after delivery, with the chloasma disappearing altogether.

NERVOUS SYSTEM AND PSYCHE

Changes in the nervous system are manifest as changes in disposition (see Chap. 2). Most changes are very mild, but in rare instances a pregnant woman may develop a true psychosis.

Occasionally during pregnancy some women develop cravings for unusual foods or strange combinations of foods, or even for items that are generally not considered edible. A craving for nonfood substances, such as starch, clay, or mothballs, is known as *pica*. Although satisfying some food cravings is usually harmless, pica involving large amounts of starch can cause ptyalism (profuse salivation), while consumption of mothballs can cause serious blood problems. Ingestion of large amounts of clay may interfere with iron absorption or cause fecal impaction.

CLINICAL REVIEW

ASSESSMENT. Karen and Ken became acquainted at a social function during the spring of Ken's second year in college. After a whirlwind courtship they were married early in June. Karen, an only child, was a junior majoring in home economics. She would have been a senior had she not taken 1 year out to reign as the beauty queen of her state. Ken, the youngest of four sons, was majoring in hotel management. In planning their future, Ken and Karen decided to complete their college education. Karen's scholarship would cover most of her expenses; their parents agreed to pay the remainder for both of them.

Karen's menstrual periods came regularly every 28 days. She had periods beginning June 15, July 13, and August 10. On September 5 she and Ken started back to school. She was due to begin her period on September 7 but she did not. When she missed her period in October also, Karen decided to see a physician. She told him about her missed periods and the weight loss she had experienced in recent weeks. She thought the loss of weight was probably due to her lack of appetite and the nausea and vomiting she experienced when she got out of bed in the mornings.

When the physician examined Karen he noted that the vagina was a purplish color and that the cervix was soft. He decided to do a pregnancy test. When the test was positive, he concluded that she was pregnant.

1. Complete the nursing care plan for Karen and Ken using the data available.

Potential Nursing Diagnoses	Interventions	Expected Outcome

2. In addition to amenorrhea, nausea and vomiting, what other presumptive signs of pregnancy might Karen experience?
3. Which of the probable signs of pregnancy did the doctor find when he examined Karen?
4. Why is a positive diagnosis of pregnancy difficult to make at this early date?
5. How soon can the doctor make a positive diagnosis of pregnancy?
6. With this pregnancy, Karen is a gravida ____, para ____.
7. Her EDC might be____.
8. How might Ken react to this pregnancy? Why?

9. How do you think Karen might be affected psychologically by pregnancy?
10. Karen must live with the changes that occur within her body as a result of pregnancy. These changes may influence her daily routine, her eating habits, her style of dress, her walk, her appearance, and her feelings. Tell how you think she might be affected by each of the following:
    a. increased vaginal secretions
    b. enlarging uterus
    c. horizontal position of the stomach
    d. enlarging breasts
    d. chloasma
    f. mobility of the pelvic joints
    g. edema of the feet
    h. weight gain
    i. varicose veins

BIBLIOGRAPHY

Brunner LS, Suddarth DS: The Lippincott Manual of Nursing Practice, 3rd ed, pp 984–994. Philadelphia, JB Lippincott, 1982
Jensen MD, Bobak IM: Maternity Care: The Nurse & the Family, 3rd ed, pp 263–264, 309–331. St. Louis, CV Mosby Co, 1985
Pritchard JA, MacDonald PC, Gant NF: Williams Obstetrics, 17th ed, pp 181–206. New York, Appleton-Century Crofts, 1985
Reeder SR, Martin LL: Maternity Nursing, 16th ed, pp 283–297. Philadelphia, JB Lippincott Co, 1987

fetal development 7

BEHAVIORAL When the goals of this chapter are reached, the student will
OBJECTIVES be able to:

○ State the number of chromosomes in each body cell of human beings.

○ Explain why the number of chromosomes in a mature germ cell differs from the number of chromosomes in a body cell.

○ Explain when and how the sex of an individual is determined.

○ Describe what happens to the ovum from fertilization to implantation.

○ Explain the function of the trophoblast in relation to the fertilized ovum.

○ Name the two membranes that surround the embryo.

○ List four or five functions of the amniotic fluid.

○ Name the three germ layers and list two or three structures that develop from each.

○ Describe the placenta and list three of its functions.

○ Describe the composition of the umbilical cord and tell its function.

○ State at which month of pregnancy the following would be present in the fetus: all organs in rudimentary form, tooth buds, meconium, sex apparent, lanugo, quickening, fetal heartbeat audible, vernix caseosa.

○ Describe fetal circulation and tell how it differs from circulation after birth.

○ Discuss the differences between identical and fraternal twins.

○ Define: gamete, zygote, fertilization, trophoblast, decidua, chorion, villi, amnion, amniotic fluid, Wharton's jelly, meconium, lanugo, vernix caseosa, ductus venosus, foramen ovale, ductus arteriosus.

MATURATION OF SEX CELLS

All living organisms are made up of tiny structural units called cells. The cells within the human body are of two types: soma cells, which are found throughout the body, and germ or sex cells, the cells involved in reproduction, which are found only within the reproductive glands. Germ cells do not mature until puberty and are not capable of functioning until then.

CHROMOSOMES AND GENES

Within the nucleus of each cell are structures called chromosomes, which occur in pairs. Each species of animal and plant life has a specific number of chromosomes, which remains constant and is typical for that species. In human beings, there are 23 pairs or a total of 46 chromosomes in each body cell. In order to maintain a constant number of 46 chromosomes, the number in each mature germ cell must be one-half the number in all other body cells. The reduction in the number of chromosomes in the germ cell occurs as the cell is maturing. During maturation, then, the number of chromosomes in the germ cell is reduced from 46 to 23. This process is called *meiosis*. Each mature male germ cell, called a spermatozoon, contains 23 chromosomes, and each mature female germ cell, called an ovum, contains 23 chromosomes. The new cell that is formed when the sperm unites with the ovum contains 46 chromosomes.

A mature sex cell is called a *gamete*. When two gametes unite, one from the male and one from the female, the new cell formed is called a *zygote*.

The chromosomes contain many *genes*. Genes carry the factors responsible for the characteristics or traits of individuals. Genes for each trait or characteristic occur in pairs in all soma cells, but the gamete contains only one gene for each trait. The zygote contains a pair of genes, one from the male and one from the female, for each characteristic or trait. Not all characteristics of each parent are inherited, since the ovum and sperm contain only one-half of the chromosomes possible. All inherited characteristics and traits are determined at the time the spermatozoon fuses with the ovum.

SEX DETERMINATION

The sex of the individual is determined at the time the sperm unites with the ovum. Two of the 46 chromosomes in human beings are sex chromosomes. In the female these are designated XX, and in the male they are XY. After maturation the ovum always contains an X chromosome; the sperm may contain an X chromosome or a Y chromosome. When a sperm containing an X chromosome unites with an ovum, the child will be a girl (XX). When a sperm containing a Y chromosome unites

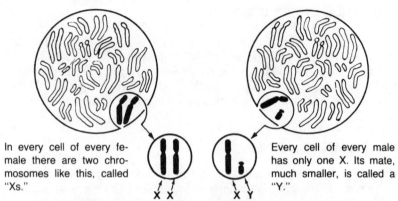

In every cell of every female there are two chromosomes like this, called "Xs."

Every cell of every male has only one X. Its mate, much smaller, is called a "Y."

For reproduction, a female forms eggs, a male sperms, to each of which they contribute only HALF their quota of chromosomes, or just one of every pair.

Since a female has TWO Xs, each egg gets one X, so in this respect every egg is the same:

But as the male has only ONE X, he forms TWO kinds of sperms:

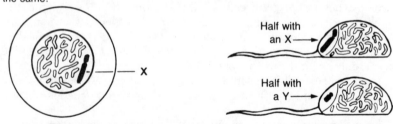

Thus: If an X-bearing sperm enters the egg, the result is an individual with TWO Xs:

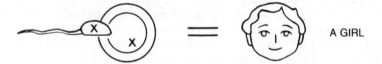

A GIRL

But if a Y-bearing sperm enters the egg, the result is an "XY" individual.

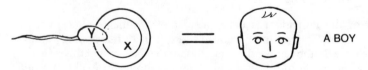

A BOY

FIG. 7-1. *Sex is determined at the time the sperm and ovum unite. (Scheinfeld A: Your Heredity and Environment. Philadelphia, JB Lippincott, 1965, p 44).*

with an ovum, the child will be a boy (XY). It is apparent that the sex of the new individual depends on the type of sex chromosome contained in the sperm that fertilizes the ovum. Since half of the sperm contain an X chromosome and half contain a Y chromosome, there is always a 50:50 chance that the child will be a girl and a 50:50 chance that it will be a boy (Fig. 7-1). Although individual families may vary in the proportion of girls to boys, in the total population about 106 males are born to every 100 females.

Even though some parents may want their unborn child to be of a certain sex, there is no known way to ensure that it will be so. Until recently there was no definite way of knowing the sex of the child before birth. Now, however, through studies of the amniotic fluid (*amniocentesis*) the sex of the fetus can be determined. This information is of value in figuring the probability that the fetus will be affected by a sex-linked genetic disorder, but the risks involved in amniocentesis preclude it as a means of merely satisfying the curiosity of eager expectant parents. This procedure is further discussed in Chapter 9.

FERTILIZATION AND IMPLANTATION

Fertilization, or *conception,* is the union of the sperm from the male with the ovum from the female. Following ovulation, the ovum is swept upward into the fallopian tube, where it may be met by sperm. Although millions of sperm are deposited at ejaculation, only one sperm is necessary to fertilize the ovum. Fertilization usually occurs while the ovum is in the outer half of the fallopian tube (Fig. 7-2). The ovum is believed to be fertilizable for 48 hours after ovulation; the sperm is believed to be capable of fertilizing the ovum for several days after ejaculation.

Immediately after fertilization the ovum divides into two cells, then four cells, eight cells, sixteen cells, and so forth, a process known as *mitosis*. Meanwhile, the movement of the cilia lining the wall of the tube and the peristaltic action of the tube propel the ovum toward the uterus. This journey through the tube to the uterus takes 3 to 6 days. During this time the ovum becomes a mass of cells called a *morula,* because of its resemblance to a mulberry. As the cells continue to divide, they arrange themselves in two layers with a cavity in the center. The outer layer of cells is called the *trophoblast* and the inner layer is known as the *inner cell mass.* The trophoblast obtains nourishment for the inner layer, from which the fetus will develop. Fluid accumulates in the cavity. At this stage the ovum is called a *blastocyst* or a blastodermic vesicle.

Two or three days after the ovum reaches the uterus, it begins to embed or implant itself in the thick, rich endometrium. Implantation of the fertilized ovum in the endometrium is also known as *nidation.* Just where the ovum implants is a matter of chance, but usually it is in the front or back of the upper portion of the uterine cavity. The endometrium

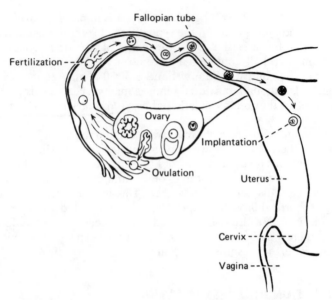

FIG. 7-2. *The ovum travels from the ovary to implantation in the uterus. Note the area where fertilization occurs.*

becomes very thick and is called *decidua*. As the ovum settles into the decidua, the trophoblast digests or liquefies the tissues with which it comes in contact. In this way it eats away the walls of the small blood vessels in the decidua where the ovum has implanted, so the ovum is then resting in a small pool of maternal blood. The trophoblast, which has now become a membrane called the *chorion*, becomes covered with a growth of rootlike projections called *villi*. Within the chorionic villi are blood vessels that are connected to the embryo. The villi on the chorion nearest the decidua dip into the pool of maternal blood. By osmosis, oxygen and nourishment from the maternal blood pass into the blood vessels in the villi to the embryo. The villi nearest the decidua develop into the placenta, but the villi on the remainder of the chorion disappear.

DEVELOPMENT OF THE EMBRYO AND SUPPORTIVE STRUCTURES

MEMBRANES AND AMNIOTIC FLUID

Soon after implantation, two membranes form around the embryo (Fig. 7-3). The outer membrane is the *chorion* (discussed earlier) and the inner membrane is the *amnion*. In addition to the fetus, the amnion contains an almost clear fluid, termed amniotic fluid, which is 98% water. It also

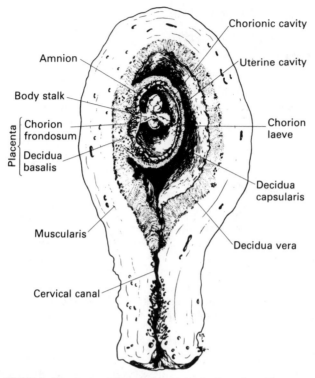

FIG. 7-3. *Pregnant uterus shown in sagittal section. The embryo is about 1 month of age.*

contains fetal urine, sebaceous material, epithelial cells, lanugo hairs, albumin, lecithin, sphingomyelin, bilirubin, fat, fructose, inorganic salts, a few leukocytes, and various enzymes. The amniotic fluid is neutral to slightly alkaline (pH 7.0 to 7.25). It is continually being absorbed and renewed at a rapid rate. The volume increases at an average rate of 25 ml per week from the 11th to the 15th weeks of pregnancy and 50 ml per week from the 15th to the 28th weeks. Although the amount of amniotic fluid present at term varies, about 1 liter is average; more than 2 liters (hydramnios) or less than 300 ml (oligohydramnios) is usually accompanied by fetal disease or abnormality. When a break occurs in the amnion, the fluid escapes through the vagina. This is the "breaking of the bag of waters," or rupturing of the membranes.

From the time of implantation to the end of the fifth week the rudiments of all the main organs of the body are laid down. During this period, the developing organism is called an *embryo*. Throughout the remainder of pregnancy to birth, while the organs and systems are developing and growing, it is called a *fetus*.

FUNCTIONS OF AMNIOTIC FLUID

- Prevents the amnion from adhering to the fetus
- Permits the fetus to move about freely
- Keeps the temperature surrounding the fetus constant
- Protects the fetus from injury from external causes
- Provides nourishment for the fetus, which is believed to drink 6 to 7 oz (180 to 210 ml) of the fluid each day

THREE GERM LAYERS

By about the 16th day after fertilization the inner cell mass begins to differentiate into three layers: the ectoderm, the mesoderm, and the entoderm. From each layer specific structures of the embryo develop. From the *ectoderm* develop the skin, nervous system, nasal passages, crystalline lens of the eye, pharynx, and mammary and salivary glands. From the *mesoderm* develop muscles, circulatory system, bones, reproductive system, connective tissue, kidneys, and ureters. From the *entoderm* develop the alimentary tract, respiratory tract, bladder, pancreas, and liver.

PLACENTA

The placenta is usually developed following the third month after fertilization. It is the structure that supplies oxygen and nourishment to the fetus and through which fetal waste products are eliminated. It is important to note that there is no mixing of maternal blood with fetal blood. During the first 12 weeks of pregnancy, the maternal and fetal circulation are separated by two layers of cells: the *cytotrophoblast* (inner layer of the trophoblast) and the *syncytiotrophoblast* (outer layer of cells covering the chorionic villi of the placenta). After this time, the cytotrophoblastic cells become fewer and widely separated, so that during the second and third trimesters, only one layer of cells separates them. This layer of cells constitutes the so-called placental barrier, which obviously is only a partial barrier and can provide only limited protection to the fetus. The oxygen and nourishment from the maternal blood pass through the vessel walls in the placenta into the vein of the umbilical cord. Likewise, the waste products from the fetus pass through the vessel walls of the placenta into the circulation of the mother. The placenta also produces three hormones: human chorionic gonadotropin, estrogen, and progesterone. At the end of pregnancy the placenta is flat and round, about 6 to 8 inches (15 to 20 cm) in diameter, about 1 inch (2.5 cm) thick, and usually weighs about one sixth of the baby's weight. The maternal side of the placenta is attached to the uterus, is rough and irregular, and is made up of 15

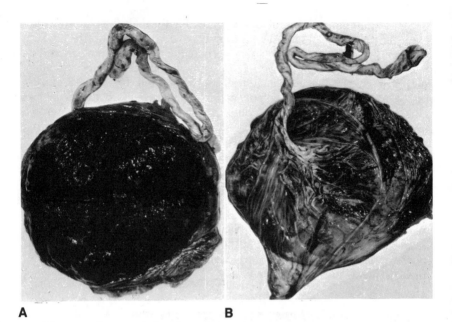

A   **B**

FIG. 7-4. (A) *The maternal surface of the placenta is rough and irregular. (B) The fetal surface of the placenta is smooth and shiny.*

to 20 segments called *cotyledons* (Fig. 7-4). The fetal side is covered with the amniotic membrane, is smooth and shiny, and contains many blood vessels branching off from the umbilical cord.

UMBILICAL CORD

The umbilical cord is the connecting link between the fetus and the placenta. It extends from the umbilicus of the fetus to the center of the fetal side of the placenta. The cord contains two arteries and one vein but has no nerves. The blood containing oxygen and nourishment is carried through the vein from the placenta to the fetus. Blood containing waste products is carried through the two arteries from the fetus to the placenta. At term, the cord is usually 20 to 22 inches (50 to 55 cm) long and is surrounded and protected by a whitish, gelatinous substance called *Wharton's jelly.* The membrane covering the cord is an extension of the amnion.

At birth, the physician or nurse checks the cord to see if there are two arteries and one vein present. In approximately 1% of newborns only one artery and one vein are present; about 10% of these infants have some kind of anomaly.

In addition to oxygen and nutrients, undesirable substances also may reach the fetus via the placenta and umbilical cord. Many drugs that gain access to the maternal circulation pass readily through the placenta and enter the fetal circulation, where they may have a devastating effect. Likewise, many viruses and other disease-producing organisms may cross the placenta and infect the fetus. Examples of viruses capable of reaching the fetus via the placenta include those responsible for rubella, chickenpox, measles, mumps, smallpox, vaccinia, poliomyelitis, cytomegalic inclusion disease, and western equine encephalitis. In untreated maternal syphilis, *Treponema pallidum* may cross the placenta and produce congenital syphilis in the fetus. Similarly, the malaria parasite and the tubercle bacillus may cause infection in the fetus.

SUMMARY OF MONTHLY FETAL GROWTH

Because each fetus grows at its own rate, the following are only rough estimates of fetal development at the various stages of pregnancy. Each phase of development is completed at the end of the period given. (Metric measurements are given in the box.)

MEASUREMENTS (APPROXIMATE EQUIVALENTS)

Length 1 inch = 2.5 cm
Weight   1 oz = 28.35 g
     16 oz = 1 lb = 453.6 g
     1000 g = 1 kg = 2.2 lb
Liquid measure 1 fluid oz = 30 ml

Fourth week (first lunar month). The embryo is approximately 0.2 inches (0.5 cm) long from crown to rump. All organs are present in rudimentary form. The head is very prominent, accounting for about one third of the entire embryo. At this time the heart consists of a tube that pulsates and propels blood through microscopic arteries. The ears, eyes, and nose are just beginning to form. The arms and legs are mere nubbins.

4 weeks

Eighth week (second lunar month). The length is approximately 1.2 inches (3 cm) and the weight $1/30$ oz (0.9 g). Because of the rapid development of the brain, the head appears very large in comparison to the trunk. The fetus has a human face and

8 weeks

arms and legs with fingers, toes, elbows, and knees.

Twelfth week (third lunar month). The centers of ossification appear in most bones, and the teeth are forming under the gums. The length is 2½ to 3½ inches (6.3 to 8.8 cm) and the weight is ½ to 1 oz (14 to 28 g). Rudimentary kidneys are present and secrete small amounts of urine. The fingers and toes have become differentiated. The external genitalia are beginning to show definite signs of male or female sex.

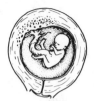

Twelfth week

Sixteenth week (fourth lunar month). The fetus weighs approximately 3½ to 4 oz (99 to 113 g) and is 4 to 6½ inches (10 to 16.3 cm) long. A black, tarry, fecal material called *meconium* is present in the bowels. The sex of the fetus becomes obvious at this time.

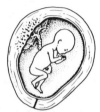

Sixteenth week

Twentieth week (fifth lunar month). This is midpoint in pregnancy. By now the mother has felt movement by the fetus (quickening), and the fetal heartbeat can be heard with a stethoscope. The length is 7 to 10½ inches (17.5 to 26.3 cm) and the weight is about 10 oz (284 g). Downy hair called *lanugo* is present on the skin, and there is hair on the head. Due to lack of fat deposits the skin is wrinkled.

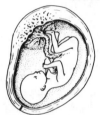

Twentieth week

Twenty-fourth week (sixth lunar month). The fetus is about 11 to 14 inches (27.5 to 35 cm) long and weighs approximately 1 lb 4 oz (567 g). A white, cheesy material, called *vernix caseosa*, appears on the skin. This substance protects the skin while it is submerged in water. If given expert care, a fetus born at this time might have some chance of survival.

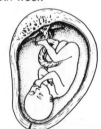

Twenty-fourth week

Twenty-eighth week (seventh lunar month). The length is 14 to 15 inches (35 to 37.5 cm) and the weight is over 2 lb (907 g).

Thirty-second week (eighth lunar month). The length of the fetus is approx-

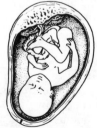

Twenty-eighth week

imately 16½ inches (41 cm) and the weight is about 3 lb 9 oz (1616 g). If the fetus is born at this time, its chance of survival is much better than if it is born earlier.

Thirty-sixth week (ninth lunar month). The chance of survival is excellent. Fat deposits under the skin give the fetus a more pleasing, plump appearance. The average length at this time is 18 inches (45 cm) and the average weight is 5 lb 4 oz (2381 g).

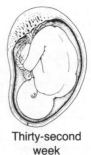 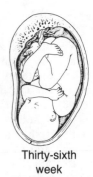

Thirty-second week

Thirty-sixth week

Fortieth week (tenth lunar month). The fetus has matured to the point that it no longer needs to remain in the uterus. The average length of the fetus is 20 inches (50 cm) and the average weight is 7 lb (3175 g).

Postmaturity (beyond 42 weeks). Any infant born more than 2 weeks after the expected date of delivery is considered to be postmature. However, since it is not always possible to know the expected date of delivery, an infant may be thought to be overdue when it is not. The effects of postmaturity vary. Some fetuses continue to gain weight as the pregnancy progresses, thus increasing the possibilities of difficult labor and cesarean section. Others lose weight because the placenta fails to function efficiently as the pregnancy continues. Typically, the postmature infant has long nails, an abundance of hair on its head, a diminished amount of vernix, and amniotic fluid that is meconium-stained. There is a progressive rise in the stillbirth rate as the pregnancy goes beyond term.

FETAL CIRCULATION

The path the blood follows after birth is different from the path it follows in the fetus, because the lungs are collapsed in the fetus and do not function. Their function of supplying oxygen to the blood and taking carbon dioxide from the blood is performed by the placenta, and it is not necessary for all the blood to pass through the lungs of the fetus as it is after birth. Consequently, certain structures exist in the circulatory system of the fetus and disappear after birth, namely the *ductus venosus*, the *foramen ovale*, and the *ductus arteriosus*. The function of these structures becomes apparent as the circulation of the fetus is observed (Fig. 7-5).

A brief review of the circulation of the blood as it occurs after birth may be helpful in understanding fetal circulation. Following birth, venous blood (that is, blood from which the oxygen has been used) from the lower part of the body flows through the inferior vena cava into the right atrium. Venous blood from the upper part of the body flows through the superior vena cava into the right atrium. Blood from the right atrium passes into the right ventricle and out through the pulmonary artery to the lungs. In

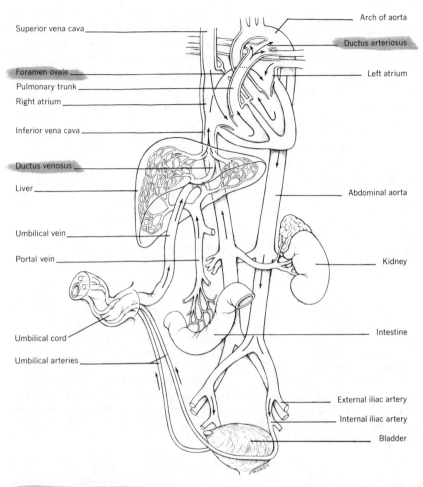

FIG. 7-5. *Diagram of the fetal circulation shortly before birth; course of blood is indicated by arrows.*

the lungs it gives up carbon dioxide and receives oxygen. From the lungs the oxygenated blood passes through the pulmonary veins into the left atrium, from which it passes into the left ventricle and out through the aorta to all parts of the body.

In the fetus, oxygenated blood from the placenta flows through the umbilical vein in the cord. After the umbilical vein enters the fetus it is joined by the ductus venosus. Most of the blood from the umbilical vein passes into the ductus venosus and then into the inferior vena cava. The remainder of the blood from the umbilical vein flows into the portal vein and into the liver; from the liver it passes through the hepatic vein into the inferior vena cava and through the inferior vena cava into the right atrium, along with blood from the superior vena cava. Since the lungs are not functioning, most of the blood from the right atrium passes directly to the left atrium through an opening called the foramen ovale; from the left atrium it passes into the left ventricle and on out through the aorta to all parts of the body. Some of the blood from the right atrium passes into the right ventricle and out through the pulmonary artery. A small amount of this blood goes to the lungs for their nourishment; the remainder leaves the right ventricle through the pulmonary artery, bypasses the lungs, and enters the aorta through the blood vessel, the ductus arteriosus.

Used blood collects in the hypogastric arteries, which become the umbilical arteries after they enter the cord. The blood passes through the umbilical arteries to the placenta. In the placenta, carbon dioxide and other waste products pass through the walls of the chorionic villi and into the maternal circulation. Oxygen and nutrients from the maternal blood pass through the walls of the chorionic villi and into the umbilical vein, continuing the cycle. Again, it is important to note that there is no mixing of maternal blood with fetal blood; the fetus makes its own blood and does not receive blood from the mother.

At birth, the lungs expand as the baby begins to breathe. The umbilical cord is no longer needed and ceases to function. Gradually the ductus venosus and the ductus arteriosus become obliterated. The foramen ovale closes and the baby's circulation becomes the same as that of an adult.

It is apparent that in fetal circulation, oxygenated blood from the ductus venosus mixes with used blood in the inferior vena cava. This mixing of oxygenated blood with used blood dilutes the concentration of oxygen in the circulation of the fetus. The fetus is able to survive in this lowered oxygen concentration (*hypoxia*) until its lungs begin to function at birth. The bluish pink color of babies at birth is due to the hypoxia of intrauterine life.

MULTIPLE PREGNANCY

A multiple pregnancy is one in which more than one fetus develops in the uterus at the same time. The most common multiple pregnancy is twins (Fig. 7-6). Twins occur about once in every 93 white births and once in 73 nonwhite births. Other multiple births occur less frequently: triplets approximately once in 9,400 births and quadruplets once in 620,000. The incidence of multiple fetuses is greater with the use of infertility agents such as gonadotropin and clomiphene.

TYPES OF TWINNING

There are two types of twins: monozygotic (identical) and dizygotic (fraternal) (Fig. 7-7).

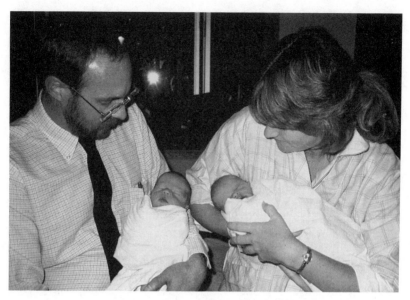

FIG. 7-6. *Fraternal twins, Matthew and Andrew.*

✓FIG. 7-7. *Twin pregnancy. (A) Fraternal twins with two placentas, two amnions, and two chorions. (B) Identical twins with one placenta, one chorion, and two amnions.*

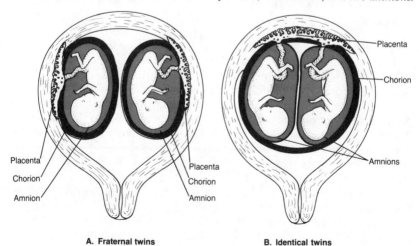

Placenta
Chorion

Placenta
Chorion
Amnion

Placenta
Chorion
Amnion

Amnions

A. Fraternal twins

B. Identical twins

Monozygotic twins result from a single ovum fertilized by one sperm. The ovum divides into two identical parts soon after fertilization. When this division occurs within 72 hours after fertilization, there are two amnions and two chorions; there may be two placentas, or one placenta that is fused. When the division occurs between the fourth and eighth days, there are two amnions and one chorion. When it occurs about 8 days after fertilization, there is one amnion and one chorion; when it occurs later, the fetuses are combined, resulting in so-called Siamese twins. Monozygotic twins occur much less frequently than dizygotic twins, and their appearance is not influenced by factors such as race, heredity, maternal age and parity, or therapy for infertility. Monozygotic twins are always of the same sex.

Dizygotic twins result from fertilization of two ova by two sperm. These twins may or may not be of the same sex and may resemble each other no more than other siblings. The occurrence of dizygotic twins appears to be influenced by race, heredity, age and parity of the mother and infertility agents. Fraternal twins are most prevalent in blacks, with the mother being responsible for transmitting this trait. The frequency of twins increases as maternal age advances to about 37 years and parity to seven. The use of infertility drugs increases the incidence of multiple pregnancy by increasing ovulation. Not only is there an increase in dizygotic twins with the use of these agents, but triplets, quadruplets, quintuplets, or sextuplets may occur.

DIAGNOSIS AND MANAGEMENT

Multiple pregnancy is suspected when a pregnancy is larger than it should be for the gestational age. Diagnosis may be made by abdominal palpation, by hearing two differing fetal heart rates, or by ultrasonography or radiography of the abdomen. However, radiographs may not reveal a multiple pregnancy if the films are of poor quality or the mother is very obese, or if one fetus moves just as the film is exposed.

The perinatal mortality is higher for twins than for single pregnancies. The fetal age is shorter, and most twins have a lower birth weight. Problems frequently encountered with multiple pregnancies include hydramnios, premature labor, uterine dysfunction, abnormal presentations, prolapse of the umbilical cord, and premature separation of the placenta. Postpartum hemorrhage immediately following delivery is to be expected unless appropriate preventive measures are employed.

The labor of a woman with a multiple pregnancy should be closely observed by skilled personnel. The fetal heart rate of each fetus should be continuously monitored by the best means available. An intravenous infusion with a needle or catheter capable of administering blood should be maintained throughout labor and delivery and for several hours postpartum. Whole blood should be cross-matched and available for use. The mother may need a tremendous amount of support because of her concern for the infants, her own physical discomfort, and because analgesia may be limited or withheld completely in order to minimize the risk to the infants.

Prior to delivery, all necessary resuscitative and supportive equipment should be made ready. Adequate numbers of skilled personnel should be available during delivery to care for the mother and each of the infants. An anesthesiologist should be present to administer anesthesia should it be necessary.

CLINICAL REVIEW

1. The two types of cells in the human body are:
   a. Gametes and zygotes
   ✓b. Soma cells and germ cells
   c. Chromosomes and genes
   d. Immature cells and mature cells

2. Mrs. Brown is pregnant for the fourth time. Her other children are girls. What is the chance that this baby will be a boy? Why?

3. In a conversation with you, Mrs. Brown confides that she hopes this baby will be a boy because her husband became very angry with her each time she gave birth to a girl. What can you tell Mrs. Brown about how the sex of the baby is determined?

4. Why might a decrease in oxygen intake of a pregnant woman be harmful to the fetus, although it might not be harmful to the mother?

BIBLIOGRAPHY

Chaffee EE, Lytle IM: Basic Physiology and Anatomy, 4th ed, pp 563–566. Philadelphia, JB Lippincott, 1980
Jensen MD, Bobak IM: Maternity Care: The Nurse & The Family, 3rd ed, pp 245–265. St. Louis, CV Mosby, 1985
Pritchard JA, MacDonald PC: Williams Obstetrics, 17th ed, pp 79–175, New York, Appleton-Century Crofts, 1985
Reeder SR, Martin LL: Maternity Nursing, 16th ed, pp 146–168. Philadelphia, JB Lippincott, 1987

Prenatal Assessment and Management

4

health care during 8 pregnancy

BEHAVIORAL OBJECTIVES When the goals of this chapter are reached, the student will be able to:

○ List three or four things the physician looks for in the complete physical examination on the first prenatal visit.

○ Discuss why the blood pressure is taken on each prenatal visit.

○ Name four laboratory tests done on the first prenatal visit and explain why they are done.

○ Conduct a rollover test and interpret its results.

○ List four or five danger signs to be reported immediately by the pregnant woman.

○ List three signs of labor the expectant mother should report to the physician.

○ Identify the components of a balanced daily diet.

○ Name three minerals and three vitamins that need to be increased during pregnancy, tell the contribution of each, and list their sources.

○ Discuss the types of employment not recommended for pregnant women.

○ Describe nipple care during pregnancy.

○ Explain how the nurse can help to establish a desirable relationship with the expectant mother.

○ Describe how the nurse can help the expectant mother relax during the antepartal examination.

○ List five or six points the nurse should remember when counseling the expectant mother regarding nutrition.

○ *Give dietary suggestions that would be helpful to the underweight or under-nourished mother, the overweight mother, and the teenage mother.*

○ *Describe Dr. Grantly Dick Read's theory concerning the pain of childbirth.*

○ *Name nine or ten minor discomforts of pregnancy and suggest simple remedies or preventive measures.*

The health care the expectant mother receives during pregnancy is called *antepartal* (ante = before, partal = birth) care, or prenatal care. Prior to this century antepartal care as such did not exist. Pregnant women endured the risks of pregnancy as best they could: those in poor health often succumbed and the heartier survived, although their health status may have been somewhat lessened by the process.

Then, in 1901, nurses from the Instructive Nursing Association in Boston began making a single home visit to some of the expectant mothers who were to be delivered at the Boston Lying-In Hospital. Gradually, the number of these visits increased to three per patient. As the value of the visits became apparent and interest in them was aroused, individuals and organizations were influenced to provide funds so that they could be continued. Consequently, the work spread so that at one time, a limited number of mothers under the care of physicians and hospitals were being visited as often as every 10 days. At each visit the mother's blood pressure was taken and a urine test was done. Thus, antepartal care, one of the most important achievements in maternity care in this century, was begun.

Antepartal care today is different in several respects from that in the early days of its inception. Women who can pay for their care now go to the physician's office, while those with lower incomes may receive care in clinics, hospitals, or public health departments. Most of the care is provided by physicians and nurses, but laboratory technicians, dentists, radiologists, nutritionists, social workers, and dental hygienists may also be involved. The care includes

Evaluating the health status of the expectant mother early in pregnancy
Correcting any health problems present
Preventing the development of other health problems
Promoting positive health

The purpose of antepartal care is twofold:

To protect and promote the health and well-being of the expectant mother
To safeguard the health and well-being of the unborn infant

Ideally, the woman's health at the end of pregnancy should be as good as or better than it was at the beginning. Ideally, each pregnant woman should give birth to a vigorous, healthy infant. If she is in perfect health when she becomes pregnant and remains healthy throughout pregnancy and childbirth, these goals are likely to be realized. But, unfortunately, this degree of health is possessed by only a small percentage of women who become pregnant. For many women the demands of pregnancy may result in their own or the fetus' illness or even death unless they receive early and continuous medical care and supervision throughout pregnancy. Antepartal care has proved helpful to all expectant mothers and has saved the lives of many.

Prenatal Physical Examination

B.P.: _____ Height: _____ Weight: _____ Usual Weight: _____

General Appearance: _____

General Examination: _____

Head: _____ Eyes: _____ Pharynx: _____ Teeth: _____

Thyroid: _____ Skin: _____ Adenopathy: _____ Breasts: _____

Lungs: _____ Heart: _____

Extremities: Varicosities: _____ Edema: _____

Other: _____

Obstetrical Examination:

Abdominal Scars: _____ Masses: _____ Herniae: _____

Uterus: McDonald's measurement: _____ cm. F.H.: _____

Presentation: _____ Duration of gestation (estimated). _____ wk

Abnormalities noted: _____

Pelvic examination: Introitus: _____ Vagina: _____

Cervix: _____ Corpus; Contour: _____ Size: _____

Adnexa: _____

Clinical Pelvimetry:

Examiner	Consultant
Subpubic angle: _____	Subpubic angle: _____
Bi-ischial: _____	Bi-ischial: _____
Diagonal conjugate: _____	Diagonal conjugate: _____
Sacrum: _____	Sacrum: _____
Ischial spines: _____	Ischial spines: _____
S.S. notch: _____	S.S. notch: _____
Clinical Classification:	Clinical Classification:

_____ Examiner

_____ Consultant M.D.

Laboratory Examination:

V.D.R.L. _____ G - C Culture _____

Chest X-Ray: _____ Tine Test - Date _____ Results _____

Hgb: _____ Hct: _____ Blood Group: _____ Rh Type: _____

Rubella titer: _____ Antibody screen: _____ Husband's Rh Type: _____

Urinalysis: Protein: _____ Glucose _____ Culture _____

Pap Smear _____

Other _____

Additional Comments: _____

_____

_____ M

Name: _____ P.F.# _____

FIG. 8-1. *A sample data sheet for the prenatal physical examination.*

istory of Previous Pregnancies (Include abortions)

a. Year	Labor				Delivery			Child at Birth			Duration of nursing	Present health of child	Complications of pregnancy, labor, delivery, puerperium
	Spont.	Induc.	wks a EDC wks p	Hours	Method	Perineum	Place	Weight	Condition	Sex			

amily History: (Underline positive items and elaborate below): 1) Congenital anomalies 2) Diabetes 3) Heart disease 4) Hypertension 5) Renal disease 6) Tuberculosis 7) Convulsions 8) Multiple pregnancies 9) Psychiatric 10) Other _____

_____

_____

ast History: Operations and Injuries _____

nderline positive items and elaborate below): 1) Transfusions 2) Drug sensitivities 3) Asthma, Hay fever 4) Allergies 5) Diabetes 6) Rheumatic fever 7) Heart disease 8) Hypertension 9) Tuberculosis 10) Urinary tract disease 11) Vascular sease 12) Venereal disease 13) Psychiatric disease 14) Other _____

_____

_____

_____

enstruation: Menarche _____ Age of Cycle _____ Duration of Flow _____ Amount Pain _____ IMB _____

story of Present Pregnancy

miting usea _____ Urinary Symptoms _____ Date of Quickening _____ LMP _____ } Normal Abnormal

adache ritus Abdominal Pain _____ Bleeding _____ PMP _____

ucorrhoea _____ Edema _____ Constipation _____ EDC _____

dications _____ Other _____

e _____ yrs. M S W D Sep Race: BL _____ Wh _____ Y _____ Br _____ Religion _____

sband: Age: _____ yrs. Ht _____ Wt _____ Significant medical history _____ Husband's Occupation _____

ity: Prior pregnancies _____ Full term _____ Premature _____ Abortions _____ Living children _____

erviewed by _____ Physician _____ M.D.

ate	Wt.	Urine	BP	Weeks	MCD	Position	FHT	Quickening	Return

HEALTH CARE PROVIDED BY THE PHYSICIAN

The physician is the leader of the health team providing health care during pregnancy. He prescribes and supervises the care that the expectant mother receives throughout her pregnancy. To do so he must know his patient as an individual and as a member of her family. He must decide what care she needs based on her health status at the beginning of pregnancy and the demands that pregnancy will make upon her.

EVALUATING HEALTH STATUS

As soon as she suspects that she is pregnant—usually after she has missed one or two menstrual periods—a woman should see her physician. On the first visit the physician obtains her medical history and does a complete physical examination, which includes a pelvic examination and laboratory tests. Some physicians also order a chest radiograph on the first visit.

Medical history

The medical history includes information concerning the patient's family history and her personal and obstetric history. The family history is important because certain health problems, such as diabetes, tuberculosis, and some hereditary diseases, could affect the course and outcome of pregnancy. The woman's personal health history gives the physician information on the state of her health in the past. The obstetric history is important if this is not a first pregnancy. It includes such information as the number of previous pregnancies, the weight of previous babies at birth, the length of labor with each, and what, if any, problems arose during pregnancy, labor, delivery, and the puerperium. This information helps the physician know what may be expected during the present pregnancy. Prenatal forms are used by most facilities to record this information as well as information gained from continuing visits throughout the pregnancy (Fig. 8-1).

Physical examination

In the physical examination, the physician looks for any defects that need correction. These may include dental caries, dietary deficiencies, overweight or underweight conditions, or any other condition that might interfere with health. The patient is weighed and her blood pressure taken on the first visit and each visit thereafter, and the findings are recorded on her chart (Fig. 8-2). By keeping a record of her blood pressure and weight, the physician can determine any blood pressure elevation or rapid weight gain from one visit to the next. A sudden or gradual increase in the blood pressure or a sudden excessive weight gain is a symptom of pregnancy-induced hypertension, a serious complication of pregnancy (see Chap. 16).

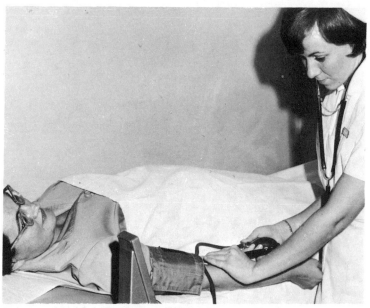

FIG. 8-2. *The mother's blood pressure is taken during each visit to the doctor.*

Pelvic examination. The physician performs a pelvic examination to determine the condition of the reproductive organs and the birth canal. He must know if there are tumors or other abnormalities present that could interfere with the birth of the baby. He also measures the pelvis to find out if it is large enough to permit the passage of an average size baby.

With the woman on her back on the examining table, knees drawn up, legs apart, and feet resting in stirrups, internal palpation of the pelvis is done to determine the height of the symphysis pubis, the shape of the pubic arch, the mobility of the coccyx, the inclination of the anterior wall of the sacrum and the side walls of the pelvis, and the prominence of the ischial spines. Then measurements of the pelvis are obtained.

Pelvic measurements. One of the most important internal pelvic measurements is the conjugata vera, or *true conjugate*. This is the distance between the sacral promontory and the posterior aspect of the symphysis pubis. Since this measurement cannot be made directly except from radiographs, it is made indirectly by measuring the length of the diagonal conjugate. The diagonal conjugate is the distance between the sacral promontory and the lower border of the symphysis pubis. This measurement is obtained by passing two fingers into the vagina and pressing inward and forward until the middle finger reaches the sacral promontory. The point on the top of the hand just under the symphysis is then marked

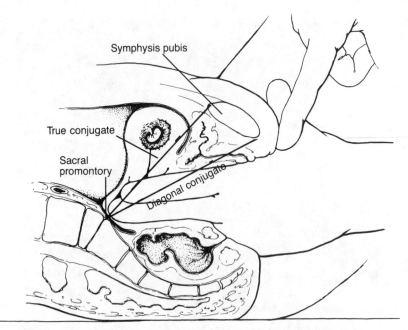

FIG. 8-3. *Method of obtaining diagonal conjugate diameter (12.5 cm).*

by putting the index finger of the other hand on the exact point (Fig. 8-3). The two fingers are then withdrawn and the distance from the tip of the middle finger to the marked point is measured; this is the length of the diagonal conjugate. If the diagonal conjugate is more than 11.5 cm, the pelvic inlet is considered of adequate size for childbirth. The size of the true conjugate is then estimated by subtracting 1.5 cm (or 2 cm if the symphysis pubis is high) from the length of the diagonal conjugate.

Another important measurement made at this time is the distance between the ischial tuberosities. This is the transverse diameter of the outlet of the pelvis and is referred to as the tuberischii diameter (TI), biischial diameter, or intertuberous diameter. An instrument such as Williams' pelvimeter (Fig. 8-4) or Thom's pelvimeter is used to obtain this measurement, or sometimes the closed fist is pressed between the tuberosities to estimate the size. The distance measured is from the innermost and lowermost aspect of the ischial tuberosities on a level with the anus. A diameter of more than 8 cm is considered adequate.

X-ray pelvimetry is the most accurate means of obtaining pelvic measurements. However, since exposure of mother and fetus to irradiation is undesirable, this procedure is performed only when absolutely necessary. It is indicated when

Manual measurements reveal a small pelvis

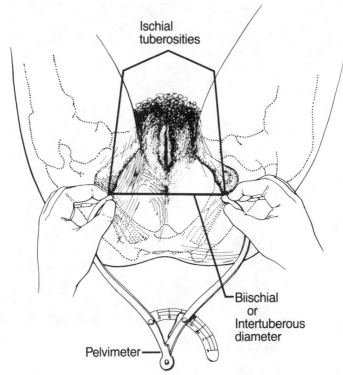

Ischial
tuberosities

Biischial
or
Intertuberous
diameter

Pelvimeter

√ FIG. 8-4. *Method of measuring tuberischii, or intertuberous, diameter of outlet.*

The patient has a history of difficult labors

Cephalopelvic disproportion is suspected because of failure to progress in labor

The presenting part is breech in term pregnancy

The usual procedure for x-ray pelvimetry consists of exposing two films: one from front to back with the woman on her back, and the other laterally with the woman on her left side or standing (Fig. 8-5). Slight distortion of size occurs on the radiographs. To correct for this, a metal ruler with centimeter markings is positioned near the perineum during the first exposure and in the gluteal fold during the second exposure. Since the same degree of distortion occurs with the ruler as with the patient, the centimeter markings of the ruler on the x-ray film are used to measure the diameters of the inlet, midpelvis, and outlet. Another method used to compensate for the distortion is to remove the patient after exposure of the first film and place a lead plate or grid containing centimeter perforations on the area previously occupied by the inlet of the patient. The same film is then exposed a second time.

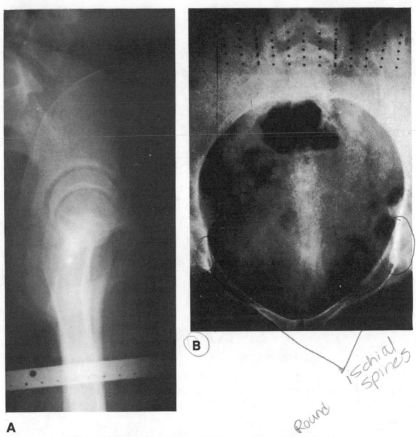

FIG. 8-5. *X-ray pelvimetry (A) Lateral view. (B) Inlet view.*

Laboratory tests and x-rays

Laboratory tests include a complete urinalysis and blood tests for syphilis, Rh factor and blood type, and hemoglobin and hematocrit readings.

Urinalysis. The urinalysis is done to find out if infection is present in the urinary system and to detect the presence of sugar or albumin. Sugar in the urine could be a symptom of diabetes and must be reported to the physician so that he can order further tests if he feels they are indicated. Albumin in the urine could be a symptom of pregnancy-induced-hypertension and must be reported to the physician.

Blood tests. Syphilis is a venereal disease that can be transmitted from an infected mother to the fetus. Untreated syphilis in the mother may result in deformities or death of the fetus, so every expectant mother should have a blood test (VDRL or other) for its detection.

The Rh factor is an antigen found in the red blood cells of some human beings. (This factor is abbreviated *Rh* after the rhesus monkey, which also contains the same antigen in its blood.) People whose blood contains the Rh factor are said to be *Rh positive*, and those whose blood does not contain the Rh factor are said to be *Rh negative*. About 85% of the white population and about 95% of the black population are Rh positive; the remainder are Rh negative.

The Rh factor is an inheritable characteristic. When the expectant mother is Rh negative, the Rh of the husband should be determined. Problems can arise with the baby when a mother is Rh negative and her husband is Rh positive (see Chap. 16 and Chap. 20).

There are four main groups or types of human blood. They are classified as A, B, AB, or O. Individuals requiring a blood transfusion should be given blood that is compatible with their own. This means that a person whose blood type is A should be given type A blood, while a person whose blood type is B should be given type B, and so on. Sometimes it is necessary to give the infant a transfusion immediately after birth; the mother's type of blood may be used in such emergencies, since the infant cannot produce antibodies at this early age.

If the mother's blood type is O, the husband's blood type should also be determined. If his blood type is A, B, or AB, then the potential for an ABO incompatibility in the infant exists (see Chap. 20).

The hemoglobin and hematocrit are checked on the first prenatal visit and periodically throughout pregnancy to find out if the levels are sufficiently high to provide the necessary iron to the mother and fetus. The hemoglobin and hematocrit levels become slightly lower as they become diluted by the increased blood volume. A hemoglobin of at least 12 g and a hematocrit of at least 35% should be maintained. Lower levels than these are symptoms of anemia.

Pap smear. The physician may also do a Papanicolaou smear (Pap smear). In this test a drop of the vaginal or cervical secretions is placed on a glass slide and spread out in a thin layer and stained. Then it is examined under the microscope to see if there are any precancerous cells present.

Chest radiographs. Some physicians order chest x-ray films for all their pregnant patients to determine the possibility of tuberculosis. Others order chest films only if other members of the family have tuberculosis or if the mother has recently been exposed to it. Some physicians prefer to have a tuberculin skin test done first; if it is nonreactive, chest films are not necessary. When a chest radiograph is obtained in a pregnant woman, the abdomen should be shielded to prevent possible damage to the fetus.

CORRECTING EXISTING PROBLEMS

The findings from the physical examination and from the laboratory tests help the physician identify health problems that need to be corrected.

If the mother needs dental work, the physician will recommend that she see her dentist. Likewise, before doing extensive dental work on the expectant woman the dentist will consult her obstetrician. During pregnancy, as at other times, the teeth need to be in good condition so that the food eaten can be well masticated. Teeth in poor condition may become foci of infection.

If the laboratory tests reveal the presence of syphilis, the physician will prescribe appropriate treatment, which usually consists of a series of penicillin injections. Treatment given early in pregnancy prevents the fetus from becoming infected.

Expectant mothers whose hemoglobin and hematocrit levels are lower than those recommended for pregnancy are treated for anemia. The physician usually prescribes iron tablets or injections.

Mothers with nutritional problems, such as dietary deficiencies or over-weight or underweight conditions, must be helped to select appropriate diets. If a nutritionist is not available, it probably will become the responsibility of the nurse to give this help (see below).

Other corrective measures are taken as the need arises.

PREVENTING ADDITIONAL PROBLEMS

Health care during pregnancy includes the prevention of health problems by careful supervision of the expectant mother throughout her entire pregnancy. To ensure adequate supervision, the mother must be seen at least once each month until the seventh month, then every 2 weeks until the last month, then every week until the baby is born. If problems arise, she is seen at more frequent intervals.

On each of these visits the physician inquires into the general well-being of the mother and checks carefully for early signs of complications. He questions her as to whether she has had swelling of the fingers or face, bleeding, constipation, headaches, or indigestion. She is given opportunity to ask questions that she may have about her pregnancy, her feelings, or anything else that concerns her. The mother is weighed; her urine is examined for albumin and sugar; her abdomen is palpated and, after they are audible, the fetal heart tones are listened to; and her blood pressure is taken.

Often, no weight is gained during the first trimester of pregnancy; some mothers actually lose weight during this time. The average weight gain during the second trimester is about one-half pound a week. During the third trimester it is about a pound a week.

The physician can determine if the fetus is growing at a normal rate by palpating the abdomen and measuring the height of the uterus (Fig. 8-6). Hearing the fetal heart tones is evidence that the fetus is alive. Vaginal and rectal examinations are done periodically and, along with abdominal examinations, indicate whether or not the pregnancy is progressing normally.

When a prenatal visit is scheduled, whether at a physician's office or

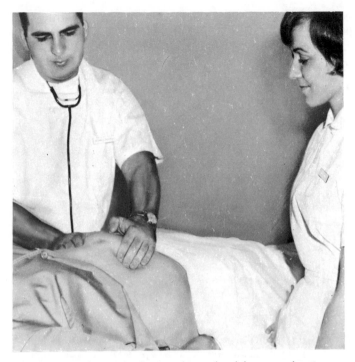

FIG. 8-6. *At each visit the doctor palpates the abdomen and measures the height of the fundus of the uterus.*

other health-care facility, the expectant woman should not have to wait long before being seen. Many women are discouraged from seeking care because of tiresome waiting. It is also important that the visit be scheduled to allow adequate time for her to discuss with the care-giver, in a relaxed atmosphere, any problems or questions she has related to her pregnancy. Enterprising nurses in some health-care facilities utilize the waiting time of expectant parents for brief teaching sessions.

In these sessions, and in all contacts with the expectant parents, nurses and other health-care providers should be sensitive to verbal and non-verbal clues from the parents indicating their feelings regarding the pregnancy and the expected child. It is believed that bonding between parents and child begins in pregnancy; nurses and other health-care givers in pre-natal care facilities are in a key position not only to assess whether bonding appears to be occurring, but also to promote it. The nurse and others may have limited time with the expectant parents, but they see them periodically over weeks or months, and if they are "tuned in" to the parents and their feelings, they may be able to provide much-needed help to the parents in coping with the pregnancy and developing a positive attitude toward the unborn child.

When subtle or obvious rejection of a pregnancy is detected by a health-care provider, steps should be taken to assist the parents to work toward coping in an acceptable and nondestructive manner. In attempting to do this, one must begin with the parents where they are and utilize the resources available to them; if these are not adequate to bring about the desired coping, then external resources may need to be involved. Health-care providers need to understand the positions of rejecting parents in order to help them. Many different backgrounds and experiences are represented by the expectant parents seen in a physician's office or other health-care facility. Each person perceives the pregnancy and the unborn child from her (his) own particular background of experiences. This perception is real and valid to the individual, and the health-care giver must try to understand it in order to be of help.

Rollover test.   This is a controversial test used by some physicians to help decide if a patient is likely to develop *pregnancy-induced hypertension* (PIH; see Chap. 9). PIH is characterized by an elevation of 30 mm Hg or more in the systolic blood pressure or 15 mm Hg or more in the diastolic blood pressure above what is considered normal for a specific woman. Usually this elevation in blood pressure occurs after the 28th week of pregnancy in a woman who has previously had a normal blood pressure.

The rollover test is done in the physician's office on women with normal blood pressure who are in the 28th to 32nd weeks of pregnancy. The patient lies on her left side and her blood pressure is taken approximately every 5 minutes until a constant reading is obtained. Then the patient is turned onto her back and her blood pressure is taken immediately and again in 5 minutes. If there is an elevation of 20 mm Hg or more in the diastolic pressure when she is turned onto her back, the test is positive.

The rollover test is controversial. Some authorities believe it is 90% reliable. Others believe it is not valid because when an individual with a normal blood pressure rolls over from the left lateral recumbent position, there is often a rise in blood pressure, and this rise cannot be related to subsequent PIH.

Immunizations.   Immunizations to prevent some health problems may not be desirable during pregnancy because they may have adverse or unknown effects on the fetus. These include immunizations for mumps, measles, poliomyelitis, smallpox, and rubella. If a pregnant woman must travel in areas where she may be exposed to cholera, typhoid, or yellow fever, she should first be immunized against these diseases. However, it would be preferable to avoid such travel during pregnancy. She should also avoid large crowds where exposure to infections is greatest. Tetanus and diphtheria toxoids as well as the tuberculin and histoplasmin tests are considered safe during pregnancy.

High-risk pregnancies.   Women who have had serious problems with previous pregnancies or who have problems with this pregnancy that may jeopardize their lives and their pregnancies are classified as "high risk."

High-risk mothers are seen at more frequent intervals during pregnancy and are also supervised more closely during labor, delivery, and the period following delivery (see Chap. 17).

Signs to be reported. All expectant mothers can help prevent additional problems by reporting to the physician immediately if they experience any of the "danger signs." Each pregnant woman should be instructed to notify the physician regarding these signs, but she should be told in such a way as not to alarm her unduly.

DANGER SIGNS TO REPORT TO THE PHYSICIAN

- ○ Bleeding or leakage of fluid from the vagina
- ○ Rapid weight gain
- ○ Swelling of the hands and face
- ○ Persistent headache
- ○ Dizziness
- ○ Visual disturbances
- ○ Persistent vomiting

In the last weeks of pregnancy, the mother is told to notify the physician of signs that labor is starting. These signs include:

A pink, mucous vaginal discharge (show)

A trickle or gush of fluid from the vagina (rupture of the membranes)

Intermittent, regular contractions of the uterus

PROMOTING POSITIVE HEALTH

NUTRITION

Adequate nutrition during pregnancy means that the intake of nutrients equals the needs of the mother and her fetus. These nutrients can be obtained in a balanced diet.

For many years, the pregnant woman was cautioned to restrict her caloric intake in order to minimize her weight gain during pregnancy. This was believed necessary to prevent PIH, since it was thought that PIH was most likely to occur among the overweight pregnant population. However, studies have shown that PIH is more prevalent among the markedly underweight. Also, a definite relationship has been found between the underweight woman and the birth weight of her infant. Infants born to malnourished women may suffer from neurologic damage and mental retardation as well as low birth weight, because the primary phase of brain cell development occurs during the fetal period. Low birth weight is associated with an increased incidence of neonatal mortality. Weight reduction programs are discouraged during pregnancy because of the possible damage to the fetus.

Current nutritional guides recognize that there is an increased need for calories during pregnancy to provide energy for building fetal and placental tissues and for sustaining the maternal tissues. To provide these energy requirements, the pregnant woman should usually increase her caloric intake by 300 calories per day over what she normally eats. These calories should be in foods that can provide the additional minerals, vitamins, and protein needed during pregnancy. A weight gain of 2 to 4 lb (1 to 2 kg) during the first trimester and 0.9 lb (0.5 kg) per week during the remainder of pregnancy is recommended, even for overweight women. A total weight gain of 25 to 30 lb (11 to 13 kg) is considered compatible with desirable pregnancy outcomes.

A balanced diet during pregnancy consists of the daily intake of 1 quart of milk; two or more servings of meat, fish, poultry, eggs, or cheese; four or more servings of vegetables and fruits; and four or more servings of breads and cereals. In addition to these basic food groups, the expectant mother should drink at least six to eight glasses of fluids daily.

The milk can be used as a beverage or in cooking or it can be combined with cereals and bread. When it is combined with cereals and bread it makes the protein in these foods more useful to the body. Skim milk may be used in place of whole milk when there is a need to reduce the fat intake; however, it should be fortified so that it is not lacking in vitamin A.

Occasionally, dried beans, peas, nuts, or peanut butter can be substituted for meats, fish, or poultry. When this is done, it is a good practice to serve milk at the same meal since the protein in it will make the vegetable protein more useful to the body.

Dark green, leafy vegetables or yellow vegetables and yellow fruits should be included in the vegetables and fruits group three or four times a week so that sufficient amounts of vitamin A will be obtained. Citrus fruits, tomatoes, or other sources of vitamin C also should be included in the diet each day.

When buying cereals and breads, the woman should choose those made with enriched flour or whole grains. This will add minerals and vitamins to the diet.

A woman who normally eats a balanced diet will need to make a minimum of changes to obtain proper nutrition during pregnancy. These changes consist of increasing her intake of the foods that will add to the dietary supply of minerals, vitamins, and proteins.

Minerals. Minerals that need to be increased during pregnancy are calcium, phosphorus, and iron. Calcium and phosphorus are essential components of bones and teeth. During pregnancy a whole new skeletal system, as well as the foundation for the permanent and temporary teeth of the fetus, is formed—thus the need for calcium and phosphorus. Calcium is also necessary for normal clotting of the blood, for normal contractility of the muscles, and for maintenance of the heartbeat. The mother's reserve of calcium, which is stored in the long bones, may be used up to supply the needs of the fetus if her intake of calcium is insufficient. During pregnancy the mother's intake of calcium should be 1.2 g/day.

Since phosphorus is found in foods rich in calcium, its requirements are also met when the calcium requirements are met. Milk is the best source of calcium; 1 quart of milk contains 1.4 g of calcium. Cheese and green leafy vegetables also contain calcium. To ensure a sufficient intake, the physician may prescribe supplementary medicinal calcium.

Additional iron is needed for the formation of hemoglobin and for transporting oxygen and carbon dioxide for the fetus. During the first few months after birth the infant's diet contains very little iron. Therefore, during the last trimester of pregnancy, the fetus stores enough iron to last for 5 months after birth.

To meet the demands of pregnancy, the mother's intake of iron should be 15 to 20 mg each day. Dark green, leafy vegetables, dried fruit, red meat, liver, eggs, legumes, and enriched or whole grain breads and cereals are good sources of iron. Medicinal iron is often prescribed to supplement that obtained through the diet.

Vitamins.   Foods containing all the vitamins should be included in the diet. However, the intake of vitamins A, C, and D especially needs to be increased.

Vitamin A affects vision and tooth formation and is important in reducing susceptibility to infection. The added intake of vitamin A is important primarily to the mother and to the preservation of the pregnancy, since this vitamin does not cross the placental barrier. The infant has a poor supply of vitamin A at birth, but breast-fed infants obtain it through the colostrum and the breast milk, which are rich in it.

Sources of vitamin A are dark green, leafy vegetables, deep yellow vegetables, yellow fruits, cod-liver oil, animal liver, eggs, butter, and cheese. If the doctor prescribes mineral oil to relieve a problem of constipation, the mother should be reminded to take it at bedtime instead of at mealtime, because mineral oil destroys the fat-soluble vitamin A in her food.

Vitamin C is found in citrus fruits, cantaloupe, strawberries, green pepper, broccoli, cabbage, potatoes, raw vegetables, and tomatoes. Vitamin C helps make the walls of the blood vessels, aids in the healing of wounds, and is necessary for the development and maintenance of normal connective tissue in bones, muscles, and cartilage.

Vitamin D is necessary for the absorption and utilization of calcium. The expectant mother's diet should contain 400 International Units (IU) of vitamin D daily. It is found in fish-liver oil, fortified milk, eggs, butter, cheese, and fresh green vegetables. Vitamin D is produced in the body on exposure to sunlight.

Protein.   Protein is a building material and is essential to the development of the new muscles in the uterus. It is also essential to the formation of the embryo and for the growth and development of the fetus. Protein is needed for the manufacture of hormones and is a constituent of blood. The increased production of hormones and the increased blood volume of the mother, along with the development of a whole new circulatory system in the fetus, create a demand for protein.

To meet her needs and those of the developing fetus, the expectant mother should increase her daily intake of protein by about 30 g. Eggs, milk, lean meat, fish, poultry, beans, peas, cheese, bread, potatoes, and cereals are sources of protein.

OTHER HEALTH GUIDELINES

Clothing. By about the third month of pregnancy, the enlarging uterus begins to rise out of the pelvis and causes a bulging of the lower abdomen. Shortly afterward, the woman begins to notice that her clothes are becoming too snug, so she shops for clothing that is more comfortable and more practical.

For greatest comfort, maternity clothes should hang from the shoulders and allow for the expansion of the growing uterus. The enlarging breasts should be well-supported by a wide-strap bra that gives support without pressure.

The woman should avoid wearing such articles of clothing as panty girdles, round garters, and knee socks, which cause circular constriction of the legs. When constriction of the blood vessels in the legs occurs, the formation of varicose veins is encouraged.

Girdles and corsets specially designed for pregnancy are available. When properly worn, they give support without compressing the uterus. It is wise for the woman to check with her physician about wearing a girdle or a corset, since some physicians object to their use during pregnancy.

During pregnancy, the woman's posture changes. The enlarging uterus extends forward and the shoulders are held backward to maintain balance, resulting in a swayback posture. This posture is further exaggerated by wearing shoes with high heels. Wearing shoes with broad heels aids in preventing falls and also helps prevent backache.

Rest. Rest and sleep are essential to replenishing the body's energy. During pregnancy one tends to tire more quickly, and the need for renewed energy is more apparent. The pregnant woman should plan rest periods in her daily schedule so that she is sure to get the rest she needs. If possible, she should lie down to rest and stretch out comfortably while her mind and all parts of her body relax completely. During the latter part of pregnancy she can add to her comfort by using a small pillow to support her abdomen while she rests on her side. If she cannot lie down to rest, she should sit as comfortably as possible with her feet and legs elevated. Throughout the day she should sit whenever possible as she performs her household or other duties. Although activity is important to her health and well-being, she should use moderation in all that she does and stop before becoming tired in order to avoid exhaustion.

Activity. Daily outdoor exercise contributes to good health and a sense of well-being anytime and is especially beneficial during pregnancy. Breathing deeply in the fresh air improves the mother's circulation and increases the oxygen supply to the fetus. Exercise in the outdoors refreshes the mind and promotes sound sleep.

The type of exercise the woman undertakes should be consistent with what she did before pregnancy. Strenuous exercises and those in which falls could occur should not be continued unless approved by her physician. Brisk walking in the fresh air is one of the best exercises. Although many women get sufficient exercise while performing household chores, they still need to spend some time each day outdoors. Furthermore, each woman should have some form of diversion that she enjoys. The diversion can be reading, music, movies, sporting events, church functions, entertaining friends, and the like. The father can contribute greatly to the happiness of the expectant mother by arranging for and sharing in the social activities.

Moments of anxiety occur when the expectant parents anticipate the responsibilities accompanying the birth of the baby. Fears concerning labor and the possibility that the child may not be "normal" increase their anxiety. A proper balance between work, exercise, rest and sleep, and diversion can minimize anxiety and promote a happy, wholesome attitude toward life and pregnancy.

Travel. Traveling for short distances is not contraindicated during pregnancy. Prior to traveling the woman should inform her physician of her plans, especially if a long trip is contemplated or if she is near term. She should choose a mode of travel that is comfortable for her and that permits her to walk about at least every 2 hours. This will help stimulate her general circulation and avoid fatigue. If she travels by car, seat belts adjusted for comfort should be worn. She should be aware of the risk that a complication of pregnancy might develop while she is far from a facility equipped for treating it.

Employment. The woman should consult her physician if she has questions concerning her employment during pregnancy. Although many occupations can be continued, those jobs involving fine balance, climbing, or assuming positions where a misstep could result in a fall should not be continued. Prolonged standing or sitting not only can be very tiring but also can slow down the return flow of blood from the feet and legs, thereby favoring the development of varicosities. Jobs requiring these positions should allow frequent rest periods during which the woman can change her position and, when possible, elevate her legs for a few minutes.

Bathing. The increased activity of the sweat and oil glands of the skin, along with the increased vaginal secretions, make daily bathing very important. Tub baths and showers may be continued throughout pregnancy. Since the posture of pregnancy makes it easy for the woman to lose her balance, she must be very careful getting in and out of the bathtub. Douches should be omitted unless specifically prescribed by the physician.

Nipple care. If the expectant mother plans to breast-feed her baby, special attention should be given the nipples. Secretions from the breasts may form a crust on the nipples, causing the skin beneath to become tender. Cracks in the skin are avenues for the entrance of infections. Unless the crust is removed, this area remains tender and is likely to crack when the infant nurses. Daily cleansing with a washcloth and warm water is usually adequate to remove these secretions and the crusting. Soaps and other astringent materials should not be used unless recommended by the physician, since they may do harm by removing the protective skin oils. The physician may suggest some type of hydrous lanolin preparation to prepare the nipples for nursing. Following the bath each day, the woman places a small amount of the lanolin on her thumb and index finger, then grasps the nipple with the same fingers and gently works the cream into all the nipple creases.

Sexual relations. The physician usually counsels the couple regarding sexual relations during pregnancy. Many physicians think that sexual relations may be continued throughout pregnancy, but others think they should be discontinued during the last month of pregnancy because of the danger of rupture of the membranes, premature labor, or infection. To lessen the possibility of spontaneous abortion, some doctors advise against intercourse in the early months of pregnancy at the time the woman normally would have her menstrual period.

Smoking. Cigarette smoking has been shown to be a health hazard. A definite relationship has been found between smoking and heart disease and lung cancer. Smoking has also been found to have such harmful effects on the outcome of pregnancy as lower birth rates, higher rates of prematurity, and higher neonatal mortality.

The *time* smoking is done during pregnancy and the *number of cigarettes* smoked appear to be significant in relation to the effects of smoking on pregnancy.

Smoking seems to be most harmful during the last 6 months of pregnancy when the central nervous system is still forming. Among women who smoke, the stillbirth rate is 30% higher and the perinatal mortality rate is 26% higher than among nonsmokers. Among women who stop smoking by the fourth month of pregnancy, the rates are the same as for nonsmokers.

The number of cigarettes smoked by the mother during pregnancy appears to have a direct affect on the infant's birth weight: the more cigarettes smoked, the lower the birth weight. Although the exact way smoking produces its effects is not known, lower birth weights may be due in part to lower caloric intake by smoking mothers. Moreover, it is believed that nicotine causes constriction of the peripheral blood vessels, resulting in changes in the heart rate, the blood pressure, and the output of the heart. These changes have a detrimental effect on the development and health of the fetus. Also, because of the higher concentration of carbon monoxide in the bloodstream of smokers, there is a decrease in the amount of oxygen; this apparently affects the fetus.

In addition to these effects, cigarette smoking seems to be even more dangerous in mothers who are considered high risk for other reasons.

Alcohol use. Chronic alcoholism may result in malformations of the fetus, an increased perinatal mortality rate, and prenatal and postnatal growth retardation. Babies born to alcoholic mothers may have withdrawal symptoms soon after birth, such as extreme hyperactivity, sweating, tremors, and generalized twitching of the face and extremities. These children tend to have a low IQ and impaired fine and gross motor function.

Medications. It is extremely important that the woman not take any drugs during pregnancy that are not prescribed by a physician who knows she is pregnant. This includes such common household items as aspirin. Prescribed medication should be taken in the smallest effective dosage and should be discontinued as soon as possible. These precautions are necessary to protect the embryo and fetus against both known and unknown effects of drugs that cross the placenta.

ROLE OF THE NURSE

NURSING STRATEGIES

Nursing assessments. As a result of her many contacts with the mother throughout the pregnancy, the nurse has the opportunity to get to know the mother and to obtain data that are essential to helping her meet the patient's needs. The data are obtained through interviews, observations, listening, and review of medical records. It is important that the plan of care developed from the data be adapted to fit the needs of the individual.

Included in the data needed is information on the woman's physical condition, her support system, her perceptions and feelings about the pregnancy, and her coping mechanisms.

Data on her physical condition are obtained during the physical examination and history taking and include height, weight, habits (such as use of drugs, alcohol, tobacco, etc.), and a history of any health or obstetric problems that could affect her and the fetus during this pregnancy.

Information on the expectant mother's support system can be obtained by talking with her and observing her. Her support system consists of family members and friends; their positive attitudes toward the pregnancy can enhance her own feelings. A steady source of income can also be considered part of her support system.

The expectant mother's feelings about her pregnancy depend on many factors: whether it was planned or unplanned, wanted or unwanted; her attitude toward sex and how it is affected by pregnancy; her feelings about the way the pregnancy is affecting her appearance; the affect the pregnancy will have on her present and future plans for a career; her living accommodations; finances; the number and ages of other children; her relationship with her spouse or partner; her expectations of herself as a person and as a parent; and her expectations of the infant. The attitudes and feelings of her spouse or partner and her support group also influence her feelings toward the pregnancy.

The expectant mother's coping mechanisms involve her knowledge of pregnancy and childbirth, her decision-making ability, and her ability to handle stress. These can be assessed through interviews and observations.

Potential nursing diagnoses:

Ineffective individual coping related to lack of support system

Ineffective individual coping related to the woman's perceptions and feelings regarding the pregnancy

Knowledge deficit related to procedures and why they are done

Anxiety related to the condition of the infant and her own health

Alterations in nutrition, less than body requirements for pregnancy and developing fetus

Alterations in comfort: pain related to the pregnancy

Nursing interventions.   In meeting the expectant mother's needs, the nurse may be called on to be teacher, counselor, resource person, friend, and support person. If the expectant mother trusts the nurse and has confidence in her, she will be more likely to express her needs and cooperate in meeting these needs.

First impressions are often important in laying the foundation for a cooperative relationship. Since the nurse is usually one of the first persons the mother sees on her initial visit to the doctor, she can begin right away to make the mother feel comfortable and at ease by greeting her in a warm, friendly manner and by introducing herself. If the nurse is obtaining the information for the medical history, she should provide privacy, assure the mother that the information will be kept confidential, and explain the reason the information is needed.

The nurse should remember that this experience may be a new one for the expectant mother and that she may be fearful of what will be done to her. The nurse can show her concern for the mother's feelings by explaining the procedures before they are done, by providing privacy, by avoiding unnecessary exposure of the mother's body during the procedures, and by assuring the mother that she will remain with her during the physical examination.

On subsequent visits the nurse can reinforce her relationship with the mother by greeting her warmly and calling her by name. Thus, the mother will be made to feel that she is known and appreciated.

Nursing referrals. The nurse can often be of assistance to the expectant mother by answering her questions concerning the layette (see Chap. 2) for the baby and in making plans for care of the family during her hospital stay and the first week she and the baby are home. She should acquaint herself with the community facilities for meeting such family needs and make referrals as approved by the physician.

ASSISTING THE PHYSICIAN

The nurse weighs the mother (Fig. 8-7) and obtains a urine specimen. On the first visit a complete urinalysis is done; on each subsequent visit the urine is tested for albumin and sugar. Often these tests are performed by the nurse. One of the simplest methods of determining the presence of albumin in the urine is to dip the end of a strip of treated paper into the urine; the end is then compared with a color code chart. The presence of albumin is indicated by a change in color of the strip (Fig. 8-8). A similar test can be used to determine the presence of sugar in the urine. The nurse records the mother's weight and the urine test results on the chart.

The nurse assists the mother onto the examining table and positions her. During the examination she assists the physician as necessary. When a pelvic examination is done, she encourages the mother to breathe normally and to keep her back flat against the table. If the mother seems

FIG. 8-7. *The nurse weighs the mother at each visit.*

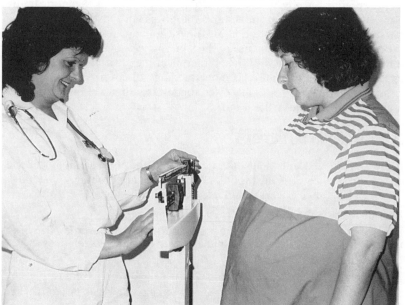

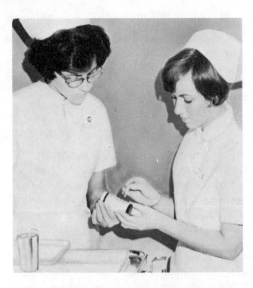

FIG. 8-8. *The mother's urine is tested for albumin at each visit.*

tense, the nurse may hold her hand or take other measures to help her relax and thus minimize her discomfort. Following the examination, the nurse helps the mother down from the table and, if a pelvic examination has been done, provides her with tissue so that she can wipe off the lubricant that was used.

Interpreting the physician's instructions.   A mother may confide to the nurse that she does not understand the physician's instructions, or the nurse may suspect she does not. The physician may also ask the nurse to explain the instructions to the mother. In any case, it is a good practice for the nurse to go over with the mother all of the physician's instructions so that she can correct any misunderstandings, discover how the mother intends to carry them out, and offer suggestions that will make it easier for the mother to carry them out.

COUNSELING ON NUTRITION

If the services of a nutritionist are unavailable, the physician may depend on the nurse to counsel the mother regarding dietary problems. The nurse is more likely to be successful in her counseling if she:

First develops a relationship of trust with the mother

Begins her counseling early in the pregnancy before the woman has been influenced too greatly by the opinions of her friends and relatives

Learns the present eating habits of the mother

Helps the mother to see why changes in her diet are important

Actively involves the mother in the diet planning and helps her to use her present resources more efficiently

Gives specific, detailed instructions in language the mother can understand

Recognizes the effects such factors as age, religion, race, socioeconomic status, and cultural background have on diet

Realizes that the amount of calories the mother needs will be influenced by her activity and metabolism

Takes into consideration the likes and dislikes of the mother and her family

Allows the mother choices when this can be done without sacrificing the desired goals, and gives firm guidance when needed

The mother may need help in using her food budget more efficiently. In such cases, the nurse should point out the value of inexpensive sources of protein such as dried beans, peas, and peanut butter. When milk or cheese is served with these vegetable proteins, the animal protein makes the vegetable protein more useful in the body. The budget can be further stretched without loss of valuable nutrients if fortified skim milk, evaporated milk, or dried milk is used in place of fresh, whole milk.

Selection of food can also be important when the budget is limited. By reading labels on breads and cereals and choosing those made with whole grain or enriched flour, the mother can obtain more nutrients for the same price. Tomatoes may be less expensive at certain times of the year than citrus fruit and are a good source of vitamin C. However, it takes twice the amount of tomatoes to supply the same amount of vitamin C obtained from citrus fruit.

The way foods are prepared affects their nutritional content. Food values and flavors can be preserved by cooking vegetables quickly in small amounts of water. Many vegetables can be eaten raw, thereby assuring consumption of their complete mineral and vitamin content as well as adding to the dietary roughage, which is important to elimination.

Counseling may be directed to a mother who shuns milk because she dislikes it or because it is constipating. Because of its value as a source of calcium, phosphorus, and protein, milk must not be left out of the diet. However, it is not essential that she *drink* a quart of milk each day. She can drink one or two glasses of milk and take the remainder in other ways, such as in soups, puddings, custards, or combined with fruits, cereals, and breads. Flavoring added to milk makes it more palatable. Evaporated milk, dried milk (whole or nonfat), or foritified skim milk can be used in cooking.

If a woman refuses to drink milk because it is constipating, she should be encouraged to try to correct the problem by other means than leaving milk out of her diet. For example, she could eat more fresh fruits and raw vegetables, drink more of other fluids, and get more exercise. If these measures are not effective, it may be necessary for the doctor to prescribe treatment for constipation.

The mother who begins pregnancy with dietary deficiencies or who is underweight or overweight also may need counseling on nutrition. The desirable weight gain during pregnancy depends on the individual and is influenced by her nutritional status and weight at the beginning of pregnancy.

If the mother has dietary deficiencies or is underweight, she is urged to eat more and larger servings of the four food groups included in a balanced diet. In order to do this, she may need to plan for between-meal snacks at intervals during the day. She can increase her mineral and protein intake by adding dried milk to mashed potatoes, meat loafs, and cereals. Also, special high-protein preparations such as Meritene can be added to the milk she drinks, or she can make eggnogs or milkshakes.

Ways to eliminate unnecessary calories from the diet are to:

Avoid fried foods

Eliminate candy and soft drinks

Substitute fortified skim milk for whole milk

Reduce the intake of sugar

Eat fresh fruits and raw vegetables for between-meal snacks instead of sugary foods

Limit or omit the use of rich sauces, gravies, etc.

Decrease serving size

Teenage patients.   Counseling the teenage expectant mother about nutrition presents added problems, because a teenage girl often has the poorest eating habits. Her diet may consist largely of such items as hamburgers, pizzas, pickles, potato chips, and soft drinks. She is often so "figure conscious" that she skips meals, particularly breakfast, and eats sparingly at other times. However, because of the important developments occurring within her body during these teen years, she needs more of the essential nutrients than at any other time of her life except during pregnancy and lactation, when added nutrients must be provided for herself and her child.

To compound the problem, the teenager is also making a psychological adjustment from childhood to adulthood. During this time she is seeking to establish her own identity and to become independent, and she wants to make her own decisions. Consequently, she may resent and resist efforts on the part of others to influence her food choices. Furthermore, her cooking skills are probably limited.

The nurse must help the teenage expectant mother see the importance of a proper diet to herself and her infant. The mother should realize that through an adequate diet she will have healthier skin and hair. Her weight will be easier to control if she eats regular meals, because she will not be hungry continually and will therefore have fewer temptations to eat foods that are less nourishing yet contain more calories. The mother must realize, too, how her nutrition affects her unborn baby. Studies have shown that there is a definite relationship between the diet of the mother and the health of the infant. For example, an inadequate intake of protein by the mother during pregnancy can cause mental deficiency and low birth weight in the infant.

In her contacts with the teenage mother, the nurse should look for opportunities for giving encouragement and praise. When done in sincerity, this will help to motivate the girl to reach the desired health goals. She should be especially commended for any skills she develops in the planning and preparation of meals.

Unconventional diets. Vegetarian diets have been adopted by some individuals. These diets are of three main types:

Strict vegetarian, consisting entirely of plant foods

Lactovegetarian, which includes dairy products as well as plant foods

Lacto-ovovegetarian, which consists of eggs, dairy products, and plant foods

Probably the biggest problem associated with vegetarian diets is obtaining adequate amounts of the essential amino acids. This is not as difficult with the lactovegetarian and lacto-ovovegetarian diets as with the strict vegetarian. With careful planning, the strict vegetarian diet need not be deficient. Some suggestions for assuring adequate nutrition on a strict vegetarian diet include:

Combining grains, which are low in lysines, with legumes, which are adequate in lysines, at the same meal

Adding wheat germ, or, when appropriate, soy flour, to recipes

Combining sesame, pumpkin, or sunflower seeds with legumes at the same meal

Combining sesame seeds with rice

The use of fortified soy milk will help assure an adequate intake of vitamin B_{12} and vitamin D.

Fad diets are not new and, as a rule, they are harmless. One exception is the Zen macrobiotic diet. This diet, predominantly vegetarian, places great emphasis on whole grain cereals and stresses limiting the intake of fluids as much as possible. Advocates of the macrobiotic diet believe that a diet of natural foods is the treatment for all diseases. The opposite has been true for some who have followed this diet, for they have developed scurvy, anemia, hypoproteinemia, hypocalcemia, malnutrition and emaciation due to starvation, and loss of kidney function due to restricted fluid intake. Death has resulted in some cases. The implications for pregnancy of adhering to this diet are obvious.

TEACHING EXPECTANT PARENTS

Early in the prenatal period, the expectant parents usually make known the type of childbirth experience (Lamaze or other natural method, or medicated) that they desire. The type they desire will be a factor in deciding whether or not they will attend classes for expectant parents and also the type of facility (home, hospital, alternate birthing center, for example) they will use, and whether the birth will be attended by a certified nurse-midwife or a physician.

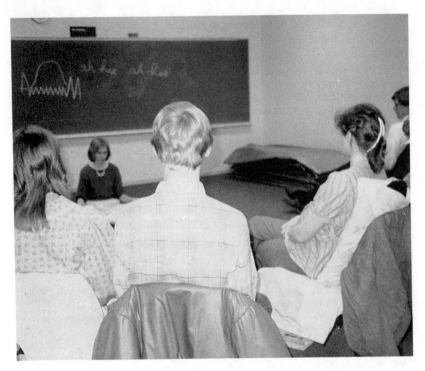

A

FIG. 8-9. *(A) Classes for expectant parents; (B) and (C) Breathing and relaxation techniques are practiced; (D) Expectant parent classes include instruction on infant care.*

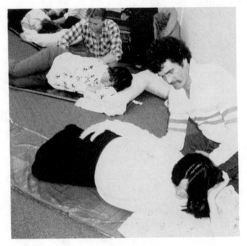

B

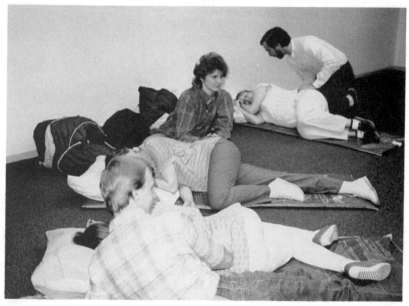

C

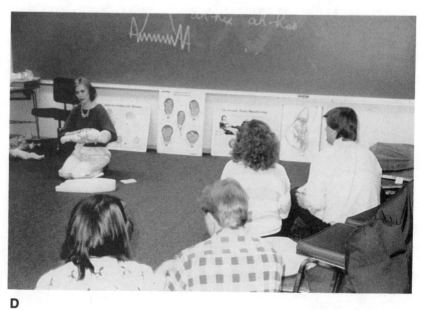

D

The nurse has an important function in helping to meet the expectant parents' need for information concerning pregnancy, childbirth, and the care of the newborn. She can do this in incidental conversations with the mother as interest is expressed as well as in planned classes for expectant parents. Such classes are offered by the Red Cross, by some physicians, by hospitals, and by other community agencies. The nurse usually conducts the classes, although an obstetrician and a pediatrician may also participate at times (Fig. 8-9).

The time and frequency of the classes are factors determining attendance by expectant parents. Because of occupational, family, and social commitments, there is no one time suitable for all. Generally, evening classes are better attended by both parents than those held during the day. When both morning and evening classes are held twice a week, opportunity to attend is provided for those who work evenings and nights as well as for those who work days. Also, if a choice of two mornings or evenings is offered, the couple can select the day and time best suited to their schedules. The content of the classes is usually repeated every four to six weeks. Thus a class that is missed can be made up in a later series.

Classes for expectant parents usually include a review of anatomy and physiology of human reproduction; a discussion of dietary needs during pregnancy and lactation; a talk and film on labor and delivery; a discussion of the care of the newborn, including a demonstration baby bath; and a tour of a hospital maternity department. In some classes, the topics for discussion are selected and planned in advance; in others, the topics discussed are those the expectant parents bring up.

When the topics for discussion are planned in advance, the content can be organized so that it is pertinent to the stage of pregnancy the women have reached. By attempting to meet the specific needs of expectant parents at each stage of pregnancy, optimal learning is promoted.

Thus, classes in early pregnancy, when the expectant parents are getting used to the idea of pregnancy, can focus on pregnancy and the physical and emotional changes that normally accompany it. In midpregnancy, when the attention is centered on the baby, information concerning fetal growth and development, along with nutritional needs of mother and infant, is appropriate. Also at this time the woman's weight increases, and the uterus becomes an abdominal organ causing changes in her body contour, appearance, and balance. Therefore, suggestions concerning appropriate clothing, recreational activities, employment hazards, and good body mechanics are suitable.

Later in pregnancy, expectant parents' interest is focused on preparation for labor and delivery and care of the infant after birth. Content dealing with those subjects can be presented at this time.

Classes dealing with birth usually include information about maternal anatomy and the physiology of the birth process as well as specific suggestions for helping the parents cope with labor and delivery in a satisfying manner.

Methods of preparation for childbirth

In recent years there has been a growing interest in "natural" childbirth. Dr. Grantly Dick Read of England was active in promoting natural childbirth. He believed that fear of labor created tension in the woman and the tension resulted in pain. By teaching women what to expect and how to help themselves during labor, he endeavored to eliminate the fear and thereby lessen the tension and pain. Classes in natural childbirth are directed toward helping the woman cooperate with the normal process of labor so that she remains in control of herself and can actively participate in the birth of her child. To accomplish this, women learn to perform exercises that strengthen the muscles involved in the birth process, and learn breathing techniques that are used to help them to relax during labor. Husbands are taught how to assist their wives during labor and delivery. In many hospitals, husbands who so desire are permitted to be present at the birth.

Among the many methods of natural childbirth being taught in this country today, perhaps the most popular are the Bradley method and the Lamaze method.

Bradley method. The Bradley method is named for its founder and promoter, Dr. Robert A. Bradley of Denver, Colorado. This is a physiological approach to childbirth which, like the Read method, stresses that labor is a normal process. In the latent phase of labor the mother is encouraged to be up and about or to engage in diversional activities such as playing cards with her husband. Tailor sitting is the position of choice when she is not ambulating (Fig. 8-10). Many patients continue this type of activity and position throughout their labor, which is often quite short.

FIG. 8-10. *The tailor sitting position is used when the mother is not ambulating.*

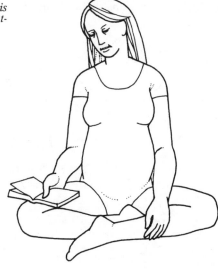

A patient who elects to labor in bed during the active phase is taught to:

Assume the Sims' position with one pillow under the head and chest and another under the forward leg (Fig. 8-11)

Simulate sleep during each contraction: close her eyes, let each muscle in her body relax

Breathe (through her mouth) slow, deep abdominal breaths throughout each contraction

During each contraction her husband places his hand lightly on her abdomen and quietly reminds her to breathe slowly and deeply while whispering words of encouragement: between contractions he rubs her lower back if she so desires or visits with her in an entertaining, supportive way

The Bradley method also advocates breast-feeding the baby immediately after birth while mother and baby are still in the delivery room. Users of this method of childbirth generally have a shorter hospital stay. This is probably due primarily to the mental attitudes developed through the classes, which emphasize the normalcy of labor and birth, and perhaps to the confidence instilled in the couple in their ability to cope with labor and to care for their infant.

Lamaze method. The Lamaze method of childbirth, named for Dr. Ferdinand Lamaze of Paris, is based on the Pavlov conditioned reflex theory. This is a psychoprophylactic (mental prevention of pain) method in which the woman is taught to substitute the usual responses to pain, such as restlessness, fear, and loss of control, with more useful behavior.

Originally the Lamaze method incorporated rapid, superficial panting during contractions, but this has been eliminated because it tended to cause hyperventilation. Hyperventilation is undesirable because it may cause alkalosis in the mother with subsequent acidosis in the fetus. There are several variations of the Lamaze method of childbirth, all aimed at

FIG. 8-11. *Pillow arrangement with patient in Sims' position.*

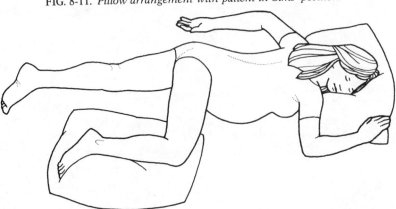

assisting the couple to learn ways of meeting their goals for labor and birth.

One example of this method is as follows. Before labor begins the couple selects some small object that will be used as a focal point for the woman during labor. This may be an object in the labor room or, more likely, an object cherished by the couple, such as a picture of a rose or a photo of their other child. This is placed where it can easily be seen by the mother.

When labor is established, the woman is positioned on her side with two pillows under her head and one pillow between her knees. When the contraction starts, she takes a deep, cleansing breath, focuses her entire attention on the focal point and breathes slow, deep chest breaths. At the end of the contraction she again takes a deep, cleansing breath. During the contraction the husband may count softly aloud in a regular, even cadence to assist her in maintaining regular, slow breaths so that she does not hyperventilate. As labor intensifies and the slow chest breathing becomes less effective, she may modify her breathing so that she starts with slow chest breathing, then switches to shallow, effortless breathing as the contraction nears its peak, then returns to slow chest breathing as the contraction diminishes. Instead of counting as labor advances, the husband may time the contraction, relaying to his wife, at 15-second intervals, the length of time the contraction has lasted so far. Throughout labor the husband gently, or firmly should the need arise, reminds his wife to relax.

Hypnosis. Hypnosis is another psychological method of inducing relaxation of the voluntary muscles during labor so that the uterus can work more efficiently. The success of this method depends on the suggestibility of the individual and the skill of the hypnotist in inducing a state of insensibility to outside impressions. When hypnosis is selected for labor, the hypnotist, who is usually an obstetrician with special training in the method, conducts several conditioning sessions with the patient during the latter part of pregnancy. During labor, the environment is kept dimly lighted with a minimum of extraneous noise and activity.

Pain relief. Although some patients who attend childbirth education classes are able to go through labor without receiving medication for pain, many cannot, nor should they be told that they must. It must be remembered that pain thresholds vary with individuals. Also, some couples who have been to classes have the misconception that labor is painless; when the contractions become painful they lose control. Still others put off practicing the exercises and preparing until labor starts, and they then have difficulty doing what they are only partially prepared to do. In spite of faithful attendance at classes and dedicated practice, a few couples lose control when the wife experiences pain and the husband is so emotionally involved that he cannot maintain his composure and provide the firm coaching that may be indicated. Unless the couple has been taught that accepting pain medication is an indication of failure, a small dose of analgesia, accompanied by supportive nursing care, can help the mother stay in control and thereby expedite the labor process. Thus, administration of pain medication at the proper time can mean the difference between a satisfying feeling of being able to cope successfully and a feeling of failure at being unable to cope. A feeling of failure to cope satisfactorily during the stress of labor and birth may have negative effects on the husband-wife relationship as well as on their attitudes toward the infant and future pregnancies.

ASSISTING THE UNWED MOTHER

For generations in many societies the unwed mother was considered a disgrace. She had committed a transgression against society, if not against the laws of the land, and her baby was labeled illegitimate. The daughter who became pregnant out of wedlock was often pressured into marriage or rejected by her parents and asked to leave her home to face her pregnancy and its outcome alone. The important thing was to save the family name. The health and even the lives of the woman and her unborn child were not considered.

In desperation many women sought and obtained abortions at the hands of the ignorant and unskilled. Infection and hemorrhage took their toll of lives; many who survived became sterile.

Those unable or unwilling to escape by abortion sought anonymity in various ways. Many moved away, obtained any kind of work they could, and were often exploited. The infant, if alive when born, was often relinquished for adoption. Some women were able to stay with relatives in a distant town until after the baby came and was placed for adoption. Others sought shelter in homes for the unwed and usually, because their stay terminated shortly after the birth of the baby and they had no way of supporting themselves and the child, they too gave up the child for adoption.

In spite of remarkable advances in almost all areas of learning and technology, some segments of society still attach a stigma to the unwed mother, causing her and her innocent unborn child to suffer as a result. Because of the stigma, many of these women, especially among the teenage group, do not seek antepartal care. Often when they do seek care it is late in pregnancy after a complication has developed and is in an advanced stage. The medical care they do get is frequently inadequate. Consequently, unmarried pregnant women have more complications of pregnancy and a higher rate of prematurity with a higher risk of death than do married pregnant women and present a special challenge to nursing care.

Despite the availability of effective methods of contraception, the trend toward early marriages, and the legalization of abortions, the rate of out-of-wedlock births continues to increase. Out-of-wedlock birth occurs in all walks of life and among all childbearing age groups; however, the highest rate is among women in their teens and 20s and in the lower socioeconomic group.

The nurse may find that she has strong feelings against the unwed mother whether she does or does not keep her baby. It is well for the nurse to recognize these feelings and to understand why she has them. However, to be effective in her care she must not be judgmental. She should be supportive and endeavor to develop a trusting relationship with this mother also, so that she can be of the most help to her. Often it is her responsibility to assist the unwed mother and father and their families by directing them to other members of the health team who can give them needed counseling and guidance. In her interactions with the unwed mother the nurse should do all in her power to preserve the dignity and respect of the individuals involved.

NORMAL DISCOMFORTS OF PREGNANCY

Although pregnancy is a normal process, some of the changes it brings about cause a certain amount of discomfort to some women. These discomforts are usually temporary and can often be relieved or prevented by simple measures. In instances where nothing can be done to relieve discomfort, the woman may be reassured to know that such changes are normal.

Nausea and vomiting.   Probably the most common discomfort experienced by pregnant women is a feeling of nausea with or without vomiting during the early part of pregnancy. Usually the nausea is felt on arising in the morning, but it may occur at any time of the day. It usually subsides after 2 to 6 weeks. Nausea and vomiting may be due to physiologic changes of pregnancy or to emotional factors.

Although not successful in all cases, many women obtain relief by eating dry toast or a cracker about one-half hour before getting up in the morning. Other relief measures may include getting plenty of rest, fresh air, and sunshine; maintaining a positive frame of mind; omitting greasy foods from the diet; and eating five or six small meals a day instead of three large ones.

Urinary frequency.   Early in pregnancy the enlarging uterus puts pressure on the bladder. This decreases the capacity of the bladder and causes frequency of urination. After about the second or third month of pregnancy this pressure is relieved as the uterus rises upward into the abdominal cavity. The urinary frequency subsides then, but it returns near the end of pregnancy when lightening occurs and the fetal head exerts pressure on the bladder.

Heartburn.   The crowding and decreased motility of the stomach during the latter part of pregnancy cause some of the stomach contents to spill back into the esophagus. This causes irritation of the lining of the esophagus and is felt as a burning sensation behind the lower part of the sternum upward along the esophagus. Although this discomfort is called *heartburn,* the heart is not involved. Preventive measures consist of eating frequent small meals instead of three large ones, reducing the amount of fat in the diet to a minimum, and avoiding fatigue. Antacid preparations prescribed by the physician are usually effective in relieving heartburn. The patient should be cautioned against taking baking soda as a remedy, because it contains sodium, which causes retention of fluids in the tissues.

Constipation. Constipation is a common problem among pregnant women. The major cause of this discomfort is decreased peristalsis of the intestine caused by pressure from the growing uterus. Decreased tone of the stretched abdominal muscles may also be a factor. Measures that the woman can take to prevent or relieve this discomfort include exercising daily; drinking plenty of fluids; eating a diet containing fruits, vegetables, dark breads, and coarse foods; and having a regular time each day for elimination. Other measures, such as laxatives and enemas, should not be taken unless prescribed by the doctor.

Flatulence. Flatulence is attributed to relaxation of the bowel during pregnancy and to undesirable bacterial action that results in the formation of gas. The woman who has this problem should eat small meals, chew her food well, omit foods from her diet likely to form gas, and be regular in elimination.

Shortness of breath (dyspnea). During the latter part of pregnancy, as the enlarging uterus rises upward and crowds the diaphragm, the woman may experience shortness of breath. This discomfort may be particularly annoying when the woman is attempting to sleep. She can usually obtain temporary relief by stretching both arms above her head for a few minutes while lying flat on her back, after which she can usually turn onto her side, relax, and go to sleep. After lightening occurs, the pressure on the diaphragm is relieved and this discomfort disappears. Shortness of breath experienced before the uterus has enlarged enough to cause pressure on the diaphragm may be a symptom of heart disease and should be reported to the doctor.

Backache. The normal postural changes occurring during pregnancy as the body attempts to maintain its balance, along with the relaxation of the sacroiliac joints and symphysis pubis that accompanies pregnancy, may cause backache for many pregnant women. In addition, a woman with weak abdominal muscles may experience severe backache because of the pronounced forward protrusion of the abdomen as the uterus grows.

To lessen the amount of backache, the expectant mother should begin to practice good body alignment early in pregnancy. In good alignment, the body is erect with no slumping, and has no marked curvatures of the spine and a minimal forward tilt of the pelvis. Insofar as possible, the mother should arrange her work areas at a proper height to minimize stooping and lifting. When she must stoop or lift she should squat, bending at the knees while keeping the back straight and the feet wide apart (Fig.

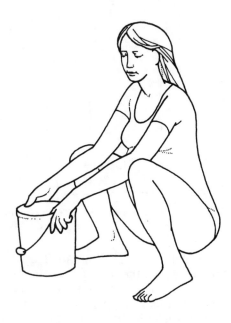

FIG. 8-12. *The squatting posture is the preferred method of lifting or reaching for low objects during pregnancy.*

8-12). Exercises (Figs. 8-13 and 8-14), abdominal supports, and adequate rest also help to relieve backache.

Varicose veins. Varicose veins (varicosities) are veins overdistended with blood. The legs are common sites for varicosities, but the rectum and vulva may also be involved during pregnancy. Varicose veins are undesirable not only because they are unsightly and cause leg ache, but also because they may develop into serious complications such as throm-

FIG. 8-13. *The knee–chest position is helpful in relieving lower backache.*

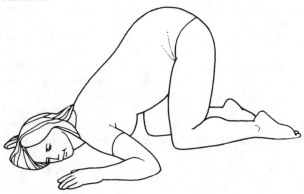

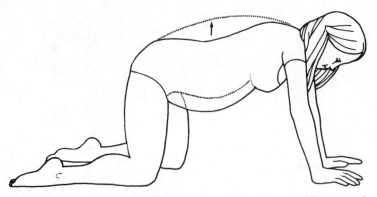

FIG. 8-14. *The pelvic tilt strengthens the muscles of the abdomen and lower back.* Good for dysmenorrhea also.

bophlebitis and embolism. Anything that interferes with the return flow of blood from the feet and legs may favor the development of varicose veins, especially if the vessel walls are weak. Standing or sitting for long periods of time, wearing round garters or tight bands, and pressure from the enlarging uterus on the pelvic veins all tend to slow circulation in the legs. If the woman must spend much time on her feet, she should have frequent rest periods when she can lie down or sit with her feet elevated. Elevating the legs at right angles to the body against a headboard or against a wall for 5 to 10 minutes three or four times a day helps to drain the blood from the veins and to prevent varicose veins (Fig. 8-15). If the legs ache even though varicosities are not visible, the physician may prescribe elastic stockings or elastic bandages to support the vessel walls. These are put on upon arising in the morning before the veins become distended, and they are removed before retiring at night (Figs. 8-16 and 8-17).

Varicose veins of the rectum are called *hemorrhoids*. They are not only painful but also may itch and bleed. Measures taken to prevent or relieve constipation also are helpful in preventing hemorrhoids, because straining at stool is largely responsible for their development. Varicose veins of the vulva may be relieved by lying down with the buttocks elevated several times a day.

Swelling of feet (edema).   During the latter part of pregnancy, many women have swollen feet and ankles by the end of the day. This swelling is due to seepage of fluid through the walls of the distended veins of the legs and will disappear following a night of rest. If it persists in spite of rest, it may be a sign of PIH, and the physician should be notified. Measures effective in preventing varicose veins are also effective in relieving this edema.

Leg cramps.   Leg cramps are among the more annoying discomforts of pregnancy because of the pain they cause and also because they usually

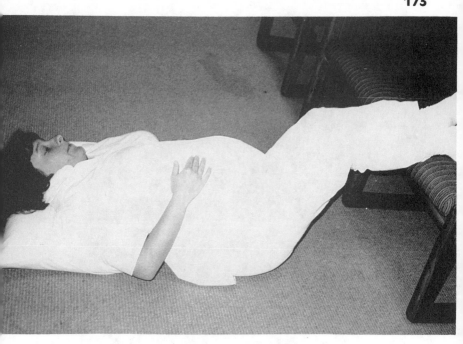

FIG. 8-15. *Elevating the legs promotes return flow of blood from the legs and helps to prevent varicosities.*

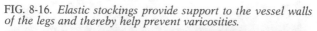

FIG. 8-16. *Elastic stockings provide support to the vessel walls of the legs and thereby help prevent varicosities.*

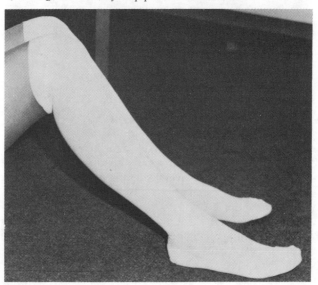

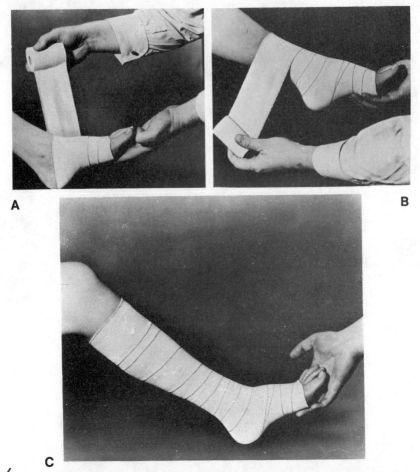

A

B

C

✓ FIG. 8-17. *(A and B) For varicosities or edema of the legs, sometimes an Ace bandage is applied as shown. (C) The bandage is applied firmly, adjusting the stretch to produce the amount of compression desired, each turn overlapping to avoid gaps.*
Not too tight though, don't pull.

occur when the mother is resting. They are believed to be caused by tension, by circulatory impairment resulting from pressure of the gravid uterus on the pelvic veins, by overstretching of the muscles and fascia of the legs, and, in some instances, by a lack of calcium. Relief is usually obtained by standing up; if this is not possible, the leg should be extended with the ankle flexed and the toes forcibly pointed toward the knee. Massaging the leg and applying heat to it are also helpful.

Vaginal discharge. Vaginal discharge increases considerably during the latter months of pregnancy. It usually creates no real problems, although it may distress the woman who is meticulous about personal hygiene. Douches should not be used unless prescribed by the physician. If the discharge becomes profuse and causes itching and burning, the woman should notify her physician, because it could be due to an infection caused by *Trichomonas vaginalis, Candida albicans,* or the gonoccocus organism.

Vaginal infections caused by *Trichomonas vaginalis* produce a profuse, irritating, yellowish green, foamy vaginal secretion with an unpleasant odor. Itching is intense. The doctor may prescribe treatment consisting of a vinegar douche followed by the insertion of a metronidazole (Flagyl) suppository into the vagina.

A yeast infection, moniliasis (also called candidiasis), is caused by *Candida albicans.* It produces a profuse, white, curdy, watery discharge that is extremely irritating to the vagina and vulva. A baby born to a mother with this infection may become infected as it passes through the birth canal; infection of the mucous membrane of the infant's mouth by *Candida albicans* is called thrush. Yeast infections are usually treated with nystatin (Mycostatin) or with methylrosaniline chloride (gentian violet).

A gonorrheal infection also produces a profuse, yellow vaginal discharge. Burning and frequency of urination are usually present. If untreated, this infection may be transmitted to the infant as it passes through the birth canal. Gonorrheal infections usually respond to treatment with penicillin.

Itching. Itching is a rather common discomfort among pregnant women. It may be due to dryness of the skin, which seems to accompany pregnancy; to irritating materials secreted by the skin glands; or to an excessive use of soap when bathing. Relief may be obtained by bathing the affected areas with a solution of soda bicarbonate, or by taking a starch or oatmeal bath. Increasing the fluid intake may also help by diluting the irritating materials secreted by the skin glands. Using a bland soap, or avoiding all soap, and oiling the skin following a bath may also give relief.

CLINICAL REVIEW

ASSESSMENT. Nancy is a 26-year-old nurse who is pregnant for the first time. Her husband Jim is a 30-year-old pharmacist at the same hospital where Nancy is the Charge Nurse on the postpartum unit of the maternity department. Nancy is 5 feet 2 inches tall and weighs 150 lb (68 kg). Before becoming pregnant she weighed 120 lb (54 kg). Neither Jim nor Nancy smokes or uses controlled drugs. Both have always been in excellent health. Nancy is the oldest child in a family of three girls and two boys. Jim has an older sister and brother and a younger brother. Both Jim and Nancy are excited about this pregnancy, which was planned and welcomed. Both families share Jim and Nancy's enthusiasm about the pregnancy.

So far, this pregnancy has been "a breeze," as Nancy says. However, now that she is in her eighth month, she is experiencing some shortness of breath, particularly at night when she is trying to sleep; she is also awakened frequently by leg cramps. Lately she has been bothered by backache and swelling of her feet and ankles.

1. Using the above information, list some nursing diagnoses that would be appropriate in a care plan for Nancy. What nursing interventions would you propose?
2. How would you evaluate Nancy's support system?
3. How do you think Nancy might perceive this pregnancy? How might Jim perceive it?
4. In what areas would you expect Nancy to have the most knowledge?

BIBLIOGRAPHY

American Academy of Pediatrics Committee on Nutrition: Nutritional aspects of vegetarianism, health foods, and fad diets. Pediatrics 59:460, 1977
Bolik B, Foley MK: Developing a community-based parent education support group. J Obstet Gynecol Neonatal Nurs 10:197, 1981
Bradley RA: Husband-Coached Childbirth, 3rd ed. New York, Harper & Row, 1981
Council on Foods and Nutrition: Zen macrobiotic diets. JAMA 218:397, 1971
Dohrmann KR, Lederman SA: Weight gain in pregnancy. J Obstet Gynecol Neonatal Nurs 6:446–453, 1986
Jensen MD, Bobak IM: Maternity Care: The Nurse & The Family, 3rd ed, pp 321–400. St. Louis, CV Mosby, 1985
Reeder SR, Martin LL: Maternity Nursing, 16th ed, pp 313–422. Philadelphia, JB Lippincott, 1987
Roberts JE: Priorities in prenatal education. J Obstet Gynecol Neonatal Nurs 5:17–20, 1976

assessment of the fetal **9** condition

BEHAVIORAL OBJECTIVES When the goals of this chapter are reached, the student will be able to:

○ List three or four methods available for assessing the condition of the fetus during the antepartum period.

○ Give an example of a chromosomal disorder that can be detected by amniocentesis.

○ Prepare the patient for amniocentesis.

○ Recognize normal-appearing amniotic fluid and the significance of meconium-stained amniotic fluid.

○ List two or three conditions in which determination of maternal estriol levels is of value.

○ Discuss the use of x-ray films in assessing the condition of the fetus.

○ Prepare a patient for ultrasound. Discuss the advantages of ultrasound over roentgenography during pregnancy. What information can be obtained about the fetus and placenta by use of ultrasound? Tell what is meant by "real-time ultrasound," and what information it provides.

○ Explain the purpose of the oxytocin challenge test (OCT).

○ List three or four conditions in which the OCT would be indicated, and two or three in which it would be contraindicated.

○ Describe how the OCT is administered and interpreted.

○ Describe the fetal activity test.

○ List three or four factors that could affect the fetal heart rate during labor.

○ Discuss the instruments available for fetal monitoring.

○ Describe the advantages and disadvantages of external and internal fetal monitoring.

○ Define the terms commonly used in electronic fetal monitoring.

○ *Describe the intervention indicated when fetal heart rate patterns suggesting fetal hypoxia occur.*

○ *Explain how fetal blood studies may be helpful.*

Until recently the methods of assessing the condition of the fetus were limited to measuring the height of the uterus and listening to the fetal heartbeat with a stethoscope. Although valuable information is obtained by these methods (*i.e.*, whether the fetus is alive and growing at a normal rate), more precise information is sometimes necessary to determine the quality of life of the fetus and to ensure its continued well-being. The need for information regarding the status of the fetus (for example, that the risk of its remaining within the uterus is greater than the risk of its being born prematurely) has led to considerable research in this area. Consequently, numerous methods of assessing the condition of the unborn infant are presently available, including ways of treating the fetus in utero and of detecting chromosomal disorders.

ASSESSMENT DURING PREGNANCY

Methods used in assessing the condition of the fetus during pregnancy include amniocentesis, determination of estriol levels in the maternal urine or blood, x-ray studies, ultrasound scanning, stress tests such as the oxytocin challenge test, and nonstress tests such as the fetal activity test. Sometimes only one of these tests may be done; usually, however, findings from more than one add emphasis and valuable supportive data to confirm a suspected diagnosis.

AMNIOCENTESIS

Amniocentesis is the withdrawal of some of the amniotic fluid surrounding the fetus. This procedure, which usually takes only about 5 minutes, can be performed safely in the physician's office after the placenta has been located by ultrasound (see below) and the position of the fetus has been determined by abdominal palpation. Usually by the 15th or 16th week of pregnancy, a sufficient amount of amniotic fluid has been produced to permit the performance of amniocentesis.

Indications

Approximately 75% of amniocenteses are performed to detect Down's syndrome. Most of the women tested are in the older age group or have had a child with Down's syndrome. Studies may also be indicated when a member of the family has been born with a genetic defect other than Down's syndrome or when population screening studies have identified a couple as carriers of a disease. If the parents are carriers of Tay-Sachs disease, for example, enzyme assays can be done on the fetal cells to detect an affected fetus.

Fetal cell studies can also reveal the sex of the infant. This information is pertinent to sex-linked defects such as Duchenne's muscular dystrophy.

The presence of an open neural tube defect, such as anencephaly or meningomyelocele, can be discovered by assay of the amniotic fluid for α-fetoprotein. Closed neural defects are not detected by α-fetoprotein assessment.

Other indications for amniocentesis include suspicion of intrauterine growth retardation or postmaturity, determination of fetal maturity, and Rh sensitization.

It is important to note that, although certain genetic abnormalities (Down's syndrome, Tay-Sachs disease, and others) can be detected through amniocentesis, the majority of birth defects cannot. Therefore, even though the presence of certain conditions may be ruled out, there is no guarantee that the child will be born normal. However, when defects are discovered early in pregnancy, the couple can have the pregnancy terminated if they so desire.

Method

The preparation for amniocentesis is simple: the patient is requested to empty her bladder, the position of the fetus is confirmed by abdominal palpation, and the site for injection is selected. The site is then cleansed with a preparation such as iodine, and a local anesthetic is injected. Using aseptic technique, the physician inserts a sterile needle through the abdominal and uterine walls into the amniotic sac. The first 1 or 2 ml of fluid obtained is usually discarded, since it may contain maternal cells. Then, approximately 20 to 25 ml of fluid is withdrawn, the needle is removed, and the site is covered with a Band-aid (Fig. 9-1).

FIG. 9-1. *Technique of amniocentesis indicating the direction of the needle in relation to the fetal position, to avoid injury.*

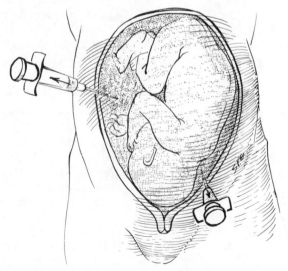

Virtually painless

The discomfort associated with this procedure is caused by injection of the local anesthetic; a sensation of pressure deep in the pelvis may also be experienced by some patients. Possible risks involved in amniocentesis include needle puncture of the fetus, bleeding due to perforation of the placenta, and infection. The danger of pricking the fetus is considered small since it is surrounded by a large amount of fluid in which it floats freely, and it actually tends to move away from the needle. Prior localization of the placenta by ultrasound scanning decreases the chances of puncturing it and causing bleeding, while careful asepsis reduces the risk of infection. There does seem to be about a 1% risk that amniocentesis will cause a spontaneous abortion.

After the procedure, the patient is kept in the physician's office for about one-half hour. If she experiences no ill effects during that time, she is permitted to go home and continue her normal activities. She may have mild uterine cramps for several hours. She is instructed to go to bed and to notify the physician immediately if she has any vaginal spotting or leakage of fluid.

Interpretation

After the sample of fluid is obtained, much information can be derived by examining its color, cells, creatinine levels, phospholipids, and bilirubin content.

Color. The amniotic fluid is normally clear in appearance. When the fetus has a bowel movement, the meconium causes the fluid to turn green. A decrease in the oxygen supply to the fetus results in increased peristaltic action of the fetal intestines and relaxation of the anal sphincter with subsequent evacuation of meconium into the amniotic fluid. Thus, meconium-stained fluid with a fetus in a vertex presentation is considered an indication of an episode of fetal distress. Meconium staining with a fetus in a breech presentation is common and is due to pressure. In instances of intrauterine growth retardation and postmaturity, the amniotic fluid is usually highly stained with meconium; amniocentesis can be helpful in confirming these diagnoses.

Cells. The cells in the amniotic fluid are the main source of information in studies of chromosomal disorders. Although the fluid contains cells from the amnion and the fetal urinary, gastrointestinal, and respiratory tracts, those of primary importance are the squamous cells shed from the fetal skin.

Samples of fetal squamous cells from the amniotic fluid are grown in tissue culture; then chromosomal studies (karyotyping) and biochemical analysis can be done. Amniocentesis for the detection of some genetic abnormalities can be done as early as the 14th week of pregnancy if a sufficient amount of fluid is present. However, it takes an average of 3 weeks before the cells in the tissue culture grow to the point where chromosomal studies can be performed. It takes an average of 4 weeks before chemical studies can be done, since more cells are needed for these.

[handwritten: Look at: lungs, renal, placental fouling]

The foregoing discussion has dealt with information regarding *fetal well-being.* Information on *fetal maturity* may also be obtained by studying the fetal squamous cells. During the 34th or 35th week of gestation, squamous cells containing fat appear for the first time in the amniotic fluid; these increase in number as the pregnancy reaches maturity. These cells are easily detected by mixing a fat stain (nile blue sulfate) with a sample of amniotic fluid and making a smear. Generally the fetus is mature when 15% to 20% of the cells appear orange on the smear, indicating that they contain fat.

Creatinine. The creatinine level in the amniotic fluid is another indication of fetal maturity. As the fetus matures, its kidneys function and it urinates in the amniotic fluid, thus causing the concentration of creatinine in the fluid to increase. At maturity the creatinine level in the amniotic fluid is more than 1.8 mg/dl. If the creatinine in the amniotic fluid is compared to that in the maternal serum, the ratio is more than 2:1. *[handwritten: normal]* *[handwritten: = mature renal system.]*

Phospholipids. Studies of the amniotic fluid can also be done to determine the lecithin/sphingomyelin ratio. Lecithin and sphingomyelin are phospholipids present in the amniotic fluid in increasing amounts as pulmonary maturity is reached. When pulmonary maturity is attained, the danger of respiratory distress syndrome occurring is lessened. It has been found that when the lecithin/sphingomyelin ratio in the amniotic fluid is 2:1, pulmonary maturity is such that respiratory distress syndrome is not likely to occur even though the infant is born prematurely. *[handwritten: L/S ratio; at 35; lecithin; sphingomyelin]*

Determination of fetal maturity is of particular importance in instances when the life of the fetus is in jeopardy if it remains in the uterus, and yet survival is questionable should it be delivered (*e.g.,* in severe cases of pregnancy-induced-hypertension in pregnancies that are between 31 and 37 weeks' gestation).

Bilirubin. Early in pregnancy a blood sample from the Rh-negative patient is tested (by the indirect Coombs test) to find out if she has antibodies against the Rh factor (D). The findings are reported as a negative or positive titer. If the titer is positive, the highest dilution in which it is positive is also reported (*e.g.,* 1:2, 1:4, 1:8, 1:16, etc.). If the titer is negative, it is repeated at 30 and 36 weeks' gestation; if these titers are also negative, it is assumed that the fetus is not affected. If the titer is positive, it is repeated in a week or so to see whether it is rising. If so, amniocentesis is indicated to find out how severely the fetus is affected.

The amount of bilirubin in the amniotic fluid has been found to be an accurate index of how severely the fetus of an Rh-sensitized mother is being affected by antibodies from the maternal circulation. When the quantity of bilirubin in the fluid is high, the fetal hemoglobin is low.

Spectrophotometry is used to determine the amount of bilirubin in the amniotic fluid. An optical density peak at 450μ is produced by bilirubin, and it is the height of this peak, or the OD_{450}, which is used to assess how affected the fetus is.

Most Rh-sensitized mothers are candidates for amniocentesis. The first amniocentesis is usually done at 24 to 25 weeks' gestation because intrauterine transfusion is not practicable before that time. However, if there is a history of perinatal death due to erythroblastosis, or if the antibody titer is rising, amniocentesis may be done at 20 to 22 weeks' gestation. It may be necessary to repeat the amniocentesis weekly if the bilirubin levels are high.

MATERNAL ESTRIOL LEVELS

There are three basic estrogens that increase progressively in the blood and urine of the mother during a normal pregnancy. These are estradiol, estrone, and estriol. Of these, the estriol levels increase the most. The precursors of estriol are formed in the fetal adrenals and converted to estriol by the placenta; to have normal amounts the fetus and placenta must function normally. Determination of estriol levels can be done on a 24-hour urine sample (Fig. 9-2) or on blood samples. In order for the 24-hour urine estriol levels to be normal, the placenta and the maternal renal system must function normally. Using a blood sample is more convenient, and the findings are not affected by maternal renal function. However, it has been found that estriol levels in the blood vary with the time of day: they are high in the morning and lower in the afternoon. This means that the blood samples should be drawn at the same time each day.

Since estriol levels are a reliable indication of whether or not the placenta is functioning normally, their determination is of greatest value in cases where placental insufficiency is most likely to occur, such as in diabetes, hypertension, and suspected postmaturity.

In diabetes the disease may affect the blood vessels and cause premature aging of the placenta. Although this does not happen in every case of diabetes, when it does the life of the fetus is jeopardized because the placental function is insufficient. Therefore, before research revealed the

FIG. 9-2. *Pattern of urinary estriol excretion in normal pregnancy.*

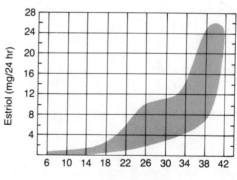

value of estriol levels in assessing placental function, it was considered necessary to deliver infants of diabetic mothers 3 or 4 weeks before the estimated due date to prevent stillbirths or neonatal deaths. This practice no doubt saved some lives, but in some cases it resulted in prematurity, which caused deaths. By doing 24-hour urinary or blood estriol determinations it is now possible to detect the diabetics with placental insufficiency and deliver them. Diabetics with normal placental function are permitted to continue to term.

In severe hypertension, placental insufficiency may develop rapidly, resulting in failure of the fetus to grow or death of the fetus. Determination of estriol levels can be helpful in deciding what action to take.

In suspected cases of postmaturity, the estriol levels, along with amniocentesis, can assist the physician in evaluating the condition of the fetus. If the estriol levels are low and the amniotic fluid is scanty and meconium-stained, the pregnancy is probably postmature.

X-RAY STUDIES

X-ray studies have long been useful in evaluating the condition of the fetus. Although they are not usually done to diagnose pregnancy, whenever an x-ray film shows the bony outline of the fetus, it is positive evidence of pregnancy. Fetal death and some abnormalities can be diagnosed from x-ray films. A few days after fetal death occurs, the characteristic overlapping of the fetal skull bones (Spalding's sign), the exaggerated curvature of the fetal spine, and gas in the fetus appear on roentgenograms. Hydrocephalus and anencephaly are abnormalities of the fetus that can be detected on x-ray studies.

Late in pregnancy x-ray measurements of the maternal pelvis (pelvimetry) are valuable in diagnosing cephalopelvic disproportion or other problems that may make vaginal delivery difficult or impossible. X-ray studies are also useful in determining fetal maturity. When the films show calcification of the distal femoral and/or proximal tibial epiphyses, the fetus is considered to be at term.

Recently amniography has been helpful in evaluating the condition of the fetus. In this procedure a water-soluble dye is injected into the amniotic fluid. The dye outlines the nonbony structures such as the placenta, cord, soft tissue, and uterine anomalies. A fetal GI series can also be done since the fetus drinks the dye. In suspected cases of hydrops fetalis, amniography can be helpful by outlining the soft tissues.

ULTRASOUND SCANNING

Ultrasound scanning is a recently developed means of measuring the size of internal structures (A-mode), such as the fetal head; providing a visual cross-sectional picture of an internal structure (B-mode), such as the placenta, so that its size, shape, and location can be determined; and observing actual movements of internal structures (real-time), such as fetal heartbeat. The fetal heartbeat has been shown as early as 7 weeks' gestation with the use of real-time. Ultrasonography involves sending intermittent high-frequency sound waves into the body by passing a transducer over the skin of the body part to be examined. The sound waves pass through the soft tissue until they encounter structures of differing tissue densities; then some of the energy, proportional to the density of the structure encountered, is reflected, or echoed, back to the transducer (Fig. 9-3). The location of body structures is determined by measuring the time it takes for ultrasound waves to reach the structure, be reflected at the point of increased density, and return to the transducer. A special transducer is used in real-time scanning that produces multiple pulse-echo systems that are activated in sequence and thereby detect movement, such as cardiac action, vessel pulsations, and breathing. Ultrasound scanning is probably the safest, most accurate, and most useful tool to be added to the practice of obstetrics in many years.

When the physician orders ultrasound (or ultrasonography or sonography, as it is also called), the nurse explains the procedure to the patient and requests that she drink plenty of fluids and *not* empty her bladder. A full bladder displaces the uterus upward, making the fetal head more accessible for measurement. The test should be performed as soon as pos-

Drink at least 1 qt. if possible.

FIG. 9-3. *Equipment for ultrasound scanning.*

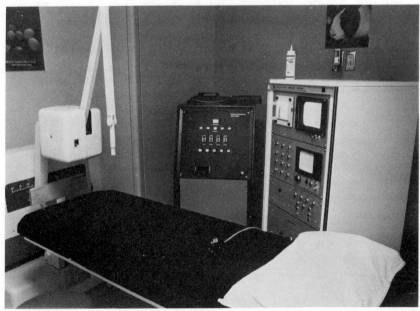

sible after the patient's bladder is full to prevent unnecessary discomfort to her. If the patient cannot take fluids by mouth, a Foley catheter can be inserted and the bladder can be filled through it. As soon as the procedure is completed the bladder can be emptied and the catheter removed.

The procedure is simple and painless. With the patient in the supine position and the abdomen exposed, a thin layer of mineral oil is rubbed over the abdomen. This reduces friction and increases conductivity. The ultrasound transducer is then passed over the skin of the abdomen (Figs. 9-4 and 9-5).

Ultrasound scanning usually takes about 20 minutes but may take longer, depending on the position and activity of the fetus. As soon as the procedure is completed, the patient should be permitted to empty her bladder.

Unlike x-rays, there are no known harmful effects produced by ultrasound. Therefore, it can be used early to diagnose pregnancy, and repeatedly—weekly or biweekly—in suspected cases of growth retardation. Ultrasound is a valuable means of determining fetal age by providing measurements of the fetal head. When the fetal size is appropriate for the fetal age, it can also provide an estimate of the fetal weight. In addition, ultrasound can be used to locate the placenta, to diagnose multiple preg-

Can determine hydrocephaly & microcephaly.

FIG. 9-4. *Ultrasound scanning provides a great deal of information about the fetus without the potentially harmful effects of x-rays.*

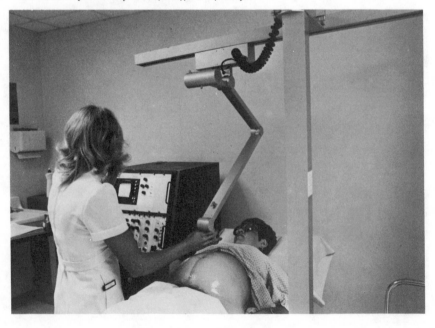

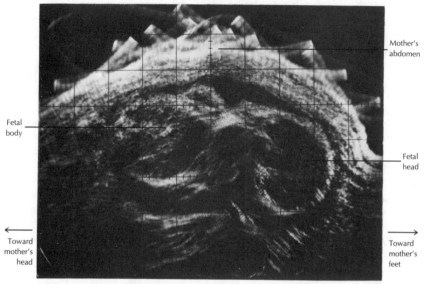

FIG. 9-5. *Ultrasound photo showing a 7-month-old fetus.*

nancies, to confirm fetal death *in utero,* and to reveal the presence of certain anomalies such as hydrocephalus, anencephaly, and hydatidiform mole.

OXYTOCIN CHALLENGE TEST *Stress test (Stress is oxytocin)*

The oxytocin challenge test (OCT) is a stress test in which the response of the fetal heart rate (FHR) to contractions is assessed. By this test, the efficiency of the "respiratory" function of the placenta can be evaluated; that is, the ability of the placenta to transfer oxygen, carbon dioxide, and essential nutrients can be indirectly measured.

Basis. It is recognized that late decelerations of the fetal heart rate during labor are due to uteroplacental insufficiency (UPI). It is also known that antepartum fetal death is commonly caused by UPI in patients with conditions such as diabetes, chronic hypertension, and preeclampsia. Therefore, it was felt that, if uterine contractions could be induced *before* labor and the response of the fetal heart rate to the contractions could be determined, it might be possible to diagnose a fetus that was encountering difficulty because of UPI. The OCT is not done to see if an infant will be able to tolerate labor; it is done to detect fetuses that are beginning to suffer because the circulation between the uterus and placenta is becoming inadquate.

Indications. OCT is indicated in those conditions in which UPI may possibly occur. These include diabetes, chronic hypertension, preeclampsia, intrauterine growth retardation, sickle cell disease, maternal cyanotic heart disease, suspected postmaturity, history of previous stillbirth, and Rh-sensitized patients with meconium-stained amniotic fluid.

Contraindications. The OCT is not done in conditions where the onset of contractions could conceivably result in rupture of the uterus, hemorrhage, or premature labor. Consequently, it is contraindicated in cases of previous cesarean section, previous therapeutic abortion by hysterotomy, multiple gestations, placenta previa, and premature rupture of the membranes.

Method. The OCT is performed in the hospital as early as the 28th week of pregnancy. A good record of the FHR and contraction pattern is absolutely essential to the interpretation of this test. The patient is positioned on her left side, the fetal heartbeat is located, and the external transducer of the fetal monitor is applied where the beat is clearest. Then the tocodynamometer is applied slightly above the umbilicus to detect contractions. Obesity, maternal or fetal activity, hydramnios, posterior position of the fetus, and bowel sounds may make it difficult to obtain a good recording of the FHR and contractions. If it is necessary to position the mother on her back in order to obtain a good tracing, then the head of the bed should be placed in a semi-Fowler's position to avoid maternal supine hypotension. The mother's blood pressure is taken before and every 10 minutes during the test.

A baseline FHR and uterine contraction pattern, if any, are obtained for a period of 10 minutes. This time allows mother and fetus to settle down. It also provides opportunity to see if the patient is already having good quality contractions, as often as three to four in 10 minutes, which last longer than 30 seconds, with interpretable FHR. This is very rare, but if it occurs, the oxytocin infusion is not given. Otherwise, an oxytocin infusion is started using an infusion pump to control the rate flow. The infusion is increased at 15- to 20-minute intervals by doubling the amount of oxytocin until the mother is having three to four contractions in 10 minutes. However, if late decelerations occur and continue for three contractions, regardless of the frequency of contractions, it is not necessary to increase the oxytocin.

Interpretation. After the contraction pattern is established at three to four contractions in 10 minutes and the fetal heart rate is recording well for a period of 30 minutes, the test can be evaluated.

When persistent and consistent late decelerations occur repeatedly with most contractions, even if the frequency of contractions is less than three in 10 minutes, the test is *positive*, indicating diminished uteroplacental reserve. When there are at least three contractions in 10 minutes and no late decelerations develop, the test is *negative*. A *suspicious* test is one in which there are inconsistent but definite late decelerations that do not persist with continued uterine contractions. If the frequency of contractions is under three in 10 minutes or the quality of the recording makes it difficult or impossible to tell if there are late decelerations, the test is *unsatisfactory*.

tractions   abnormal "late

Positive or suspicious tests are repeated in 24 hours; negative tests are repeated weekly. Unsatisfactory tests are repeated at the discretion of the physician.

After sufficient interpretable information has been obtained or the test has been ruled unsatisfactory, the oxytocin is discontinued. The fetal monitor is generally left on until the contractions diminish or stop completely. Occasionally, patients at 32 weeks' gestation or more may have continued contractions after the oxytocin is stopped; the physician may prescribe 2 oz of vodka in orange juice to stop these contractions.

FETAL ACTIVITY TEST

The fetal activity test (FAT) is a nonstress test to provide reassurance of fetal well-being. In this test fetal movement is noted as well as the response of the FHR to the movement. It has been found that the fetus that is active and whose heart rate accelerates in response to external stimuli and to fetal movements is likely to be in good condition. A nonreactive fetus may be suffering from anoxia due to diminished uteroplacental blood flow. Decreased uteroplacental blood flow can occur in such conditions as pregnancy-induced hypertension, diabetes, placenta previa, abruptio placentae, and postmaturity. Since there is no possibility that the FAT will start labor or bleeding, it can be done in patients with any of these conditions as well as in patients who have had a previous cesarean section. An FAT is often done when a woman reports that the baby is less active than previously.

Method. When an FAT is to be done, the woman is positioned on her left side with the head of the bed elevated about 30°. The external transducer of the fetal monitor is applied to her abdomen where the fetal heart is heard most clearly. The tocodynamometer is then applied even though she is not having measurable contractions. This is to record any sharp spikes or abrupt changes on the uterine contraction graph that occur when the fetus moves. In obese women these changes may not appear on the graph so that some other means of recording fetal movement must be used. This can be accomplished by having the woman, her husband, or the nurse press the test button on the monitor each time the woman feels the fetus move. Sometimes the fetus is so active that an accurate recording of the FHR accelerations is not possible. When this occurs, the woman can be kept in bed for about an hour to permit the fetus to settle down; then the test can be repeated.

Interpretation. The FAT is normal and the fetus is considered to be in good condition when three or four FHR accelerations with active fetal movements are obtained. When the fetus is inactive in spite of manual stimulation, or when FHR accelerations do not accompany fetal movements, further tests, such as an OCT, may be desirable.

Nursing considerations. An OCT or FAT is ordered when a woman is known to have, or is suspected of having, a complication that could threaten the well-being of the fetus. She is usually told by her physician why the test is being done, and may therefore be quite apprehensive about the procedure and the results. The nurse can help put the patient at ease by a kind, understanding manner and can help relieve some of the anxiety regarding the test by explaining the procedures to her before they are done. Permitting the woman and her husband to express their fears and to ask questions can also be helpful in alleviating anxiety. Because these procedures are done to determine, within their limits, the condition of the fetus, it is best for the nurse not to express an opinion about the outcome before the results of the test are known. This can both prevent the woman from building false hopes based on unfounded optimism and prevent undue concern by a pessimistic opinion.

ASSESSMENT DURING LABOR

FETAL MONITORING

Intrapartum assessment of the condition of the fetus is best accomplished by continuous monitoring of the FHR. At the present time, the FHR is the best indicator of the adequacy of fetal oxygenation. Inadequate fetal oxygenation (hypoxia), if prolonged and untreated, can result in fetal brain damage or death.

It is the purpose of fetal monitoring to detect any changes in the FHR during labor that indicate inadequate oxygenation of the fetus so that measures can be taken to prevent brain damage and death.

FACTORS AFFECTING FHR

FETAL FACTORS:

- o Compression of umbilical cord
- o Compression of fetal head
- o Intrauterine growth retardation
- o Postmaturity

MATERNAL FACTORS:

- o Drugs given to mother during labor
- o Hypotension
- o Rh sensitization
- o Diseases: diabetes, hypertension, heart disease, preeclampsia, anemia, etc.

OBSTETRIC FACTORS:

- o Placenta previa
- o Abruptio placentae
- o Hypertonic uterine contractions

Factors affecting FHR

Many factors may decrease the oxygen supply to the fetus and thereby affect the FHR. Probably the most common are those that decrease the blood flow to the uterus or to the fetus. Factors that decrease blood flow to the uterus include:

Hypertonic uterine contractions

Maternal hypotension (supine or that caused by spinal or epidural anesthesia)

Maternal diseases (diabetes, hypertension, heart disease, preeclampsia, anemia)

Obstetric complications (placenta previa, abruptio placentae)

The most common cause of decreased blood flow to the fetus is compression of the umbilical cord.

Other factors predisposing the fetus to distress that may be detected by changes in FHR include Rh sensitization, intrauterine growth retardation, and postmaturity.

Certain nervous system responses of the fetus are also reflected in the FHR. For example, stimulation of the parasympathetic (vagal) nervous system causes slowing of the FHR, whereas stimulation of the sympathetic nervous system increases the FHR. Therefore, certain drugs that affect the nervous system may, when given to the mother during labor, affect the FHR. Compression of the fetal head (which acts as a vagal stimulus) may also affect the FHR.

The degree to which the fetus is affected by these factors depends to a great extent on:

The health of the fetus and placenta

The type, severity, and duration of the particular factor causing changes in the FHR

The length of time between the appearance of the change in FHR and the birth of the infant.

A healthy fetus with a healthy placenta usually has sufficient reserves to enable it to compensate for minor stress during labor. Consequently, brief appearances of hypoxia due to one of these factors may be tolerated well with no change in the FHR. However, when either the fetus or the placenta is not healthy, the ability to compensate is diminished, and FHR signs that the fetus is in trouble may appear quickly.

If at all possible, the cause of the alteration in FHR should be discovered so that the significance of the change can be understood and appropriate action taken. In some instances, such as when the change results from compression of the fetal head, no action may be necessary. In others, such as when the change is due to compression of the umbilical cord, dire consequences may follow if immediate action is not taken.

The time relationship between the onset of FHR changes and birth may be important to the well-being of the infant. In some instances, such as when the changes are due to prolapsed cord or to uteroplacental insufficiency (UPI), it may be necessary to deliver the infant as soon as possible in order to save its life. In other instances, such as when the FHR changes occur after administration of a drug to the mother, some physicians feel there is less chance of respiratory depression in the infant at birth if corrective measures have returned the FHR to normal for a while before birth.

Instruments

The FHR can be determined during labor by listening with a fetoscope or by use of a Doppler probe or electronic monitoring equipment.

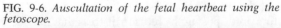

FIG. 9-6. *Auscultation of the fetal heartbeat using the fetoscope.*

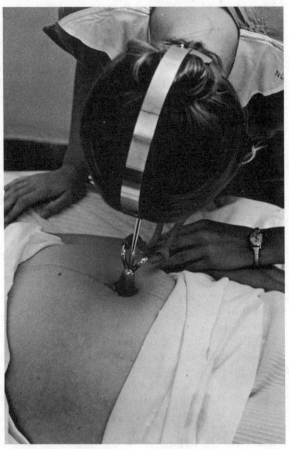

When the monitoring is done with the fetoscope, the heart rate should be listened to during and immediately following each contraction (Fig. 9-6).

The Doppler probe is a low-energy ultrasound flow probe that is capable of detecting fetal heart activity very early in pregnancy. It can also be used for external fetal heart monitoring late in pregnancy and in labor. The disadvantages to using this instrument are that it picks up the maternal pulse as well as the fetal pulse, and it requires accurate aiming and constant positioning.

ELECTRONIC FETAL MONITORING

The most satisfactory instrument for measuring the FHR during labor is the electronic monitor, which can be applied externally or internally. When this instrument is used the FHR and the uterine contractions are monitored simultaneously and a continuous, permanent recording is made. It is therefore possible not only to observe the FHR constantly throughout labor, but also to evaluate changes in FHR in relation to the contractions. The information obtained through electronic monitoring, along with other findings, such as the absence or presence of meconium-stained amniotic fluid, provides the basis for intelligent decisions regarding the need for intervention.

Indications

Some authorities believe that all labor patients should be monitored electronically; others believe that only high-risk patients and those who develop problems during labor need to be electronically monitored. Both groups stress that electronic monitoring does not eliminate or minimize the need for adequate numbers of highly qualified personnel to care for the laboring woman and her unborn child.

PATIENTS WHO MAY BENEFIT FROM ELECTRONIC MONITORING

- High-risk patients
- Those with meconium-stained amniotic fluid
- Those with unsatisfactory antepartum assessment (low L/S ratio, low or falling estriol levels, or abnormal OCT)
- Those with a multiple pregnancy
- Those with obstetric complications (placenta previa, abruptio placentae, premature labor)
- Those whose labors are not progressing normally
- Those receiving oxytocin infusions

ELECTRONIC FETAL MONITORING

EXTERNAL MONITORING

Advantages

o   It is noninvasive, that is, internal examinations and insertion of equipment are not necessary.
o   It can be done at any time; the cervix does not have to be dilated nor the membranes ruptured first.
o   The transducers can be applied by the nurse, so the physician does not need to be present.
o   A permanent record of the FHR and contractions is made.

Disadvantages

o   Uterine activity cannot be calibrated.
o   It does not record baseline FHR variability.
o   Obesity and maternal and fetal activity, as well as fetal position, affect the quality of the recording.
o   The straps or stockinette may be uncomfortable to the patient.

INTERNAL MONITORING

Advantages

o   There are minimal artifacts (interferences in the recording).
o   Baseline FHR variability is recorded.
o   Uterine activity is calibrated.
o   Recordings are not affected by obesity, maternal and fetal movement, or fetal position.
o   Abnormal FHR recordings are more easily recognized.

Disadvantages

o   The membranes must be ruptured and the cervix must be dilated 3 to 4 cm before it can be done.
o   There is a degree of risk of fetal and/or maternal infection.
o   An improperly placed electrode or catheter could conceivably cause injury to fetus or mother.
o   Although some hospitals permit RNs to apply the internal electrode and catheter, many consider it the function of the physician, thereby necessitating his presence for its initiation.

Methods

External fetal monitoring is accomplished by securing a fetal transducer (to pick up the FHR) and a tocodynamometer (to pick up the uterine contractions) to the mother's abdomen by means of elasticized straps or a piece of stockinette. The contact side of the fetal transducer is coated with a thin layer of transmission gel to promote conduction of the electrical signals it receives. Then it is placed on the part of the mother's abdomen where the FHR is heard most clearly (Fig. 9-7). The tocodynamometer is placed on the fundus of the uterus where the contractions are felt most strongly.

When external monitoring is to be used, the patient should be requested to empty her bladder first. This will add to her comfort, since the stockinette or straps used to hold the transducers in place put pressure on the bladder area. Thus the need to interrupt the monitoring soon after it has begun will be minimized. Furthermore, detection of the fetal heartbeat is easier when a full bladder is not between the transducer and the uterus.

Before the transducers are applied, the patient should be positioned as comfortably as possible, preferably on her side. If she must be on her back, the head of the bed should be elevated 30° to prevent supine hypotension. By positioning the patient before placing the transducers, the nurse can obtain a better recording with fewer adjustments of the transducers after monitoring is begun.

Internal fetal monitoring is accomplished by application of an electrode directly to the presenting part (head, buttock, etc.) of the fetus (Fig. 9-8). For safety, the electrode should never be attached to the face, fontanelles, sutures, or genital area.

With the internal fetal electrode in place, the uterine contractions can still be recorded by use of the external tocodynamometer or directly

FIG. 9-7. *Patient with external fetal monitor applied. Note that the monitor function can be observed by the patient.*

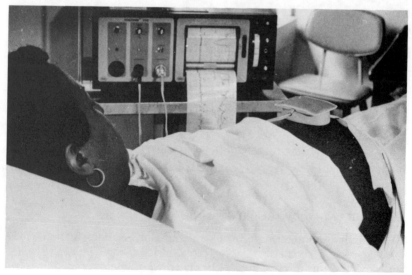

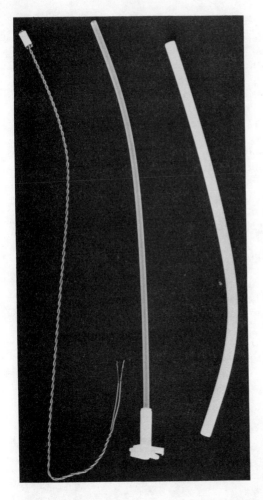

FIG. 9-8. *Scalp electrode and introducer for internal fetal heart monitoring.*

by use of a special fluid-filled plastic catheter that is inserted into the cervix and passed into the uterus above the presenting part. The end of the catheter outside the body is attached to a strain gauge on the monitor. Intrauterine pressure is passed along the fluid in the catheter to the diaphragm in the strain gauge.

Data obtained by fetal monitoring

Electronic fetal monitoring provides the most precise information available regarding the well-being of the fetus during labor. The most significant aspect of this information is associated with fetal oxygenation.

The nurse caring for the patient being monitored must have a complete understanding of the terminology used in fetal monitoring and must be able to relate it to the data obtained. Without this understanding, appropriate interpretation of the data will not be possible and the monitoring will be meaningless. (This information is summarized in Table 9-1.)

Terminology. The most common fetal monitoring terms are:

Baseline
Baseline variability
Tachycardia
Bradycardia
Accelerations
Decelerations

The *baseline* is the FHR recorded between contractioins over a period of at least 10 minutes when the internal scalp electrode is in place. The baseline FHR normally ranges between 120 and 160 beats per minute.

Internal electronic fetal monitors give a beat-to-beat recording of the heart rate. Normally there is a degree of variation, or fluctuation, from beat to beat. This *baseline variability* is a good indication of fetal well-being, whereas a loss of variability, or a smooth baseline, is a sign of fetal distress. In the normal, healthy fetus, stimulation caused by contraction or palpation of the uterus may increase the baseline variability. It is also believed that wakefulness of the healthy fetus may influence the variability. Anything that depresses the central nervous system causes loss of baseline variability; this would include drugs such as atropine, scopolamine, promethazine, sedatives, narcotics, and magnesium sulfate. Diazepam (Valium) is a most potent agent in causing loss of variability. Loss of variability due to drugs is usually temporary, and variability returns without intervention. *Hypoxia* is the most important cause of loss of baseline variability.

Tachycardia is a baseline FHR over 160 beats per minute. Tachycardia may be due to maternal fever, maternal hyperthyroidism, maternal ingestion of certain drugs that block the parasympathetic nervous system, fetal cardiac arrhythmias, fetal hypovolemia, and fetal hypoxia. Persistent tachycardia may be a sign of fetal distress, particularly if it appears in conjunction with a loss of baseline variability.

Bradycardia is a baseline FHR below 120 beats per minute. Bradycardia is rare and may be associated with congenital heart block in the fetus. Unless persistent or marked, it is not generally considered to be a sign of fetal distress.

There are two main types of pattern changes in FHR during labor: accelerations and decelerations.

Accelerations are short-term increases in FHR above the baseline. When they occur, accelerations are usually uniform in shape, begin at the same time as the contraction, and end when the contraction ends.

(*Text continues on p. 200*)

TABLE 9-1 TERMS USED IN ELECTRONIC FETAL MONITORING

TERM	DEFINITION	CHARACTERISTIC	USUAL CAUSE	SIGN OF FETAL DISTRESS?	INTERVENTION BY NURSE
Baseline	FHR recorded between contractions over a period of 10 minutes	Normally between 120 and 160 BPM	—	—	—
Baseline variability	Normal irregularity of baseline FHR	Fluctuation of FHR Abnormal = smooth baseline with loss of variability	CNS depressants UPI	No Yes	None Position on left side. Give O₂. Notify doctor.
Tachycardia	Baseline FHR over 160 BPM	—	Maternal fever May be caused by hypoxia	No Yes	None Decrease uterine activity. Correct maternal hypotension. Position on left side. Give O₂. Notify doctor.
Bradycardia	Baseline FHR below 120 BPM	Rarely occurs	Probably congenital heart block in fetus	No	None
Acceleration	Short-term increase in FHR above baseline	Usually occurs during contraction but may not Often seen in breech presentation	—	No	None
Early deceleration	Slowing of FHR that begins when contraction starts, reaches its lowest point at peak of contraction, and returns to normal by the end of contraction	"Mirrors" contraction Uniform in shape Gradual onset, gradual return to baseline FHR stays within normal range	Compression of fetal head	No	None

Variable deceleration	Slowing of FHR that bears no constant time relationship to contraction	Nonuniform Abrupt fall of FHR and rapid return to baseline Usually falls to less than 100 BPM Most common deceleration pattern seen	Compression of umbilical cord	May or may not be	Change mother's position. Decrease uterine activity, if possible. Administer O_2. Correct maternal hypotension, if present. Notify doctor if these measures do not correct.
Late deceleration	Slowing of FHR that begins at, or soon after, the peak of the contraction and does not return to normal until well after the contraction ends	Uniform in shape Gradual onset, gradual return to normal Depth of deceleration reflects intensity of contraction May be associated with decreased baseline variability and tachycardia	UPI	Yes	Position on left side. Administer O_2. Decrease uterine activity, if possible. Correct maternal hypotension, if present. Notify doctor. Prepare for birth if pattern persists.

Abbreviations: BPM = beats per minute; UPI = uteroplacental insufficiency.

They are often associated with breech presentation and are not a sign of fetal distress.

Decelerations are short-term decreases in FHR below the baseline. There are three types of decelerations, classified according to their occurrence in relation to the contractions: early, variable, and late.

Early decelerations are said to "mirror" the contraction. They are uniform in shape, that is, they are the same with each contraction. Onset and offset are gradual; decelerations start when the contraction starts and end when it ends. Usually early decelerations stay within a normal range; rarely do they fall below 110 beats per minute. Early decelerations are due to compression of the fetal head that results in stimulation of the parasympathetic (vagal) nervous system. If atropine is given to the mother, the balance between the sympathetic and vagal systems is restored and the decelerations disappear. This type of deceleration is not a sign of fetal distress.

The most common pattern of decelerations seen is that of *variable decelerations.* As the name implies, variable decelerations are not uniform in shape; they may fall abruptly and return abruptly. The depth of the fall is also variable, sometimes going as low as 60 beats per minute; however, it returns to normal by the end of the contraction. This pattern is common late in labor, although it may occur at any time, even between contractions. It is due in most instances to compression of the umbilical cord and may or may not be a sign of fetal distress.

When the following four criteria are met, this pattern is not considered a sign of fetal distress:

The heart rate does not stay down to 60 to 70 for more than 30 seconds.
It is not associated with a slow return to baseline.
It is not associated with a rising baseline heart rate.
It is not associated with a loss of variability.

Late decelerations are uniform in shape and have a gradual onset and gradual return. The deceleration begins at or after the peak of the contraction and returns after the contraction ends. The depth of the deceleration reflects the intensity of the contraction: the stronger the contraction, the slower the fetal heart rate. Late decelerations are due to fetal hypoxia caused by UPI and are a sign of fetal distress. However, late decelerations must persist for several contractions before a diagnosis of fetal distress is made. Late decelerations may be associated with decreased baseline variability and an elevated heart rate.

Interpretation.   Tremendous responsibility rests upon the nurse caring for the patient in labor. This responsibility is not diminished at all when electronic monitoring is employed. Indeed, even more responsibility then rests upon the nurse, for it is she who must not only maintain close watch over the mother and her labor but must also be able to recognize which FHR patterns indicate fetal well-being, which indicate that the fetus is beginning to have difficulty, and which show the fetus to definitely be in distress.

A normal baseline FHR with a normal baseline variability and a lack of variable or late decelerations are indications that the fetus is well oxygenated.

Decreasing baseline variability with an increasing baseline FHR or variable decelerations with normal baseline variability accompanied by meconium-stained amniotic fluid are *warning signs* that the fetus may be starting to have difficulty.

Loss of baseline variability, accompanied by late decelerations, or severe variable decelerations are *ominous signs* that the fetus is in distress.

Intervention

The nurse must recognize and interpret the various FHR patterns and communicate her assessment to the physician so that appropriate intervention can be initiated to prevent irreversible brain damage or death to the fetus. Thus her knowledge and skills are vital to the fetus, whose very life may depend on her judgment and intelligent actions.

The most significant changes in the FHR during labor (tachycardia, loss of baseline variability, severe variable decelerations, late decelerations) are caused by hypoxia. This hypoxia is most often due to maternal hypotension, compression of the umbilical cord, excessive uterine activity, or UPI. Intervention is directed toward restoring adequate fetal oxygenation as quickly as possible.

When FHR patterns suggesting fetal hypoxia occur, the following measures should be taken:

Change the mother's position, preferably to her left side; because the vena cava is on the right side, blood flow to the mother and to the uterus is best in this position. Variable decelerations are sometimes best corrected by positioning the mother on her back with the head of the bed elevated 30°.

Decrease uterine activity by discontinuing the oxytocin infusion if one is being administered.

Administer oxygen to the mother. A glucose infusion is also helpful but must be prescribed by the physician.

Correct hypotension of the mother. This can usually be accomplished quickly by positioning her on her left side and, if necessary, elevating her legs 30°.

If these measures fail to restore a normal FHR pattern within 30 minutes, the physician will want to deliver the baby by the quickest means possible. However, the nurse does not wait 30 minutes to notify the physician of these changes. She notifies him when the first changes appear so that he is aware that a possible problem exists and can make the necessary decisions.

Special nursing interventions

When monitoring equipment is first introduced into a labor and delivery department, patients and their husbands are awed by it and may associate its use with a problem with the mother or baby. This produces anxiety.

In areas where fetal monitoring equipment is widely used, there is less anxiety about it because many patients have had it used during previous labors or have heard about it from friends, or have had it explained to them in expectant parents' classes or during tours of the maternity department. Many obstetricians use a modified version of the Doppler probe, called a Doptone, in their offices to listen to the fetal heart sounds, so many patients are familiar with it before they go into labor. When a labor patient is admitted who has no knowledge of the fetal monitor, the nurse should explain its use in understandable terms to allay any anxiety the patient and her husband may have about it.

The belts or stockinette used to hold the transducers in place during electronic fetal monitoring are uncomfortable to some women. The nurse can explain that these need to be snug to prevent the transducers from slipping. However, if there are no contraindications, such as fetal distress or a physician's order to the contrary, the monitoring can be discontinued periodically to relieve the patient's discomfort. Many women and their husbands find the fetal monitor fascinating. Some women use it as an effective distractor from the discomfort of their contractions, while some husbands become so absorbed with it that they forget their coaching duties.

Some have criticized the routine use of electronic fetal monitoring because they feel it has led to unnecessary intervention by the obstetrician, with an increase in the number of cesarean section births. This is a controversial issue, with the key word being *unnecessary*. When electronic fetal monitoring is used, it is possible that data provided by it may be misinterpreted by a person unfamiliar with it so that errors in judgment may occur. It is also possible that data provided by it may *prevent* unnecessary intervention, such as cesarean sections. In considering that electronic fetal monitoring provides information concerning the status of the fetus that is otherwise not available, it seems reasonable to expect that when it is used routinely, more infants in distress will be detected than when this equipment is not used. At the same time, it would appear unwise not to act on the evidence present in the monitoring data that indicates that the fetus is in distress. Since cesarean section is usually the quickest method of delivery available in the absence of a completely dilated cervix, delivering the infant that way may be best in order to prevent further damage to it. So, although more cesarean section births may result from routine use of electronic fetal monitoring, the outcome for the fetus may be more satisfactory.

Faulty electrical appliances used in hospitals, such as lamps, radios, electric beds, and monitors, can be hazardous to patients. Although the maintenance or biomedical department is usually responsible for the safety of electrical equipment used in the hospital, the nurse shares this responsibility. Not only must she report equipment that is malfunctioning or in poor condition (frayed cords, broken plugs, cracked lamps, etc.), but the nurse is also responsible for knowing how the equipment functions so that she can operate it correctly and safely.

Electronic fetal monitoring equipment may occasionally malfunction but, according to the companies which produce it, it is constructed in such a way that even large voltages from faults cannot produce current flow to or from the patient. The patient cannot be electrocuted through the monitor. This is extremely important, since application of a faulty internal fetal scalp electrode could otherwise be very dangerous.

FETAL BLOOD STUDIES

If fetal distress is present or suspected, it may be desirable to find out if immediate action is necessary in order to save the life of the infant. If so, determination of the pH, PO_2 (oxygen tension) and PCO_2 (carbon dioxide tension) in a sample of fetal blood may provide this information. In fetal distress, when the life of the fetus is in jeopardy the pH and PO_2 fall while the PCO_2 rises. When these values remain normal, even though other symptoms of fetal distress may be present, a conservative course may be followed.

However, it is not always possible to do blood studies on the fetus because of the inaccessibility of the fetal parts for obtaining the sample. It is preferable to obtain the sample from the fetal scalp, although it is possible to get it from the buttocks. To obtain a fetal blood sample the membranes must be ruptured, the cervix must be at least 3 to 4 cm dilated, and the presenting part must be well down in the pelvis (Fig. 9-9).

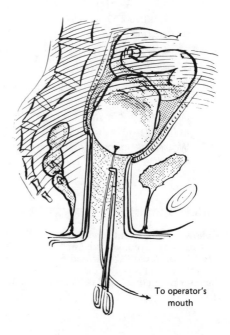

FIG. 9-9. *Technique of obtaining blood samples from the fetal scalp during labor.*

To operator's mouth

CLINICAL REVIEW

ASSESSMENT. Mrs. V. is a 30-year-old schoolteacher; her husband is a computer programmer for a large firm. He is 32 years old. They have been married for 9 years. For 1 year after they were married Mrs. V. was on oral contraceptives. Soon after she stopped taking contraceptives she became pregnant. That pregnancy ended at term with the birth of a 10-lb (4536-g) stillborn. At that time it was discovered that Mrs. V. had diabetes. Since then she has been under the care of an internist and her diabetes has been well controlled.

Mrs. V. is now in the 34th week of her second pregnancy. She has received close medical supervision from both her internist and her obstetrician. So far the pregnancy has progressed normally and her diabetes has remained under control. As her pregnancy nears term, both Mr. and Mrs. V are concerned that it not end in a stillbirth. Her doctors are also concerned that this pregnancy have a happy outcome. They realize that to accomplish this, not only must a stillbirth be avoided but also, if possible, birth of a premature infant must be prevented. In reassuring the parents, the obstetrician explains that there are ways of finding out the condition of the fetus, as well as the efficiency of the placenta, in this pregnancy that were not available with Mrs. V.'s first pregnancy.

1. What methods of determining the well-being of this fetus are available to Mrs. V.'s obstetrician?

2. Which of the following studies that can be done on amniotic fluid will be helpful to Mrs. V.'s obstetrician in deciding whether or not to terminate her pregnancy 3 or 4 weeks before her estimated due date?

   a. Color

   b. Cells containing fat

   c. Chromosome analysis

   d. Creatinine level

   e. Lecithin-sphingomyelin ratio

   f. Bilirubin concentration

3. What valuable information can Mrs. V.'s obstetrician obtain by determining her blood or urinary estriol levels?

4. Of what benefit might x-ray studies of the fetus be to the obstetrician in dealing with the problem confronting him?

5. Would continuous monitoring of the fetal heart rate be indicated when Mrs. V. is in labor? Why?

BIBLIOGRAPHY

Galloway KG: Placental evaluation studies: The procedures, their purposes, and the nursing care involved. Am J Maternal-Child Nurs 1:300–306, 1976
Lee CY, DiLoreto PC, Logrand B: Fetal activity acceleration determination for the evaluation of fetal reserve. Obstet Gynecol 48:19, 1976
Monitoring methods and equipment. Cranbury, NJ, Hoffman-LaRoche

Parer JT, Puttler OL Jr, Freeman RK: A clinical approach to fetal monitoring. Berkeley Bio-Engineering, Inc, 1974

Reeder SR, Martin LL: Maternity Nursing, 16th ed, pp 925–968. Philadelphia, JB Lippincott, 1987

Sadovsky E, Polishuk WZ: Fetal movements in utero: Nature, assessment, prognostic value, timing of delivery. Obstet Gynecol 50:49, 1977

Trieweiler MW, Freeman RK, James J: Baseline fetal heart rate characteristics as an indicator of fetal status during the antepartal period. Am J Obstet Gynecol 125:618, 1976

Werch A, Acosta A, Besch PK: The role of amniotic fluid analysis. J Obstet Gynecol Neonatal Nurs 3:43–46, 1974

Normal Childbirth **5**

process of normal 10 labor

○ *Define: labor, lightening, show, effacement, dilatation, presentation, habitus, lie, station, amniotomy.*

○ *List the signs of approaching labor.*

○ *State the chief difference between false labor and true labor.*

○ *List two possible dangers following early rupture of the membranes.*

○ *Explain the importance of the period of relaxation between contractions.*

○ *Describe how the frequency, duration, and intensity of contractions are monitored.*

○ *Name and describe the six positions the occiput may occupy in the mother's pelvis.*

○ *Tell what is accomplished in the first, second, and third stages of labor, and give the average length of time of each for primigravidas and multigravidas.*

○ *Describe the sensation the laboring patient experiences with the onset of the second stage of labor.*

○ *Name and describe the mechanisms of labor.*

○ *Explain how the skull bones of the baby adapt to the birth canal.*

○ *Name and describe three kinds of episiotomies.*

○ *Give three reasons for episiotomy.*

○ *Name the three types of perineal lacerations and tell what each involves.*

○ *Name two or three types of anesthesia that may be used for delivery, and list the advantages and disadvantages of each.*

○ *Discuss the significance of the fourth stage of labor.*

After approximately 280 days, the fetus reaches a degree of maturity at which it is able to survive outside the uterus. When this maturity is attained, a process begins by which the fetus is expelled from the uterus; this process is called *labor*. Labor is accomplished by regular, rhythmic contractions of the uterine muscles.

What causes labor to start is not known, but it is believed that more than one factor is involved. As pregnancy reaches term, the posterior lobe of the pituitary gland is thought to produce an increased amount of the hormone oxytocin. Oxytocin stimulates the uterus to contract. Also, as the gestation reaches term, the uterus becomes greatly distended. This distention, or stretching of the muscles, increases the irritability of the uterine muscles, causing them to contract.

SIGNS OF APPROACHING LABOR

When any one of the following signs is experienced by the pregnant woman, labor may start soon:

Lightening
False labor
Show
Spontaneous rupture of the membranes

Lightening.   About 2 weeks before labor starts, primigravidas usually notice that the uterus "drops" lower down in the abdomen. This "dropping" is actually the settling of the fetus into the brim of the pelvis and is called *lightening*. Following lightening, the pressure of the uterus against the diaphragm is relieved and the pregnant woman is able to breathe more easily. At the same time, the uterus once again exerts pressure against the bladder, causing frequent urination. The increased pressure in the pelvis resulting from lightening may cause leg cramps. Multigravidas may not experience lightening until labor starts.

False labor.   Some expectant mothers are annoyed by false labor as early as 3 weeks before term. The contractions of false labor are an exaggeration of the Braxton Hicks contractions, which are present throughout pregnancy. Although they are painful, these contractions are usually short and occur at irregular intervals. They do not increase in intensity and are relieved by walking. Unlike true labor, in which the contractions are felt in the lower back and abdomen, false labor contractions are usually felt only in the abdomen. The chief difference, however, between false and true labor is that in false labor the cervix does not dilate. The more pregnancies a woman has, the more likely she is to have false labor.

Show.   Shortly before actual labor starts, the pregnant woman may have a small amount of pink-tinged vaginal discharge. This discharge, called *show*, consists of the mucus plug from the cervical canal mixed with a small amount of blood. The blood is from tiny vessels in the cervix that rupture as changes occur in preparation for labor, which usually starts with 24 hours after the appearance of the show.

Spontaneous rupture of the membranes. Spontaneous rupture of the membranes occasionally occurs before labor starts. It is commonly referred to as "dry birth" by lay people. A dry birth is generally anticipated with much anxiety, since it is supposed to be much more painful than one in which the membranes rupture after labor is well established. The actuality of a dry birth is remote, however, since the mechanism that produces amniotic fluid continues to do so until the birth of the baby. The fluid that is lost initially when the membranes rupture varies in amount from a trickle to a gush, depending on how much fluid is between the presenting part and the cervix at the time and how snugly the presenting part fits against the cervix following the rupture.

Dangers associated with early rupture of the membranes include prolapsed cord and infection. In prolapsed cord, the cord is washed downward with the flow of fluid when the membranes rupture, and lodges below the presenting part. The presenting part can then put pressure on the cord, thereby cutting off circulation to the fetus. Unless the condition is diagnosed and corrected immediately, the fetus will die (see Chap. 14).

The membranes surrounding and containing the fetus and amniotic fluid act as a protective barrier against infection. When they rupture, this barrier is removed and both mother and infant become highly susceptible to infection. The danger of infection increases as the time between rupture of the membranes and birth is prolonged. When the membranes rupture early, it is important to take the woman's temperature at frequent intervals to detect a fever that would signal the onset of infection. Because of the possibility of introducing infection-producing organisms into the uterus, vaginal examinations are done only when absolutely necessary once the membranes have ruptured.

CONTRACTIONS

Contractions of the muscles of the uterus are the forces that bring about the birth of the baby. Because these contractions create a certain amount of discomfort, they are frequently called "pains" by the mother. The amount of discomfort produced by contractions varies; some mothers seem unable to tolerate even mild contractions, whereas others appear not to mind strong contractions. Because mothers do react differently to contractions, and because they also may be influenced by suggestion, it is well for the nurse to use the term "contractions" rather than "pains" when speaking to the patient. In true labor, the contractions are usually felt first in the lower back and then radiate to the front of the abdomen.

Contractions are *intermittent* and *involuntary*. They are intermittent in that each contraction is followed by a period of relaxation. This period of relaxation, or interval between contractions, provides rest periods for the mother, the uterus, and the fetus. Labor contractions produce repetitive stress for the fetus. Between contractions the pressure of the uterine arteries is about 85 mm Hg; the pressure of the uterine muscle (myometrium) is about 10 mm Hg, and the pressure of the amniotic fluid is about 10 mm Hg. During normal contractions, the pressure of the uterine arteries can be as high as 120 mm Hg, and the pressure of the uterine muscle and of the amniotic fluid can reach 60 mm Hg. Therefore, every time the uterus contracts after the mother is in active labor, the uterine blood flow is cut off and no blood gets into the intervillous spaces. The fetus thus gets no oxygen, and in effect is forced to "hold its breath" during contractions. The period of relaxation between contractions permits the uterine blood flow, and therefore the fetal oxygen supply, to return to normal. The length of the intervals between contractions may be 10 to 20 minutes at the beginning of labor. As labor progresses, the intervals become shorter.

There is no voluntary control of uterine contractions. The mother can neither start nor stop them, nor can she lengthen, strengthen, or shorten them.

There are three phrases to each contraction. The *increment* is the beginning phase during which the contraction is increasing, or building up, its strength. The *acme* is the phase in which the contraction is at its peak of strength. The *decrement* is the phase during which it is decreasing in strength.

ASSESSMENT OF CONTRACTIONS

During labor, the *frequency, duration,* and *intensity* of contractions are charted. The frequency is determined by timing from the beginning of one contraction to the beginning of the next. The frequency of contractions increases from once every 10 or 20 minutes at the beginning of labor to every 2 or 3 minutes by the end of labor.

The duration of a contraction is determined by timing the contraction from its beginning to its end. Contractions may last only 15 or 25 seconds at the beginning of labor, but they become longer as labor progresses. Toward the end of labor they usually last 45 to 70 seconds.

The intensity of a contraction is determined by placing a hand on the mother's abdomen and feeling the firmness of the uterus during a contraction. The stronger the contraction, the firmer the uterus becomes; intensity is described as mild, moderate, or strong. During a mild contraction there is very little firmness of the uterus, and it can be indented easily with the fingertips. In a moderate contraction, the uterus is firmer but can be indented a little. In a strong contraction, the uterus is very firm and cannot be indented. Contractions are usually mild early in labor but become stronger as labor progresses.

FETAL POSITIONS INSIDE THE UTERUS

Presentation. Presentation refers to the part of the fetus that is lowest in the mother's pelvis. The baby's head is the presenting part in approximately 97% of all deliveries. These are known as *vertex* presentations (Fig. 10-1). *Breech* presentations occur in approximately 3% of all deliveries. In breech presentations, the presenting part may be either the buttocks, the feet, or both parts (see Chap. 18).

Fetal habitus. The relationships of the fetal parts to one another are described by the term *fetal habitus* (or *attitude*). Because the fetus floats in water, it is able to assume many positions in varying degrees of flexion or extension. In the later months of pregnancy, however, the fetus is characteristically in an attitude of flexion. In flexion the fetal spinal column is bowed forward, the head if flexed forward with the chin on the sternum, the arms are flexed and folded on the chest, and the legs are flexed with the ankles crossed and the thighs against the abdomen. When the fetal parts are completely flexed, the fetus assumes an ovoid shape—roughly the shape of the uterus—and occupies the least space possible.

Lie. The relation of the long axis of the fetus to the long axis of the mother is called *lie*. Lie is either longitudinal or transverse. In most instances, the long axis of the fetus is parallel to the long axis of the mother (the longitudinal lie). On rare occasions the fetus lies crosswise in the uterus (the transverse lie). The shoulder is the presenting part in

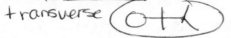

transverse

FIG. 10-1. *Vertex presentations.*

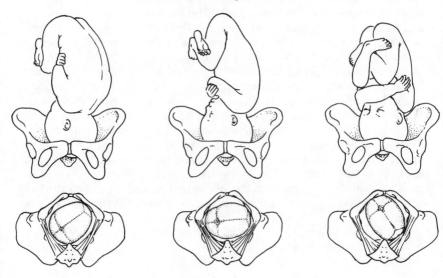

Turning baby occurs from outside.

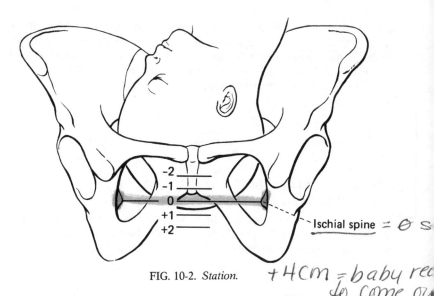

FIG. 10-2. *Station.*

[handwritten: Ischial spine = θ s]

[handwritten: +4cm = baby read to come ou]

a transverse lie. A term pregnancy with a transverse lie constitutes an obstetric complication that usually necessitates cesarean section.

Station. During labor, the relation of the presenting part to the ischial spines of the mother's pelvis is referred to as *station.* When the presenting part is 1 or 2 cm above the spines, it is at −1 or −2 station. When it is 1 or 2 cm below the spines, it is at +1 or +2 station. When the presenting part is level with the spines, it is said to be at 0 station; 0 station is considered to be the middle of the pelvis (Fig. 10-2). When the widest biparietal diameter of the baby's head is at or has entered the inlet of the pelvis, it is said to be *engaged.* Before the head becomes engaged, it is said to be *floating.*

Position. The relation of a certain point on the presenting part to the mother's pelvis is known as *position* (Fig. 10-3). In a vertex presentation,

FIG. 10-3. *Position. (A) Right occiput anterior; (B) Right occiput posterior; (C) Left occiput anterior.*

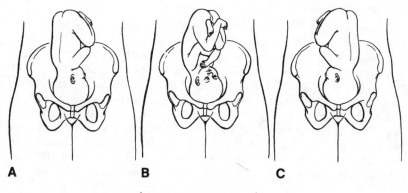

A   B   C

*[handwritten: ROA / LOA easiest
ROP / LOP hardest to deliver]*

that certain point is the back of the baby's head, called the occiput. In a breech presentation it is the sacrum. For example, in vertex presentations in which the occiput is toward the left and front of the mother's pelvis, the position is described as left occiput anterior (abbreviated LOA). There are six positions the occiput may occupy:

Left occiput anterior (LOA)
Left occiput posterior (LOP)
Left occiput transverse (occiput is directly toward the mother's side rather than toward her front or back) (LOT)
Right occiput anterior (ROA)
Right occiput posterior (ROP)
Right occiput transverse (ROT)

The LOA and ROA positions are the most common and make delivery the easiest. In LOP and ROP positions, labor may be longer and harder and the mother experiences severe backache (see Chap. 18).

STAGES OF LABOR

Labor is divided into three stages; specific developments occur in each stage. The average length of the first and second stages differs for primigravidas and multigravidas. The average length of the third stage is the same for both.

FIRST STAGE

The first contractions may occur at irregular intervals. Labor is said to start when the contractions begin coming at regular intervals. These contractions bring about two important changes in the cervix during the first stage of labor:
Complete *effacement* (shorten) of the cervical canal (no cervix felt)
Complete *dilatation* of the cervix

Effacement. At the end of pregnancy, the cervical canal is about 1 to 2 cm (about ¾ inch) long, and the circular opening of the cervix is approximately 1 cm (less than ½ inch) in diameter. Usually the first thing accomplished during the first stage of labor is the complete effacement (that is, the elimination or obliteration) of the cervical canal; effacement is a gradual process, and the amount is estimated as the percentage (such as 50%, 70%, 90%, and so forth) of effacement that has taken place. The percentage of effacement is determined by inserting a gloved finger into the vagina or rectum and feeling the cervix. The more effacement that has taken place, the thinner the cervix becomes. By the time 100%, or complete, effacement has occurred, the cervix is as thin as it will get.

SUMMARY OF STAGES OF LABOR

I	II	III

DEFINITION:

o From beginning of regular contractions until complete dilatation of cervix	o From complete dilatation of cervix to birth of baby	o From birth of baby to birth of placenta

WHAT IS ACCOMPLISHED: *100 %*

o Complete effacement and dilatation of cervix 10cm	o Birth of baby	o Separation and expulsion of placenta

FORCES INVOLVED:

o Uterine contractions	o Uterine contractions and intra-abdominal pressure (pushing)	o Uterine contractions and intra-abdominal pressure

LENGTH:

o Primigravidae: Average: 12 hours	o 1¼ hours	o 5 to 15 minutes
o Multiparae: Average: 7 hours	o 30 minutes or less	o 5 to 15 minutes

Dilatation. The cervical opening gradually increases in size (dilates) from 1 cm to 10 cm. When it is dilated 10 cm, it is said to be fully or completely dilated (see Fig. 11-4). Complete dilatation of the cervix is necessary to permit the baby to be expelled from the uterus. The amount of dilatation, estimated in centimeters, is also determined by feeling the cervix during a vaginal or rectal examination. As dilatation of the cervix progresses, there is an increase in the amount of bloody show.

Duration of first stage

The first stage of labor has been divided into two phases. The *latent* phase is the early, slow part of labor that consumes the most time. It is from the beginning of regular contractions until the cervix is about 4 cm dilated. During this phase the contractions are mild or moderate in intensity, and dilatation takes a long time to occur. In the *active* phase, the contractions are stronger and more effective, with dilatation occurring much more rapidly. This phase is shorter, lasting from 4 to 5 cm dilatation to the end of the first stage of labor. During the latent phase the mother can be encouraged to be up and about—this will often help to hasten this period. During the active phase she can be assisted into a comfortable position in bed and coached in relaxing.

When complete effacement and complete dilatation of the cervix have been accomplished, the first stage of labor ends. This stage lasts 8 to 24 hours in primigravidas, with an average of 12 hours. The average length of the first stage of labor for multigravidas is 7 hours. The first stage of labor is longer for primigravidas because these changes have never occurred before and the tissues are more resistant. The first stage of labor may often be shortened for both primigravidas and multigravidas if they can relax during contractions. Relaxation reduces tension and thereby reduces the tissue resistance, making the work of the contractions easier and more effective.

Medication during first stage

Uterine contractions may cause so much discomfort during the first stage labor that it is impossible for the mother to relax; therefore, it is important she be given medication for pain relief. However, medication that the mother receives may cross the placenta and enter the bloodstream of the baby. Some medication that is an effective analgesic for the mother may be harmful to the baby if given in large or repeated doses. Therefore, the amount of medication a mother is given during labor is usually sufficient to take the "edge" off the pain and help her to relax between contractions, but is less than would be needed to completely relieve all of her pain.

Drugs commonly used for pain relief during labor include barbiturates such as secobarbital (Seconal) and pentobarbital (Nembutal), narcotics such as meperidine (Demerol) and alphaprodine (Nisentil), phenothiazines such as promethazine (Phenergan) and promazine (Sparine), and amnesics such as scopolamine (Table 10-1).

SECOND STAGE

When the cervix is completely dilated, the second stage of labor begins. During this stage the baby is forced down the birth canal and out through the vaginal opening. This is accomplished by the combined action of the uterine contractions and intra-abdominal pressure exerted by the mother as she "bears down." When the cervix is completely dilated, the mother experiences pressure on the rectum like that felt when one has to have a bowel movement. This feeling is caused by the baby and is experienced each time the woman has a contraction. The bearing down or pushing that the mother then feels compelled to do is just like straining to have a bowel movement, but more forceful.

Rupture of the membranes. Often the membranes rupture spontaneously during the first stage of labor or at the beginning of the second stage. If they do not rupture spontaneously, the physician may insert an instrument into the cervix and rupture them. Artificial rupture of the membranes by the physician is called *amniotomy.*

Occasionally a woman mistakes urinary incontinence or vaginal secretions for rupture of the membranes. To determine if the membranes are

TABLE 10-1 DRUGS COMMONLY USED DURING FIRST STAGE LABOR

DRUG	USUAL DOSAGE	HOW ADMINISTERED	WHEN GIVEN	EFFECTS	NURSING MEASURES FOLLOWING ADMINISTRATION
HYPNOTICS (BARBITURATES) Secobarbital (Seconal)	100–200 mg (1½–3 grains)	PO, IM, rectally	Early in labor	Relieves tension Provides rest Produces sleep	Instruct not to get out of bed Side rails up on bed Provide atmosphere conducive to rest and sleep Call signal within easy reach Watch for signs of restlessness and excitement
Pentobarbital (Nembutal)	100–200 mg (1½–3 grains)	PO, IM, rectally	Early in labor	Relieves tension Provides rest Produces sleep	
NARCOTICS Meperidine (Demerol)	50–100 mg	IM, IV	After cervix 3–4 cm dilated	Relieves pain Relaxes cervix	Instruct not to get out of bed Side rails up on bed Check FHT, respirations Watch progress of labor closely Observe for effects of medication (i.e, mother's reaction to her labor)
Alphaprodine (Nisentil)	15–45 mg	IM, IV	After cervix 3–4 cm dilated	Relieves pain	
AMNESIC Scopolamine	0.3–0.4 mg (1/200–1/150 grains)	IM	With narcotic prior to general anesthetic	Amnesia Produces drowsiness Produces sleep Inhibits secretions	Same as for narcotics Watch for signs of restlessness and excitement Stay with patient
TRANQUILIZERS Promethazine HCl (Phenergan)	25–50 mg	IM	With narcotic or barbiturate	Sedative Relieve apprehension Tranquilizing action	Same as for narcotics
Propiomazine HCl (Largon)	20 mg	IM, IV	Early in labor alone, or with narcotics		
Hydroxyzine HCl (Atarax; Vistaril)	25–50 mg	IM			

[handwritten annotations: "dative", "c̄ phenergan or Nubare or Largon", "Truth serum" causes rambling", "Dries up secretions", "sedative", "not given much anymore"]

ruptured, the physician can do a speculum examination, or the fluid can be tested for acidity or alkalinity with a strip of nitrazine tape. If the membranes are ruptured, a pool of fluid can usually be seen in the vagina near the cervix when a sterile speculum is inserted in the vagina and opened to reveal the cervix. When no fluid is seen, a sterile cotton swab can be inserted into the cervical os and then withdrawn and pressed against a strip of nitrazine tape. If there is amniotic fluid on the swab, the nitrazine tape will turn a blue-green, blue-gray, or a deep blue color, indicating an alkaline reaction. If there is no amniotic fluid on the swab, the nitrazine tape will remain a yellow or olive-yellow color, indicating an acid reaction. Urine and vaginal secretions are usually acid, while amniotic fluid is alkaline. The nitrazine test is useless when blood is present, because blood also gives an alkaline reaction.

✓ Mechanisms of labor

There are four positional changes or movements the presenting part of the fetus undergoes as it passes through the birth canal. These positional changes are *flexion, internal rotation, extension,* and *external rotation.* They, with *descent* of the fetus, constitute the mechanisms of labor. More than one of these changes may be occurring at the same time. The purpose of these movements is to present the smallest possible diameter of the presenting part to the irregular birth canal so that it will meet with the least possible resistance.

✓ **Descent.** One of the first and most important movements in the birth process is descent of the presenting part. In primigravidas, engagement often occurs before labor, with no further descent until second stage labor. In multigravidas, descent usually begins with engagement.

The bones of the baby's head are soft and have not grown solidly together before birth; therefore they are able to overlap, or "mold," to fit the birth canal. The head, which is normally the largest part of the infant's body, acts as a wedge to force open the birth canal to permit passage of the baby. If the head can get through the birth canal, the rest of the body is usually able to follow without difficulty.

✓ **Flexion.** Flexion normally occurs as the descending head contacts and meets resistance from either the pelvic walls, the cervix, or the pelvic floor (Fig. 10-4). With the head flexed so that the chin is on the sternum, the smallest anteroposterior diameter (suboccipitobregmatic) is presented to the pelvis.

✓ **Internal rotation.** The fetal head usually enters the pelvis in the transverse position. Internal rotation is the movement of the head from the transverse position to the anterior position, with the occiput rotating toward the front of the mother's pelvis (Fig. 10-5). Following this movement, the occiput rests beneath the symphysis pubis. The occiput sometimes rotates posteriorly instead of anteriorly and comes to rest in the hollow of the sacrum. This results in a persistent occiput posterior position (see Chap. 18).

✓**Extension.**   The outlet of the birth canal extends upward and forward to its external opening at the vulva. Following internal rotation, the base of the occiput is in direct contact with the lower border of the symphysis publis. Until the flexed head reaches the pelvic floor, the uterine contractions force it downward. When it reaches the pelvic floor, it meets with strong resistance, which forces it upward toward the vulvar opening. Thus, the combined actions of pressure from the symphysis publis against the occiput, force of the uterine contractions, and resistance from the pelvic floor cause extension of the head. As extension occurs the occiput is born first, then the forehead, nose, mouth, and chin (Fig. 10-6).

✓**External rotation.**   After the head emerges, the occiput rotates toward the same side it occupied before birth. If it was toward the left side of the mother's pelvis, it turns toward her left; if it was toward her right, it turns to the right. This external rotation of the occiput to its previous position is known as *restitution.* External rotation of the occiput is accompanied by internal rotation of the baby's body (Fig. 10-7). The anterior shoulder is then born, followed by the posterior shoulder and the rest of the body (Fig. 10-8). When the entire body has been born, the second stage of labor ends.

✓Episiotomy

When the occiput is seen at the vaginal opening, the anesthesia agreed upon by the woman and the physician is administered (see below). As the head distends the vaginal opening (*crowns*), the physician may decide to make an incision, called *episiotomy,* into the perineum at the lower border of the vaginal opening. The episiotomy may be:

Midline (ML)
Right mediolateral (RML)
Left mediolateral (LML)

A midline episiotomy is an incision down the center of the perineum toward the anus. In a right mediolateral episiotomy, the incision is made slightly lateral toward the mother's right; a left mediolateral episiotomy is slightly lateral toward her left (Fig. 10-9). Episiotomies are done to prevent:

Undue stretching of the muscles of the perineum, which could lessen the tone of these muscles
Prolonged pressure of the baby's head against the perineum, which could damage the baby
Lacerations of the perineum, the uneven edges of which are more difficult to repair than the even edges of episiotomy

Lacerations are described as first, second, or third degree according to the extent of the tear. In a *first-degree laceration* only the mucous membrane and the skin are torn. In a *second-degree laceration,* the mucous membrane, skin, and muscles of the perineum are torn. In a *third-degree laceration,* the spincter muscle of the anus is torn as well as the tissues involved in a second-degree laceration.

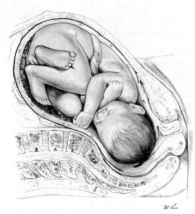

FIG. 10-4. *Normal flexion during descent in left occiput anterior position.*

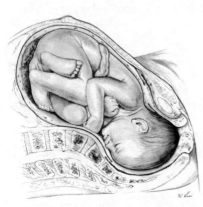

FIG. 10-5. *Internal rotation to occiput anterior position.*

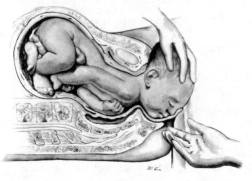

FIG. 10-6. *Birth of the head by extension.*

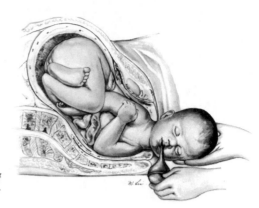

FIG. 10-7. *External rotation of the head produces internal rotation of the body.*

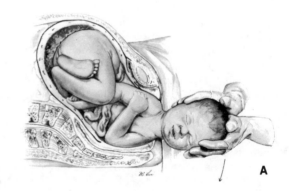

A

FIG. 10-8. *Delivery of the anterior shoulder, (A) and delivery of the posterior shoulder (B) are followed by delivery of the body.*

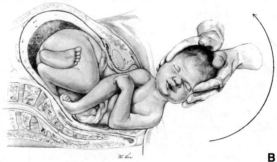

B

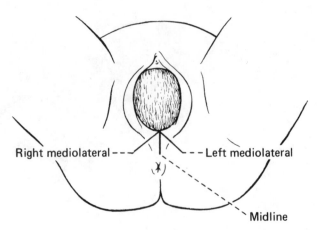

FIG. 10-9. *Types of episiotomies.*

Usually 00 or 000 chromic catgut suture is used to repair the episiotomy. This suture is absorbable and does not have to be removed. The repair is done from the inside to the outside with the vaginal mucosa and fourchet being closed first, then the fascia and muscles, and finally the subcutaneous fascia and skin. Midline episiotomies may be somewhat less painful than mediolateral ones, because they are located in a natural crease that reduces the tension on them. The discomfort due to the episiotomy varies with individuals, but it may last for several days.

Duration of second stage

The pushing that the primigravida must do is hard work. It may take 2 hours for her to move the baby down the birth canal and out; the average length of the second stage of labor is 1.25 hours. Multigravidas have less tissue resistance to overcome, because the tissues of the birth canal have been stretched before, and they usually do not have to push as long to give birth. The average length of the second stage of labor for multigravidas is 30 minutes or less.

Anesthesia

General anesthesia. Anesthesia for delivery must be safe for the baby as well as safe and effective for the mother. For mothers who wish to be asleep during delivery, inhalation (general) anesthesia is available. In inhalation anesthesia, a mask is placed over the mother's mouth and nose while she breathes the anesthetizing gas mixed with oxygen. When this type of anesthesia is anticipated, it is important that the mother not be given food or fluids by mouth during labor, to reduce the possibility of

Causes severe depression of neonate

her vomiting while anesthetized and aspirating some of the vomitus into her lungs. A drying agent, such as atropine or scopolamine, is given before the anesthetic to decrease secretions. Gases used for general anesthesia may be highly explosive; therefore, precautions must be taken to eliminate the possibility of producing static electrical charges that could ignite the gases. All equipment and personnel in the delivery room must be conductive. To be conductive, personnel must wear cotton outer garments and conductive shoes; nurses in the delivery suite must wear cotton slips or slips containing a cotton mixture. No one except the person administering the anesthesia should touch the anesthetic machine. Prolonged use of inhalation anesthesia before the baby is born may cause damage to the baby by decreasing its oxygen supply; therefore, this type of anesthesia is usually not given until the baby is ready to be born.

Regional anesthesia. If the mother wishes to be awake when the baby is born, she may have a regional or a local anesthetic. Saddle block, caudal block, pudendal block, paracervical block, and epidural block are examples of regional anesthesia. In a *saddle block,* the anesthetizing drug is injected under the dura of the spinal cord. The area anesthetized is the part of the body that comes in contact with the saddle when one rides a horse. After this anesthesia takes effect, the mother no longer feels her contractions. The mother's blood pressure is taken frequently after a saddle block. This anesthesia does not affect the baby unless there is a drop in the mother's blood pressure after its administration.

In *caudal anesthesia,* the drug is injected into the caudal space within the sacrum. A polyethylene tubing may be inserted and left in place so that additional medication can be injected as needed; this is called a continuous caudal. Caudals may be started as soon as labor is well established and continued throughout labor and delivery. The mother does not feel her contractions as long as this anesthesia is continued. The mother's blood pressure and the fetal heart tones are checked at frequent intervals following administration of a caudal.

A *pudendal block* is given after the mother is ready for delivery. The pudendal nerves supplying the perineum are injected with the anesthetizing drug (Fig. 10-10). This type of anesthesia produces marked relaxation

(*Text continues on p. 228*)

FIG. 10-10. *Pudendal block.*

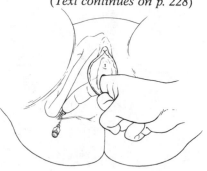

TABLE 10-2 TYPES OF ANESTHESIA COMMONLY USED FOR DELIVERY

TYPE OF ANESTHESIA	GASES OR DRUGS USED	HOW GIVEN	AREA ANESTHETIZED	EFFECTS ON BABY	CONTRACTIONS FELT?	POSSIBLE DANGERS
INHALATION (general)	Penthrane Nitrous oxide Ethylene Cyclopropane Ether	Inhaled through mask placed on face	Complete anesthesia	Prolonged use may cause respiratory depression, hypoxia	No	Explosion Laryngospasms Vomiting with aspiration of food or fluid into lungs Excessive uterine bleeding due to relaxation
REGIONAL Pudendal block	Lidocaine (Xylocaine) Procaine (Novocain) Hexylcaine (Cyclaine) Piperocaine (Metycaine) Mepivacaine (Carbocaine)	Injected into area of pudendal nerves	Perineum	None	Yes	None unless allergic reaction to drug
Saddle block (low spinal)	Tetracaine (Pontocaine) Dibucaine (Nupercaine) Drugs used for pudendal	Injected under dura of spinal cord	Pelvic region	None unless hypotension in mother	No	Hypotension

	Drugs	Method	Region	Effect on fetus		Complications
Caudal	Piperocaine (Metycaine) Tetracaine (Pontocaine) Mepivacaine (Carbocaine) Lidocaine (Xylocaine)	Injected into caudal space of sacrum	Pelvic region	None unless hypotension in mother	No	Hypotension
Paracervical block	Lidocaine (Xylocaine) Chloroprocaine (Nesacaine) Mepivacaine (Carbocaine) Piperocaine (Metycaine) Procaine (Novocain)	Injected transvaginally on either side of cervix	Relieves pain of uterine contractions (analgesia) rather than typical anesthetic effect	Occasional bradycardia of transient nature	May or may not be	Fetal bradycardia
Epidural block	Piperocaine (Metycaine) Lidocaine (Xylocaine) Mepivacaine (Carbocaine) Chloroprocaine (Nesacaine)	Injected into lumbar region of epidural space	Pelvic region	None unless hypotension in mother	No	Hypotension
LOCAL Local infiltration	Same as for pudendal	Injected into skin and tissues of perineum	Area injected	None	Yes	None unless allergic reaction to drug

of the perineum and may be used for this purpose even when an episiotomy is not done. Relaxation of the muscles of the perineum hastens delivery by reducing the resistance of the tissues to the stretching they must undergo. With this anesthesia, the mother continues to feel her contractions. The baby is not affected by a pudendal block.

Paracervical block is the injection of an anesthetic solution on either side of the cervix. A 10-ml control syringe attached to a 20-gauge, 6-inch (15-cm)-long needle is used. The needle is first inserted into a sheath that covers all of it except about 0.5 cm, the desired depth for the injection. To prevent unnecessary pricking of the patient, the needle point is kept covered in the sheath while it is passed through the vagina to the injection site. Two types of sheaths commonly used are the Kobak and the Iowa trumpet. Paracervical block analgesia may be given as a one-time dose, or a needle with a plastic catheter attached to it may be left in place on each side of the cervix so that repeated doses can be given.

Paracervical block, given to the primigravida when the cervix is 6 to 7 cm dilated and to the multigravida when the cervix is 5 to 6 cm dilated, can be very effective in relieving the pain of uterine contractions without stopping labor. The pain relief usually lasts about an hour. Temporary fetal bradycardia sometimes occurs following paracervical block. This can be avoided by reducing the dosage and the concentration of the solution.

In *epidural block*, the anesthetic solution is introduced into the epidural space through the lumbar spine. The patient is positioned on her left side with her legs partially flexed. After the lumbar region is cleansed and draped, the skin and ligamentum flavum are injected with a small amount of the anesthetic solution. Then a 16-gauge Tuohy needle is passed through the skin and ligamentum flavum into the epidural space. The position of the needle is then tested by attaching a syringe to it, and aspirating. If spinal fluid is obtained, the needle is in the wrong place and must be repositioned. If no fluid is obtained, the position of the needle is further tested by injecting 2 ml of air. If the air passes without resistance, the needle is probably in the correct position. Then a plastic catheter is threaded through the needle into the epidural space and the needle is withdrawn. To confirm the proper location of the catheter, two test doses of 2 ml of anesthetic solution are injected through it at 5-minute intervals. If the catheter is properly located, no anesthetic effects will be experienced from these small doses; if it is in the spinal canal, however, a safe, low spinal anesthesia will be produced. After confirmation of proper location of the catheter, an appropriate dose of anesthetic solution is injected and the catheter is taped in place. The patient's blood pressure, pulse, respirations, and the fetal heart tones are recorded every minute for 15 minutes after each dose of anesthetic solution is injected and every 5 minutes thereafter.

Continuous epidural block is effective as analgesia for labor and as anesthesia for delivery. However, because of the time involved in administering it, it may be more appropriate for primigravidas than for multigravidas whose labor is progressing rapidly.

✓The potential disadvantages to epidural block are:

It may cause hypotension in the mother
If given too soon, it may stop or prolong labor
It increases the frequency of forceps delivery

Epidural anesthesia is contraindicated in shock or hemorrhage because of its vasodilator effects, and it should be used with caution in PIH. Before epidural block is given, an intravenous infusion of a 5% solution of dextrose should be started. Increasing the rate of the infusion is very effective in correcting hypotension resulting from epidural anesthesia.

Local anesthesia.   When local anesthesia is used, the drug is injected into the tissues of the perineum where the episiotomy is to be made. (Fig. 10-11). The only effect of this type of anesthesia is the loss of sensation in the tissues infiltrated with the medication. The baby is not affected by local anesthesia.

THIRD STAGE

The third stage of labor extends from the birth of the baby to the delivery of the placenta. Following the birth, the placenta becomes detached from the wall of the uterus and, as a result of uterine contractions and intra-abdominal pressure, is expelled. After the baby is born, the uterine cavity decreases in size as the uterus contracts. This decreases the size of the area where the placenta was attached, with the result that the placenta begins to separate from the decidua. The two mechanisms by which separation and expulsion of the placenta occur are the Schultze mechanism and the Duncan mechanism. In the Schultze mechanism, which occurs in about 80% of cases, the placenta separates first in the center while the membranes are still attached to the decidua. The shiny fetal side is seen first as the placenta is expelled. Very little blood escapes first in the Schultze mechanism, since most of it collects behind the placenta. In the Duncan mechanism, which occurs in about 20% of cases, separation occurs first at the sides and the placenta is expelled sideways, with the

FIG. 10-11. *Local infiltration.*

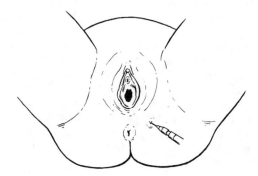

maternal side seen first. The Duncan mechanism appears to be bloodier since the blood comes out beside the placenta. Separation and expulsion of the placenta occur within 5 to 15 minutes after the baby is born. The average length of the third stage of labor is the same for primigravidas and multigravidas.

FOURTH STAGE

The first hour following the birth is often referred to as the fourth stage of labor. This is a critical period both for the parents and for the infant. Since most postpartum hemorrhages occur during this time, the mother must be observed closely and the uterus must be kept firmly contracted. The infant's airway must be kept free of mucus and the body temperature maintained. At the same time, maternal-infant bonding and paternal-infant bonding must be promoted (see Chap. 15). This period, then, requires the nurse to make skillful assessments of the physical needs of mother and infant and, at the same time, to provide opportunity for initiation of family attachments that may vitally affect the future relationships between parents and child.

THE MOTHER AND LABOR

The feelings of expectant mothers toward labor are varied. One mother may see it as a welcome event that ends a long period of waiting for a much-wanted child. Another may see it as a test of her endurance; another may see it as a terrifying ordeal from which there is no escape. Rarely does a mother regard labor with indifference.

Certain worries concerning the outcome of labor are shared by many expectant mothers. There is the fear that something may be wrong with the baby, or that it may be born dead. The mother is concerned about her own welfare. She may fear the pain of labor and worry that she may lose her own life while giving birth. The mother who is having her first baby may be afraid because she does not know what is going to happen. Such a mother may be frightened when she sees the show, when the membranes rupture, or when she feels pressure from the baby on her rectum. A mother who has had a long, difficult labor with a previous pregnancy may be afraid that this labor will be the same.

Many mothers have passed on to their daughters tales of horror and superstition concerning childbirth; daughters who are heirs to such tales are likely to be apprehensive about labor. Mothers who anticipate labor with exaggerated fears and apprehension are often more sensitive to pain and less able to tolerate labor than mothers who approach labor calmly without unnecessary fears. Ways in which the nurse can deal with such concerns are taken up in the next chapter.

CLINICAL REVIEW

ASSESSMENT: Mrs. C., a 19-year-old primigravida, was admitted to the hospital at 8 A.M. She stated that she had been having contractions off and on all night but that they had started coming 10 minutes apart at 5:30 A.M. and had stayed regular since then. Her membranes had not ruptured. After the physician examined Mrs. C., he said that the presenting part was at 0 station, the cervix was 3 cm dilated, and effacement was complete.

1. Mrs. C. is in the _____ stage of labor.
2. While admitting her, the nurse noted that Mrs. C. had contractions starting at 8:10, 8:14, 8:18, 8:22, and 8:26. These contractions lasted 40 seconds. The nurse felt Mrs. C.'s abdomen lightly with her fingertips during the contractions. The uterus felt quite firm but could be indented slightly. Tell the frequency, duration, and intensity of Mrs. C.'s contractions.
3. Mrs. C. asked the nurse how long she thought it would be before the baby was born. What should the nurse tell her?
4. About 9:30 A.M., Mrs. C. got up to the bathroom to urinate. When she got back to bed she called the nurse and told her she was bleeding. The nurse noted that the "bleeding" consisted of a pink-tinged mucus discharge. How could she explain to Mrs. C. what was happening?
5. At 11 A.M., the physician examined Mrs. C. He decided to rupture the membranes. This procedure is called artificial rupture of the membranes, or _____.
6. At 1:30 P.M., Mrs. C. stated she felt as if she had to have a bowel movement. What should the nurse suspect?
7. Examination of Mrs. C. at this time revealed that the cervix was completely dilated and the presenting part was 2 cm below the ischial spines. At what station was the presenting part? What was the dilatation in centimeters? What stage of labor is Mrs. C. in now? How did the length of her previous stage of labor compare with the average length of that stage for primigravidas?

BIBLIOGRAPHY

Nicolls ET, Corke BC, Ostheimer GW: Epidural anesthesia for the woman in labor. Am J Nurs 81:395–455, 1981

Pritchard JA, MacDonald PC, Gant NF: Williams' Obstetrics, 17th ed, pp 323–365. New York, Appleton-Century-Crofts, 1985

Reeder SR, Martin LL: Maternity Nursing, 16th ed, pp 446–456. Philadelphia, JB Lippincott, 1987

nursing care during labor 11

BEHAVIORAL When the goals of this chapter are reached, the student will
OBJECTIVES be able to:

○ Describe how the nurse admitting the labor patient can establish a rapport with her.

○ List four or five procedures commonly performed when a patient in labor is admitted, and explain why they are done.

○ Explain the procedures for giving the shave (prep) and enema.

○ List five or six ways the nurse can provide emotional support to the patient and her husband during labor and birth.

○ Explain why oral fluids and food intake may be restricted during labor.

○ List three ways in which the nurse can promote physical comfort during labor.

○ Explain how a full bladder can be detected during labor and give two reasons for preventing bladder distention.

○ List four measures that are taken to prevent infection in mother and baby.

○ List three observations made throughout labor.

○ Name three signs of fetal distress that should be reported to the physician.

○ Describe the effect meconium has on the amniotic fluid.

○ Describe symptoms that characterize transition.

○ Describe signs that indicate that birth is about to occur.

○ Describe positioning and cleansing of the patient on the delivery table.

○ List three items regarding birth that must be recorded by the nurse.

○ Name three oxytocic drugs commonly used and explain their action.

○ Describe the first thing the physician does as the baby's head is born and tell why.

- *Discuss the importance of maternal-infant bonding and tell how it can be encouraged at birth. List signs that might indicate rejection of the child by the parents.*

- *Discuss three major considerations in an emergency delivery.*

FIRST STAGE OF LABOR

When an expectant mother is admitted to the hospital in labor, she may be fearful and apprehensive, especially if this is her first experience in a hospital. It is important that the nurse admitting the mother greet her and the father warmly, introduce herself, and do all she can to make the mother feel comfortable and at ease (Figs. 11-1 and 11-2).

The nurse can help establish a desirable relationship with the mother by showing consideration for her as an individual. She does this by explaining each procedure before doing it, by providing privacy, and by avoiding unnecessary exposure of the mother during procedures. When explaining procedures or answering questions, the nurse should speak clearly and use terms that the mother understands. When possible, the nurse should assume an unhurried manner while caring for the mother.

Although each hospital has its own admission routine, there are certain procedures common to most. These include:

Obtaining the necessary information for the record

Taking the temperature, pulse, respirations, and blood pressure of the mother and listening to the fetal heart tones

Taking care of the mother's clothing and other belongings

Determining the progress of labor

Preparing the mother for labor and delivery

FIG. 11-1. *The admitting nurse greets the expectant parents warmly.*

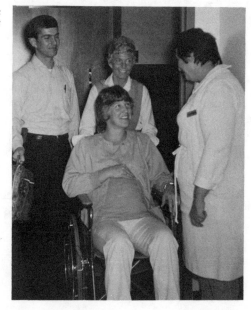

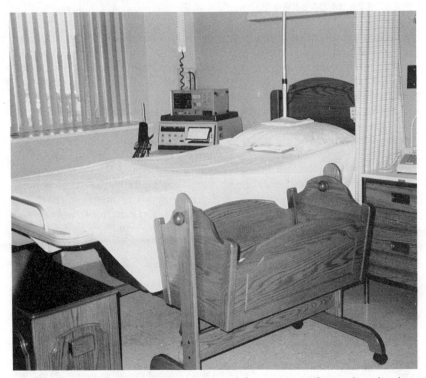

FIG. 11-2. *Labor room ready for admission of the patient. Birth can also take place in this bed.*

Information about the mother and her labor before she arrived at the hospital is needed so that intelligent care can be given. Part of this information is on the record sent to the hospital from the clinic or the physician's office; part is obtained by questioning the mother when she is admitted to the labor suite. This information includes the time her contractions started and whether the membranes are intact or ruptured. If the membranes are ruptured, the time they ruptured is recorded. When the membranes are ruptured for more than 24 hours before delivery, there is danger of infection to the mother and baby. Information concerning allergies to medications is also recorded on the chart.

In hospitals where general anesthesia is used, the nurse should find out whether the mother wears dentures or contact lenses and when she last ate. This information is needed by the anesthetist.

Obtaining a urine specimen for analysis may be part of the admission procedure. This may be a clean, voided specimen or a catheterized specimen, depending on the practice in the hospital or the physician's order. However, a voided specimen is usually not as reliable as a catheterized specimen if the mother is bleeding or if the membranes have ruptured, because blood and amniotic fluid contain albumin. In some hospitals, a catheterized specimen is obtained at the time of delivery rather than at admission.

The temperature, pulse, and respirations are taken to determine if there is evidence of infection present on admission. A blood pressure of 140/90 mm Hg or higher may be a symptom of preeclampsia and should be reported to the physician. Since the blood pressure may rise 5 to 10 mm Hg during a contraction, a reading should be taken between contractions rather than during a contraction. Fetal heart tones are an indication that the fetus is alive; they should be regular in rhythm and range in rate from 110 to 160 beats per minute. An irregular heartbeat, or a rate of less than 110 or more than 160 beats per minute, may be a sign of fetal distress and should be reported to the physician at once.

While the nurse is obtaining the admission information, she notes the frequency, duration, and intensity of the contractions. She also observes the mother's reaction to the contractions. She notes the presence and the amount of bloody show.

The mother's clothing and other belongings may be kept at the hospital or sent home. If they are not sent home, they should be labeled with the mother's name and kept in a safe place.

DETERMINING PROGRESS OF LABOR

If the physician is present, he examines the mother to find out the station of the presenting part and the amount of effacement and dilatation of the cervix. If the physician is not present, the nurse examines the mother. By these means the progress of labor is determined.

Rectal examination. To do a rectal examination, the nurse washes and dries her hands and then puts on a clean glove. Lubricating jelly is then applied to the index finger on the examining hand. After explaining to the woman what she is going to do, she requests that the woman lie on her back with both knees up and wide apart. Keeping the patient covered, the nurse slips the gloved hand under the sheet. With the thumb under the remaining three fingers, the nurse gently inserts the index finger into the rectum. After entering the rectum, the examining finger is directed upward and forward until it contacts the presenting part of the fetus (Fig. 11-3). Then it gently passes over the surface of the presenting part until the cervix, which is felt as a circular opening, is located. The diameter and circumference of the cervix are then estimated to determine the amount of dilatation (Fig. 11-4). The thickness, or depth, of the rim of the cervix is felt in order to estimate the percentage of effacement. When feeling the presenting part, one seeks to locate the sagittal suture and, if possible, the fontanelles, in order to confirm that it is vertex and to ascertain the position. When the buttock is presenting, the sagittal suture and fontanelles are not felt; also, the buttock is softer than the

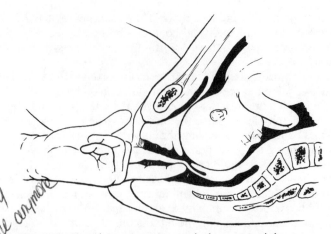

Rarely done anymore

FIG. 11-3. *Rectal examination reveals the station of the presenting part and the amount of effacement and dilatation of the cervix.*

FIG. 11-4. *Cervical dilatation in centimeters (actual size).*

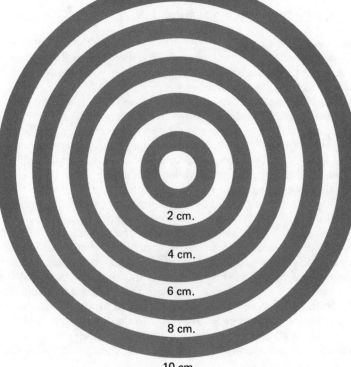

2 cm.

4 cm.

6 cm.

8 cm.

10 cm.

head. Station is determined by first locating the ischial spines of the mother, which feel like a small bump on either side of the pelvis, and then estimating how high or low the presenting part is in relation to them. Great care is taken when entering and withdrawing from the rectum to avoid contaminating the vagina with fecal material. After the examination, the anus should be cleansed to remove the lubricant and any feces present.

Vaginal examination. A vaginal examination reveals the same information as a rectal examination. When a vaginal examination is done, direct contact is made with the cervix and, if the membranes are ruptured, with the fetus. Therefore, a sterile glove is worn and sterile lubricant used. Two fingers are gently introduced into the vagina and passed upward into the cervix. Then the same steps are followed as in a rectal examination. Great care is taken to avoid contact between the vulva and the examining fingers as they enter the vagina in order to prevent contamination and subsequent infection of the birth canal.

PREPARATION FOR LABOR AND DELIVERY *Test Question* 1

The preparation of the mother for labor and delivery may include a shave (prep) and an enema; these are ordered by the physician. The prep allows the physician to see the area where he is working as he does the episiotomy, delivers the baby, and repairs the episiotomy.

Shave. The prep may be a mini-prep, a partial shave, or a complete shave. A mini-prep consists of shaving the area between the lower border of the vagina downward to the anus. This is where the episiotomy is done if one is needed. In a mini-prep the hair on the vulva should be clipped if it is very long. In a partial prep the area from the clitoris downward to and surrounding the anus is shaved. A complete shave includes this area and also the mons pubis. The mini-prep and the partial prep have replaced the complete shave in many labor and delivery departments because the woman experiences less discomfort as the hair is growing back. The shave is an embarrassing procedure for many women; the nurse should provide privacy when it is to be done.

Disposable shave kits are convenient for doing the shave. If they are not available the supplies needed are a pair of clean gloves; a container with a lathering solution, such as povidone-iodine (Betadine), soap, or pHisoHex; four 3 × 4-inch gauze sponges; two paper towels; and a razor and razor blade (disposable razors with blades assure cleanliness and sharpness).

When a shave is to be done the nurse washes her hands thoroughly and assembles the above supplies and takes them to the patient's bedside. After explaining to the patient what she is going to do and providing privacy, she positions the patient on her back with her knees up and legs wide apart. The nurse makes sure that the solution for lathering is warm. She then puts on the gloves and places the paper towels next to the patient's buttock. The towels are used to collect the hair that is removed so that it does not get on the linen. The razor is placed in the warm solution and the container is placed conveniently on the paper towel. One 3 × 4-inch sponge is dipped into the solution and squeezed just enough to prevent it from dripping, then it is used to lather the area to be shaved. The lathering strokes are begun at the highest part to be shaved and continued from side to side, working downward until the anus is reached. This is to prevent contamination by contact with the anus. After the sponge has come in contact with the anus it is discarded. The nurse then takes a dry sponge in her left hand and the razor in her right hand. Beginning at the highest point to be shaved, she holds the skin taut with the sponge while she shaves the patient. The shaving strokes are made downward and in the same direction the hair grows. The razor is rinsed in the lathering solution as necessary to remove hair from it. The area around the anus is shaved last; then the razor is not used again until it has been washed and sterilized. It is usually easier to shave the episiotomy and anal areas with the patient on her left side with her left leg flexed and her right leg drawn upward and the nurse behind her. When the shave is completed, the nurse wets a sponge in warm water and rinses the shaved area from top to bottom, then dries it with a sponge in the same manner. The paper towel with the hair and the sponges is discarded in the waste receptacle. The lathering solution is emptied into the toilet since it now contains hair (hair can clog sinks). If the container used for the lathering solution is to be used again, it can be washed and resterilized with the razor. The razor blade should be discarded in an appropriate container so that no one can be cut by it.

Enema. An enema may be ordered to empty the lower bowel. This makes more room for the baby as it comes down the birth canal and helps prevent the mother from having a bowel movement on the delivery table. An enema may also stimulate the uterus to contract. A mother in advanced labor usually is not given an enema, for two reasons: it may be only partly expelled before she is taken to the delivery room, and the remainder is likely to be expelled as the baby is born; or the baby may be born while the mother is still on the bedpan expelling the enema. In either instance, the baby may become infected as a result of contamination from fecal material.

Before giving an enema, the nurse assembles the necessary supplies, including the type of enema ordered, lubricant, and a disposable towel. She explains to the patient what she is going to do and provides privacy. If the bathroom is shared by other patients, the nurse should make sure it is available for this patient; if it is not, she should have a bedpan ready. The patient is then positioned on her left side with her left leg flexed and her right leg drawn upward. The disposable towel is placed next to her buttock. The nurse lubricates the tip of the enema tubing and, if a soapsuds enema is to be given, tests the temperature of the solution and removes air from the tubing by filling the tubing with enema solution. The tubing is then gently inserted into the rectum so as not to hurt any hemorrhoids the patient may have. Pressure from the presenting part sometimes makes insertion of the tubing difficult. If the patient is in active labor, the nurse can stop the flow during contractions so as not to add to

usually most women have mild diarrhea (1-2 episodes) before labor & don't need enema.

her discomfort. Sometimes it is possible to distract the woman's attention from the discomfort of the enema by engaging her in conversation about other things, such as the ages and names of her other children or whether she and her husband prefer a son or daughter this time. Patients who are in active labor when an enema is given should be examined as soon as possible after the enema is expelled because rapid dilatation may occur following an enema.

Potential nursing diagnoses:

Knowledge deficit related to the labor process

Knowledge deficit related to relaxation techniques

Fear related to anticipated pain of labor and birth

Alterations in comfort: pain related to labor contractions

Alterations in comfort: pain related to dryness caused by mouth breathing

Alterations in comfort: pain related to fluctuations in temperature perceptions

Alterations in comfort: pain related to full bladder

Potential fluid volume deficit related to decreased fluid intake

Alterations in comfort: pain related to exposure of body

Alterations in comfort: pain related to vaginal drainage

Ineffective individual coping related to pain and fear of labor

EMOTIONAL SUPPORT: FIRST STAGE

For a long time the emphasis in medicine and nursing was on meeting the physical needs of patients with little attention being given to their emotional needs. This situation may have arisen because physical needs are often more obvious or more demanding or easier to treat; or it may have been felt that by meeting the physical needs, one would take care of the emotional needs automatically. Now, however, both types of needs are recognized as important, and both must receive attention if care is to be complete.

Recognition of the emotional needs of labor patients has led to changes in the way normal labor is conducted in hospitals. These changes are making labor a satisfying experience rather than the terrifying ordeal it once was. Consequently, labor units are no longer noisy with the moans, groans, and screams of the occupants.

Goal. The emotional support the mother receives or fails to receive during labor can influence not only her self-image and the course of this labor, but also her attitudes toward her husband, their child, and future pregnancies. It is of the utmost importance, then, that she receive the emotional support she needs so that she is able to cope in a satisfying manner during this labor and birth.

Support by the husband. The husband gives emotional support to his laboring wife in several ways. His presence with her at this time assures her of his concern for her, and his desire to share this experience contributes greatly to her happiness and comfort (Fig. 11-5). Early in labor his efforts to keep her amused and entertained by playing cards or Scrabble or some other favorite activity, accompanied by appropriate manifestations of his wit and humor, can help her forget some of her anxieties and fears. If they have been to childbirth education classes, he can coach her in her relaxation and breathing techniques. This enables her to maintain her poise and keep control over herself so that she does not panic when the contractions become close and intense. Throughout the active phase of labor his touch and whispered words of love and praise are sources of courage to her, inspiring her to continue to do the very best job possible.

Support by the nurse. All laboring patients need some emotional support from the nurse. The amount varies widely from a few words of praise to almost continuous support with each contraction. The need for support by the nurse seems to be influenced by:

The preparation of the mother (couple) for childbirth

The performance of the mother (couple) during labor

Whether the mother has her husband or a significant other with her or is laboring alone

The type of labor previously experienced, if any

FIG. 11-5. *The presence of her husband gives emotional support to the patient in labor. Note the electronic fetal monitor, which provides a continuous record of the FHR and the contractions. The rectangular (Toco) transducer on the mother's abdomen detects the contractions, and the circular transducer detects the FHR.*

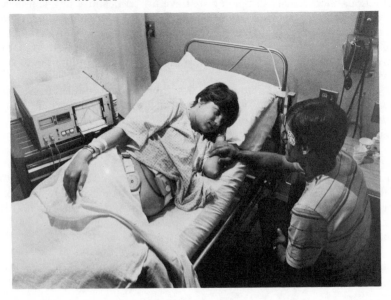

Individuals or couples who have had previous pregnancies or who have attended childbirth education classes have some idea of what to expect during labor. The true test, however, of the adequacy of preparation is in their performance during labor. Many of these patients are able to cope with varying degrees of success with minimal support from the nurse. Performance during labor by couples who have been to childbirth classes seems to be directly related to their degree of commitment to the particular method taught and whether or not they have practiced the exercises and relaxation and breathing techniques. Those who are dedicated to the method usually practice consistently and perform exceptionally well during labor with minimal dependence on the nurse for support. Those less committed, or who have not practiced consistently, may perform well during early labor but may need increasing support from the nurse as labor progresses.

A few couples who attend childbirth classes misunderstand what is presented and harbor misconceptions that are detrimental to their performance during labor. A classic example of this is the misconception that, if she does the relaxation and breathing techniques, the wife will experience no pain during labor. When the couple discovers that this is not so, they tend to panic. These couples need considerable support by the nurse.

Some expectant parents who have not had previous pregnancies or gone to childbirth classes may nevertheless be well prepared for labor. They obtain their information through reading the many books on childbirth that are available. Often they do as well during labor as those who have attended classes.

Even though couples may attend classes, not all husbands are effective coaches, and not all wives respond to the husband's coaching. Moreover, there are still husbands and wives who prefer the traditional role of the husband, where he maintains a safe distance from the labor room and does not become involved. Then there are some wives who would like to have their husbands with them during labor but whose husbands refuse. Often these women make excuses for their husbands, explaining that, "He can't stand to see me hurting," or "He doesn't like hospitals," or "The sight of blood makes him sick." Usually these husbands are content to stay in the fathers' waiting room while the wife labors. Other husbands may not be with their wives during labor because they are divorced or are separated by distance, death, or marital problems. The unwed mother, of course, has no husband. When any of these situations exists, the laboring mother may wish to have a significant other with her. This is usually possible if there is no husband or if the husband is out of town. However, some hospitals stipulate that only the husband may be with the woman during labor if he is available. Of course, if he is in the fathers' waiting room, he is "available." Thus some women are forced to labor alone. Although the nurse is a poor substitute for a husband or significant other, she must do what she can to provide all the emotional support needed by the mother who labors alone.

Occasionally the nurse will care for a multigravida who appears to be apprehensive and overreacts to mild contractions in early labor. As labor progresses the patient manifests extreme fear and the nurse has great difficulty preventing total panic. The cause of this behavior is often discovered to be related to a "bad" experience with a previous labor. It is not uncommon for the patient to say that "I was left alone for hours" or "They wouldn't believe me when I told them the baby was coming," or "I was in hard labor for 3 days and they wouldn't give me anything." Such a patient needs extra emotional support by the nurse during this labor to help replace those unpleasant memories with happy ones.

How the nurse provides support.   Before the nurse can effectively provide emotional support during labor, she needs to develop a relationship of trust with the mother (couple). Although it is easier to develop such a relationship slowly over a period of time, this is not possible for the labor nurse unless she also conducts the childbirth education classes or is a midwife or practitioner who provides continuous care throughout the pregnancy. More often the nurse sees the mother (couple) for the first time when the mother is admitted to the hospital in labor. The relationship must then be developed within a short time and under stressful conditions.

There are numerous ways the nurse provides emotional support to the laboring patient and her husband. She may make a conscious effort to supply the support needed or she may do so unknowingly as she attends to the physical needs. Emotional support can be conveyed by her manner, by her actions, and by the instruction and guidance she gives.

The nurse needs to gain the confidence and cooperation of the patient and her husband as soon as they arrive in the labor suite. By her manner and actions she conveys to them that she and they are a team working together to accomplish birth in as safe and satisfying a manner as possible. She can begin with the initial examination when they are wondering if they "came in too early." Regardless of their preparations, she can explain to them about the two things (effacement and dilatation) that have to happen to the cervix before the baby can be born. This she does in terms they can understand. Then she tells them to what extent these have progressed in the patient's cervix. The nurse can also discuss briefly with them how the contractions work to accomplish effacement and dilatation, and how labor can be hastened by the patient's relaxing during contractions. She can explain that the first 5 cm of dilatation takes the longest and the last 5 cm of dilatation occurs more rapidly.

The nurse can inform the couple that medication for pain relief is available should it be needed. The dosage is sufficient "to take the edge off" the pain so that the mother is able to remain in control, but not enough to cause harmful effects to the baby. To obtain maximum benefit from the medication the mother should continue to use her relaxation and breathing techniques.

As labor progresses, the nurse monitors the patient's response to labor. Generally it is much easier to keep a patient (couple) in control than it is to help her (them) regain control once it is lost. Furthermore, labor is shortened and the patient's self-image is enhanced if control is maintained continuously. When the husband is performing effectively as a labor coach and his wife is responding to his coaching, the nurse can remain in the background and not interfere. She must, however, be alert to indications that the patient is about to lose control so that she can reinforce the husband's coaching in time to avoid loss of control. The nurse must also be aware of the status of the labor at all times.

If, conversely, the husband is not coaching his wife, the nurse should do so. Beginning at the onset and continuing throughout the contraction, the nurse quietly reminds the mother to do her breathing as she has been taught and to let all muscles go loose. This is repeated with each contraction. Words of encouragement can be interspersed with the reminder of what to do. A progress report on the dilatation of the cervix can also be given when it is necessary to examine the patient.

Sometimes an amniotomy is performed by the physician. When this is to be done the nurse can explain to the mother that the discomfort will be no more than for a pelvic examination. The mother should be told that, after the amniotomy, she will continue to lose fluid until the baby is born. This information alleviates anxiety about the procedure and relieves any concerns the mother may have about a "dry birth." It will also keep the mother from thinking she has lost control of her bladder. The nurse should explain to the mother that her contractions will probably become more intense after the bag of waters has broken and that her labor is likely to progress more rapidly. These effects are due to the fact that the baby's head, which is firmer than the bag of waters, and therefore a better dilating wedge, can now exert pressure on the cervix. In this way the patient's fears of stronger contractions can be tempered by the knowledge that labor will be over sooner.

If the patient is laboring during a mealtime, the nurse can suggest to the husband-coach that she coach his wife while he takes a break and gets some nourishment. If he has not brought a lunch with him, she can direct him to the available facilities, such as a snack shop or vending machines. He should also be told where the nearest restroom is. Every consideration possible should be provided for his comfort as well as his wife's. By doing so, the nurse is providing emotional support for both.

THE NURSE PROVIDES SUPPORT TO THE COUPLE DURING LABOR BY:

o Being kind, friendly, thoughtful, and considerate to each of them

o Being gentle and matter-of-fact when performing examinations and procedures that may be uncomfortable or embarrassing to the patient

o Providing a quiet, private atmosphere so that the mother can concentrate on her relaxation and breathing techniques during contractions with as few extraneous interruptions as possible.

o Staying with the mother throughout the active phase of labor
o Treating husband and wife with dignity and respect
o Explaining to them what is happening and what they can expect to happen as labor progresses
o Offering encouragement in the form of praise when they are doing a good job
o Maintaining calm objectivity and being firm when the need arises in order to keep the patient in control or to help her regain control
o Anticipating the physical needs of the patient and taking care of them quickly

NURSING INTERVENTIONS TO PROMOTE COMFORT DURING LABOR

o Provide privacy; avoid unnecessary exposure of patient's body
o Keep lips and mouth moist
o Cleanse vulva and perineum
o Change underpad as necessary
o Adjust room temperature; add or remove blankets as necessary
o Provide cold, damp cloth for face as needed
o Assist to a comfortable position
o Give backrub
o Keep bladder empty

SIGNS OF FETAL DISTRESS TO REPORT TO THE DOCTOR

o Persistent tachycardia
o Severe variable decelerations or late decelerations that persist in spite of position changes of mother
o Loss of baseline variability
o Meconium in the amniotic fluid in a vertex presentation
o Irregular fetal heart rate
o Fetal heart rate that slows below 100 beats per minute during a contraction and does not return to normal within 10 to 15 seconds after the contraction ends

PHYSICAL CARE

Ambulation. Early in labor, the mother is usually permitted to ambulate as much as she desires. However, if the membranes have ruptured and the presenting part is high, the physician may order bed rest because of the danger of the cord prolapsing (see Chap. 18).

Oral intake. The food and fluid intake during labor is usually decided by the physician. Solid foods are not recommended, for two reasons. First, whatever is in the stomach when labor starts, or is eaten after it starts, is likely to be vomited. Second, if the mother receives general anesthesia for delivery, she may vomit while she is anesthetized and some of the vomitus may get into her lungs. It is well to remember that "when labor starts, digestion stops." Unless she is planning to have general anesthesia, the mother may be permitted to have fluids early in labor. But if she is in labor for several hours without food or fluids, the physician may order fluids to be given intravenously to prevent dehydration.

General comfort measures. By being alert to little things that may annoy the patient, the thoughtful nurse can find many ways to promote her comfort. For instance, the mother's mouth and lips become dry. If permitted by the physician, ice chips can be kept at the bedside to relieve the dryness. If this is not permissible, the mother can be supplied with mouthwash so that she can rinse her mouth as she desires. Petroleum jelly can be used to relieve the dryness of the lips and to prevent their cracking.

Often the membranes rupture during the first stage of labor, and the mother continues to lose fluid until the baby is born. Also, as labor progresses, the amount of bloody discharge (show) increases. These vaginal discharges make the mother feel sticky and uncomfortable. Although a perineal pad is not worn while she is in labor, because organisms that could cause infection may be carried from the anus to the vagina by the pad, a square pad can be placed under the buttocks to collect the vaginal discharges. The nurse should cleanse the vulva and change the underpad as often as necessary.

Early in labor, the mother may feel cool, especially her feet. Adjusting the room temperature or providing her with blankets will add to her comfort. As labor progresses, she may feel very warm. The room temperature may again be adjusted or the blankets removed. At this time, many mothers appreciate a cold, damp cloth applied to the face.

The nurse can further add to the comfort of the mother by helping her to relax during contractions. This is accomplished by assisting her into a comfortable position and coaching her to do slow, deep, abdominal breathing with each contraction. If the mother is relaxed during contractions, the cervix dilates faster and labor is shorter.

As the baby moves down the birth canal, many mothers experience pressure and discomfort in the lower back. Rubbing the lower back relieves this discomfort somewhat and helps the mother to relax. If the husband is present, the nurse can show him how to rub his wife's back.

Medication. As labor progresses, some mothers need medication to help relieve the pain so that they can relax. The time at which the medication is given can have an effect on the progress of labor. Medication that is given early in labor when the cervix is dilated only 2 or 3 cm may slow or even stop labor. On the other hand, medication given when labor is well established and the cervix is 4 to 5 cm dilated may speed up labor. Therefore, the progress of labor is observed very closely after medication is given. Drugs for pain relief often make the mother feel lightheaded and dizzy, so it is important that the side rails be put up on the bed and the mother be instructed not to get out of bed. The mother's respirations and the fetal heart tones are observed at frequent intervals to see if they are being affected by the medicine.

Bladder care. During labor, the mother's bladder should not be allowed to become distended. A full bladder is uncomfortable and may be injured by labor. It may also prevent the descent of the baby and interfere with uterine contractions. Since the bladder is located in the lower abdomen during labor, it is usually quite easy to see and feel when it is full. A full bladder appears as a mound rising from the symphysis upward toward the umbilicus. It feels soft and spongy, much like a partially filled hot water bottle.

Prevention of infection. While caring for patients in labor, the nurse must do all she can to protect the mother and baby from infection. She puts on a clean "scrub" dress each time she comes on duty and never wears it out of the maternity unit. No one who has an infection is permitted to take care of the mothers and babies. Furthermore, mothers who have infections must be separated from other mothers. Equipment, such as washbasins, emesis basins, and bedpans, used by one mother must be washed thoroughly and sterilized before being used by another. All personnel who care for the mother must wash their hands frequently to prevent infection.

Observations. Throughout labor, the mother is observed for signs of infection, pregnancy-induced hypertension or other problems. Her temperature, pulse, respirations, and blood pressure are taken every 4 hours. Elevations are reported to the physician. Vaginal bleeding other than show is also reported to the physician. If an electronic monitor is available for continuous monitoring of the fetal heart rate (FHR), it should be used as soon as the active phase of labor is established (Fig. 11-6). If electronic monitoring is not available, the nurse should listen to the FHR frequently, especially during and immediately after contractions. The fetal heart tones are listened to immediately after the membranes rupture to see if the cord has prolapsed. If prolapse of the cord has occurred, the heart tones may be absent or they may be slow or irregular because of pressure from the presenting part on the cord.

The nurse should report signs of fetal distress to the physician immediately. These signs include (1) persistent tachycardia, (2) severe variable decelerations or late decelerations that persist in spite of position changes of mother (see Chap. 9), (3) loss of baseline variability, or (4) meconium in the amniotic fluid with the infant in a vertex presentation. When the FHR is monitored by the nurse using a fetoscope, she would report to the physician (1) persistent tachycardia, (2) irregular FHR, or (3) FHR that slows

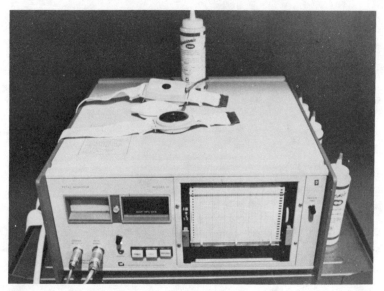

FIG. 11-6. *When available, the electronic fetal monitor is used as soon as labor is well established. External monitoring of the FHR and uterine contractions is accomplished by transducers applied to the mother's abdomen and held in place by elasticized straps. A thin layer of transmission gel is applied to the flat surface of the fetal transducer before it is positioned on the mother's abdomen where the fetal heartbeat is heard most clearly. The Toco transducer is placed where the contractions are felt most strongly.*

below 100 beats per minute during a contraction and does not return to normal within 10 to 15 seconds after the contraction ends.

Normally the amniotic fluid is quite clear, but when it contains meconium, the fluid becomes yellowish or greenish in color. When the oxygen supply to the fetus is decreased (hypoxia), the anal sphincter relaxes and meconium is excreted. In a breech presentation, meconium is commonly present in the amniotic fluid as a result of pressure on the buttocks.

The nurse notes the frequency, duration, and intensity of the contractions as labor progresses. The physician is kept informed of the progress of labor and of unusually strong contractions that last longer than a minute and a half. The nurse observes the mother's reactions to her contractions. When a mother who has been relaxing well with her contractions suddenly becomes unable to relax, the alert nurse recognizes this as a sign that the mother is probably in transition. *Transition* is the period near the end of the first stage of labor and the beginning of the second stage, when the cervix is 8 to 9 cm dilated (see Fig. 11-4). During transition, the mother usually gets the "shakes," which she cannot control. The bloody show increases, and she may have nausea and vomiting. The membranes may rupture at this time if they have not already ruptured.

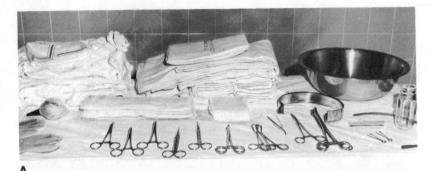

A

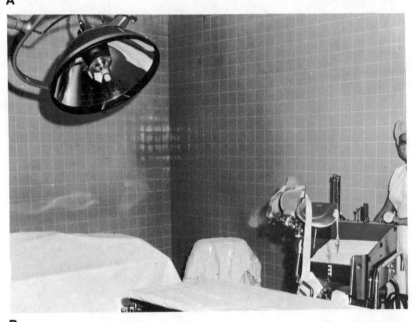

B

FIG. 11-7. *(A) Sterile supplies are arranged in readiness for delivery. (B) After the sterile supplies are prepared, they are covered with sterile drapes until the time of delivery.*

Preparation for delivery. Sometime during the first stage of labor, the nurse makes the necessary preparations for delivery. Wearing a cap to cover her hair and a mask to cover her mouth and nose, and using aseptic technique, she assembles and arranges in a convenient order the sterile supplies that the obstetrician will need for mother and baby. These supplies are then covered with a sterile drape until the mother is ready for delivery (Fig. 11-7).

The nursing-care plan for the mother during first stage labor is presented in Table 11-1.

SECOND STAGE OF LABOR

✓**Signs of the second stage.** When the cervix is completely dilated, the mother feels pressure on her rectum as if she must have a bowel movement. This feeling is caused by the baby's head pressing against the rectum as it comes down the birth canal. Often this is the first sign that the second stage of labor has begun. Other signs are involuntary bearing down and the deep, grunting sounds that may be made by the mother in reaction to this feeling of pressure. Some mothers interpret the meaning of the pressure and tell the nurse, "The baby is coming." When any one of these signs appears, the nurse should realize that birth may be about to occur.

✓**Transfer to delivery room.** When to transfer a mother to the delivery room depends on whether she is a primigravida or a multigravida and the practice in the individual hospital. The rapidity with which labor has progressed is another important factor to consider.

In some hospitals multigravidas are taken to the delivery room when the cervix is 7 to 8 cm dilated. In other hospitals they are not transferred until the cervix is completely dilated. In some hospitals primigravidas are transferred to delivery when they are completely dilated; in others they are transferred when the head is visible at the vaginal opening.

Pushing techniques. When dilatation is complete, the primigravida should be instructed to push effectively. One way is to take three deep breaths when a contraction starts. She blows out the first two breaths, holds the third, places a wrist under each knee, pulls back on her legs, and strains down as long as the contraction lasts (Fig. 11-8). If she must get another breath before the contraction ends, she lets out all of the air, takes a deep breath, holds it, and pushes until the contraction is over. She should rest between contractions. If she is on the delivery table, she can hold onto the handles on the table and pull back on them instead of pulling on her legs. Multigravidas are coached in pushing after they are in the delivery room.

The best position for pushing is the one that is most effective. This varies with the individual and will be influenced by the method of childbirth chosen. Some women push better lying on their back with the head of the bed elevated; others do better on their side or in the squatting position. The nurse should be flexible on this point and, when possible, should encourage the mother to use the position that works best for her.

Potential nursing diagnoses:

Alterations in comfort: pain related to exposure of body

Ineffective individual coping related to effort expended in pushing

Fear related to pressure on rectum

Knowledge deficit related to how to push effectively

Ineffective individual coping related to pain and seeming lack of progress

(*Text continues on p. 254*)

TABLE 11-1 NURSING-CARE PLAN FOR MOTHER DURING FIRST STAGE LABOR

ASSESSMENTS	POTENTIAL NURSING DIAGNOSES	INTERVENTIONS	EXPECTED OUTCOME
Interview patient (couple) to find out when contractions started, status of membranes, method of childbirth desired, support system, etc.; examine patient to determine effacement, dilatation, and station	Anxiety related to whether this is false labor	Assure patient (couple) that labor has begun	Anxiety relieved; patient in labor
	Knowledge deficit related to labor	Explain labor and what occurs as labor progresses	Couple understands labor process
Take vital signs, listen to FHT on admission and frequently during labor; attach electronic fetal monitor if available	Potential for injury, infection, hemorrhage related to ruptured membranes, examinations, complications during labor	Record vital signs and FHT on appropriate forms; interpret monitor strips; report abnormal findings	Condition of mother and infant remains stable during labor; complications do not develop; indications of complications are detected early
Listen to patient's complaints; observe for discomfort; anticipate needs	Alterations in comfort: pain related to dry mouth, temperature fluctuations, full bladder	Give ice chips, if permitted; provide mouth care; offer petroleum jelly for lips or remind her to use her lip balm; adjust thermostat; add or remove blankets as necessary; offer cold, wet washcloth for face; remind her to empty bladder *q.* 2–3 hr; catheterize if necessary	Mouth is moist; patient empties bladder; verbalizes comfort regarding temperature
	Anxiety related to supine hypotension	Position on left side; explain why she feels faint	Anxiety relieved; patient does not feel faint

Monitor fluid intake and output	Fluid volume deficit related to decreased intake	Give oral fluids if permitted; administer intravenous fluids as ordered	Fluid balance and adequate hydration maintained
Determine effectiveness of coaching		Assist with coaching if necessary; reinforce coaching as needed; do not interfere if coaching is effective	Coaching effective; patient remains in control
Determine quality and effectiveness of contractions and progress of labor	Potential for injury, fatigue, infection, complications of labor related to ineffectual contractions, lack of progress of labor	Time frequency, duration, intensity of contractions; examine patient periodically; inform patient of progress; inform physician of progress or lack of progress at appropriate times	Labor progresses normally
Observe patient's pain tolerance and ability to relax between contractions and to do breathing exercises during contractions	Alterations in comfort: pain related to contractions; loss of control	Encourage patient to use breathing techniques during contractions and to relax and rest between contractions; praise her for proper breathing and relaxation; encourage her to tell you what makes her comfortable; give analgesia as prescribed if patient wants it	Pain manageable; patient remains in control or regains control
Observe for increase in show, loss of amniotic fluid	Alterations in comfort: pain related to vaginal drainage	Cleanse perineal area as needed (*between* contractions); change underpad as needed; examine patient	Patient clean and reasonably comfortable; status of labor known
Observe for onset of second stage labor	Knowledge deficit related to cause of perineal pressure	Examine patient; praise her for progress; inform physician of progress; prepare for second stage labor	Patient understands cause of pressure

Can dell side-lying or on all
or on fours

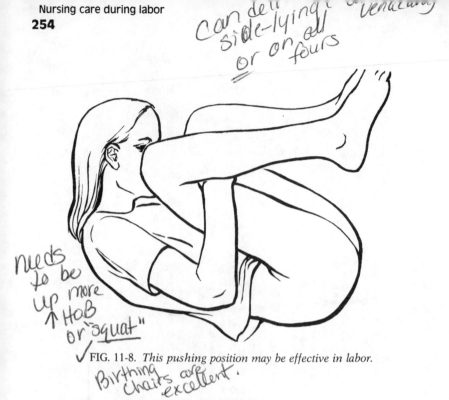

needs to be up more ↑ HoB or "squat"

✓ FIG. 11-8. *This pushing position may be effective in labor.*

Birthing Chairs are excellent.

EMOTIONAL SUPPORT: SECOND STAGE

During the second stage of labor, the nurse should stay with a primigravida as she is pushing and be generous with praise and words of encouragement. If the father is present, the nurse should assist him in coaching his wife through the delivery. This part of labor is hard physical work and requires considerable effort on the patient's part. The nurse should remind the mother to relax and rest between her contractions. The mother perspires from the exertion of pushing and usually appreciates having her face wiped with a cold, damp cloth while she is resting. If permitted, a few ice chips help to relieve the dryness of her mouth.

In order to help the mother understand why the pushing takes time and is such hard work, the nurse can explain that the birth canal is a narrow opening that has never been dilated to the extent that it must be to permit passage of the baby. In addition, the tissue surrounding the canal offers resistance to the descent of the baby. Each time the mother pushes, the baby descends a certain amount; between contractions, the baby retreats upward a certain amount. The mother should understand that long, steady pushes are more effective than short pushes, and that when the baby's head reaches a certain point (has passed under the symphysis), it will no longer retreat upward between contractions. The efficiency of long, steady pushes can be contrasted with short pushes by explaining that each time she pushes long and steadily she brings the baby down two steps. Short pushes bring the baby down only one step. Since the baby scoots back up one step between contractions, the only way to make progress is by pushing long and steadily with each contraction.

Occasionally a patient, feeling the pressure of the baby's head on the rectum and fearing that she will have a bowel movement if she pushes, may actually do her best to keep *from* pushing. The nurse must recognize when this is occurring and gently encourage the patient to push in spite of her reluctance to do so. If the patient has had an enema as part of the admission procedure, the nurse can tell her that she probably will not have a bowel movement even though she feels as though she will. Rather than causing embarrassment, the nurse can further assure her that if a bowel movement occurs while she is pushing, it is an excellent indication that she is pushing properly. The nurse can quietly and matter of factly remove the stool and cleanse the area should a bowel movement occur.

Some primigravidas tend to panic when they feel the pressure of the baby's head at the vaginal orifice. This can usually be avoided by explaining beforehand that this pressure will occur and that is is a *good* sign, a sign of progress.

The position and exposure while pushing may be distressing to a patient and may prevent wholehearted effort on her part. The nurse should be alert to this possibility and, although the position is necessary, she can avoid exposure by keeping the patient covered and by keeping the labor room door closed. If someone other than the husband is with the patient, that individual can be requested to wait in the waiting room during this stage of labor if the patient so desires.

Another cause for concern by the patient in second-stage labor is the fear that, if she pushes, the baby may arrive before the doctor does. The nurse can assure her that the doctor has been informed of her progress and that by the time he is needed he will be present.

Some patients become so tired they feel they cannot push one more time. Honest progress reports at this time act as a stimulus to greater effort. For example, the nurse can explain how far the mother had to push the baby down when she first started pushing and compare that with how far she still has to push it. Also, the mother should be told when the baby's head first becomes visible, for this is very effective in lifting her spirits and in providing added incentive for her to continue to work hard.

The nurse must watch the perineum for bulging while the mother is pushing, to determine the progress of labor.

CARE DURING DELIVERY

When the mother is taken to the delivery room, the nurse assists her onto the delivery table. Leggings are put on her so that her legs do not come into contact with the cold metal of the stirrups. Both legs are lifted into the stirrups at the same time to prevent strain on the pelvic ligaments,

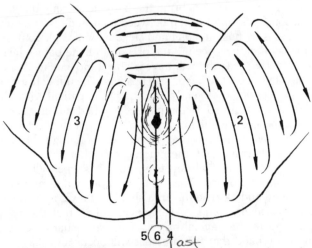

FIG. 11-9. *Several steps must be followed in cleansing the mother for delivery.*

and the stirrups are adjusted to fit the mother's legs. The short end of the delivery table is then removed. The nurse cleanses the mother's abdomen, thighs, and vulva with a cleansing solution (Fig. 11-9). Her abdomen and legs are then covered with sterile drapes and one is placed under her buttocks (Figs. 11-10 and 11-11).

FIG. 11-10. *The mother is draped, ready for delivery.*

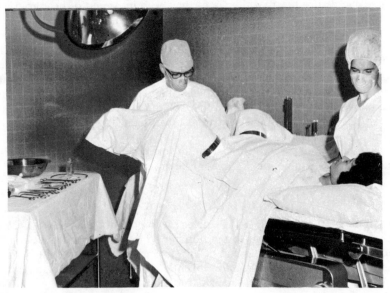

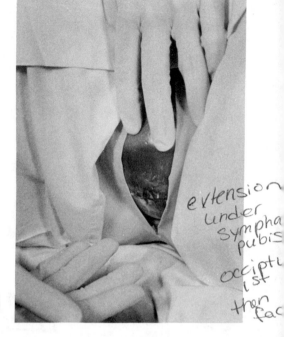

FIG. 11-11. *Draping with sterile towels also covers the anus and reveals only the bulging vagina.*

[handwritten margin notes: extension under sympha pubis occiput 1st then fac]

The nurse makes available to the physician the supplies that he needs. If the mother is not receiving general anesthesia, the nurse stays at her side and encourages her to bear down with each contraction. However, if the physician coaches the mother to push, the nurse should not do so. The nurse listens to the fetal heart tones after each contraction until the baby is born.

The nursing-care plan for the mother in second stage labor is presented in Table 11-2.

THIRD STAGE OF LABOR *[handwritten: (Placental stage) for c in 5-15 minutes All women]*

The birth of the baby marks the end of the second stage of labor and the beginning of the third stage. The nurse records on the chart pertinent information regarding the birth. This includes:

Time of birth *[handwritten: then placenta delivered.]*
Position of the baby *[handwritten: vertex, ROA, LOA, ROP, LOP (Posterior-occip takes longer back lab]*
Whether the delivery was spontaneous or whether forceps were used *[handwritten: or vacuum]*
Type of episiotomy
Sex of the baby
Condition of the baby

[handwritten: see p.332 Apgar back o baby head agai Resa Heart Rate reflex, irritability]

see p.332

TABLE 11-2. NURSING-CARE PLAN FOR MOTHER DURING SECOND STAGE LABOR

ASSESSMENTS	POTENTIAL NURSING DIAGNOSES	INTERVENTIONS	EXPECTED OUTCOME
Observe for ineffective pushing, loss of control	Knowledge deficit related to how to push efficiently	Instruct patient how to push; position her for pushing; praise her for effective pushing; instruct her to relax and rest between contractions	Patient pushes efficiently
	Ineffective individual coping related to fatigue caused by pushing		Patient remains in control
Watch for signs of impending birth: bulging perineum, membranes ruptured, presenting part visible	Anxiety related to pressure on rectum	Explain cause of rectal pressure	Patient understands cause for rectal pressure
Listen to FHT at least every 15 minutes or observe monitor strip for changes in FHR	Potential for injury, late decelerations related to compression of cord	Record FHT; report FHR that does not return to normal following contraction	FHR returns to normal between contractions; no injury to infant
Observe for excessive warmth	Ineffective thermoregulation related to being too warm	Comfort restored	
Anticipate delivery	Potential for injury, infection, trauma to mother or infant related to unsterile or uncontrolled conditions at birth	Prepare delivery room; instruct coach in delivery procedure; supply with appropriate clothing; transfer patient to delivery room; position patient for delivery; do perineal prep; prepare warm area for infant; assist physician as necessary; record FHT, BP, pertinent information on appropriate forms	Birth occurs under sterile, controlled conditions; no infection or injury to mother or infant
Monitor FHT and mother's BP			

The third stage of labor ends when the placenta is delivered. The nurse records on the chart the time the placenta is delivered and whether it was delivered spontaneously or was removed manually by the doctor.

After the placenta is expelled, the physician orders the nurse to give the mother oxytocic drugs, which cause the uterus to contract. Oxytocin (Pitocin, Syntocinon), methylergonovine (Methergine), and ergonovine (Ergotrate) are oxytocic drugs commonly used. When the uterus contracts after the third stage of labor, the open blood vessels at the site where the placenta was attached are clamped off to prevent hemorrhage. The time, the amount, and the name of the oxytocic given are recorded on the chart.

CARE OF THE BABY

As soon as the baby's head is born, the physician clears the airway by suctioning the mucus, blood, and amniotic fluid from the nose and mouth (Figs. 11-12 and 11-13). This is commonly done with a rubber bulb syringe or a De Lee mucus trap attached to a catheter. The airway should be cleared before the baby takes its first breath so that none of the fluid or secretions is aspirated into the lungs when the baby starts to breathe. After the baby is born and is breathing, the physician cuts and clamps

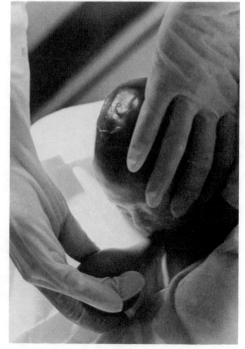

FIG. 11-12. *The neonate's mouth is suctioned at the beginning of restitution through the completion of restitution.*

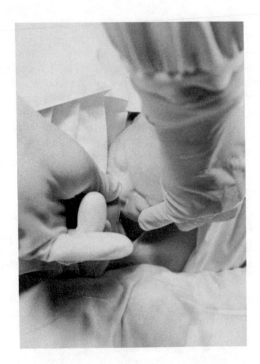

FIG. 11-13. *Suctioning of the neonate's nostrils at the beginning of external rotation.*

FIG. 11-14. *The umbilical cord of the newborn is clamped.*

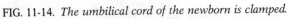

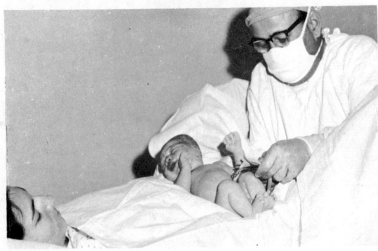

the umbilical cord (Fig. 11-14). The cord contains no nerves, so the baby is not hurt when it is cut. The cord is clamped to prevent the baby from hemorrhaging through it. If the mother is awake, the physician holds up the baby so that she can see it. The baby is then placed in a heated crib or an incubator.

Immediately after the baby is placed in the crib or incubator the nurse should dry it thoroughly, including the head, to conserve body heat and prevent cold stress. This drying is done with a soft towel or receiving blanket. At this time the nurse can also inspect the baby for abnormalities.

While the physician repairs the episiotomy the nurse cares for the baby. State laws require that medicine be put in the baby's eyes at birth to prevent gonorrheal ophthalmia neonatorum, a severe conjunctivitis that may cause permanent blindness. One drop of a 1% solution of silver nitrate is commonly used for this purpose. Two minutes after the silver nitrate is applied, the eyes are rinsed with normal saline solution, which helps prevent the silver nitrate from causing the eyes to become red and swollen (Fig. 11-15). Some hospitals use an antibiotic ointment instead of silver

FIG. 11-15. *Prophylactic eye care of the newborn is vital. Note that during initial care in the delivery room warmth is provided by means of radiant heat from above as well as by heat from below.*

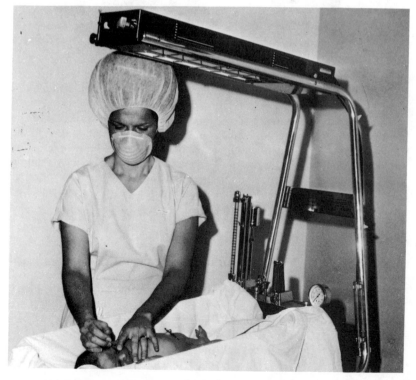

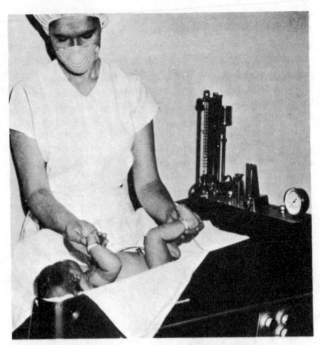

FIG. 11-16. *The infant receives identification.*

nitrate. The eye medication should be instilled within 1 hour after birth. With this time limit, the nurse can delay instilling it until the infant has had the opportunity to look around and establish visual patterns.

The nurse in the delivery room carries out measures to preserve the identity of the baby after it is separated from the mother and taken to the nursery. She may put identical bracelets on mother and baby or she may put beads, containing the mother's surname, on the baby. Footprinting the baby and thumbprinting the mother on the same record is another means of identification commonly used in addition to the bracelets or beads (Fig. 11-16).

CARE OF THE MOTHER

After the episiotomy is repaired, the drapes are removed and the vulva and perineum are washed from front to back with warm water and a towel. The area is dried in the same manner, and perineal pads and a sanitary belt or a T-binder are put on the mother. To prevent contamination, care is taken not to touch the side of the pad that touches the mother. The short end of the delivery table is put back and both of the mother's legs are removed from the stirrups at the same time. She is covered with a cotton blanket and dressed in a clean gown. Her blood pressure and pulse

Postpartum hemorrhage may occur
within 1°

are taken and the height and tone of the uterus are noted. The height of the fundus of the uterus is measured in relation to the umbilicus; it may be above, below, or even with the umbilicus. Usually the fundus is even with or below the umbilicus at the time the mother is ready to be taken from the delivery room. The tone of the uterus refers to how well it is contracted. A uterus with good tone stays contracted and feels firm to the touch; a uterus with poor tone relaxes and feels soft. Contractions of the uterus following delivery are necessary to prevent the mother from hemorrhaging; therefore, the uterus should feel firm when she is transferred to the recovery room. The recovery room nurse is given a complete report on the delivery and the condition of the patient.

FOURTH STAGE OF LABOR

As soon as possible after the birth, the mother, and the father if he is present, should have the opportunity to hold, touch, and cuddle the infant. Skin-to-skin and eye contacts between mother and infant are important to mother-infant bonding. If the mother wishes to breast-feed the baby at this time, the nurse should assist her. The nurse can protect against cold stress by wrapping the infant snugly in a blanket and by increasing the room temperature. Ample time, in an unhurried atmosphere with minimal interruptions, should be provided for the family to get acquainted and to begin to form the emotional attachments that are essential to family unity (Fig. 11-17).

The delivery nurse has opportunity to observe the parents' attitude toward the newborn at birth and to assess their interest in the bonding process. She should be sensitive to signs that could indicate possible rejection of the infant by one or both parents at this critical time. If she becomes aware of such manifestations, she should inform the obstetrician and also the nursery and postpartum nurses, and if their joint assessments confirm that the parents' attitude is one of rejection, appropriate measures can be taken to help them and to protect the infant. The mother's failure to form attachments to her infant may have devastating effects on the child and may ease the way to child abuse.

One of the ways that one or both parents may show rejection at the time of birth is by being passive and indifferent toward the infant: refusing to hold, touch, or examine it, and avoiding eye contact with it. Hostility toward the infant may be revealed through inappropriate remarks about its physical characteristics or through the way the parents look at the child and otherwise respond when the child is mentioned. If the sex of the child has been made the condition of acceptance, they may express disappointment when it is not the preferred sex. Rejection of the infant may also be seen in nonsupportive interaction between the parents.

The nurse must keep in mind that labor can be very tiring for the mother, so that she may not feel like doing more than simply checking to

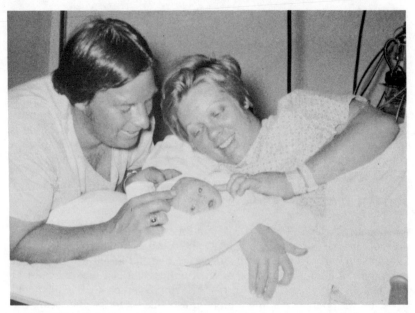

FIG. 11-17. *Baby Sara becomes acquainted with her parents soon after birth.*

make sure the baby is all right. In this case, the getting-acquainted period can be postponed until the mother has had time to rest.

While the parents are involved with the infant, the nurse can complete the delivery records. Then, when the parents are ready for her to do so, she can complete her care of the infant and take it to the newborn nursery.

The nursing-care plan for the mother in third or fourth stage labor is presented in Table 11-3.

EMERGENCY DELIVERY BY THE NURSE

Labor sometimes proceeds so quickly that the mother or obstetrician is unable to get to the hospital in time. In the absence of a physician, the nurse may be the best qualified person to deliver the baby. A rapid spontaneous delivery in which the usual preparations by the physician and nurse are lacking is called *precipitate delivery*. This type of labor is most likely to occur in multiparous women, although it occasionally occurs in primigravidas.

Because the nurse may have to deliver a baby when the physician is not present, it is important that she know what to do. The three most important things for her to do in an emergency delivery are:

ASSESSMENTS	POTENTIAL NURSING DIAGNOSES	INTERVENTIONS	EXPECTED OUTCOME
Anticipate mother's need for cleanliness, warmth, and protection from infection	Alterations in comfort: pain related to normal vaginal drainage after birth	Wash your hands thoroughly; clean perineum with warm water and dry with clean towel; apply perineal pads from front to back; avoid touching side of pad that goes next to perineum; put clean, warm gown on patient; put warm blanket on patient	Patient clean, warm, comfortable, and free of infection
	Ineffective thermoregulation related to birth		
	Potential for injury and infection related to lowered resistance following birth		
Determine status of fundus, flow, perineum, bladder, and vital signs	Potential for injury and hemorrhage related to relaxed uterus, retained placenta, or lacerations of birth canal	Record height and tone of fundus, amount of flow, condition of perineum, and vital signs every 15 min; massage fundus gently if necessary to expel clots and keep it firmly contracted; report any	Moderate flow without clots; no hematoma formation
	Alteration in patterns of urinary elimination related to birth trauma	unusual discoloration or swelling of perineum; offer bedpan or assist to bathroom periodically; record vital signs on appropriate forms; report abnormal findings	Vital signs normal
Observe parents' interaction with infant	Potential alterations in parenting related to disappointment in sex or appearance of infant	Allow opportunity for parents to hold infant and for mother to breast-feed if desired; assist with feeding as necessary; arrange *en face* position of mother and infant; do not interfere if interaction is occurring; answer questions	Couple happy with infant and satisfied with labor and birth
	Knowledge deficit related to normal behavior of infant at this time		
Anticipate mother's need for pain relief, fluids, nourishment, rest, and sleep	Alterations in comfort: pain related to involution, episiotomy, thirst, hunger, and fatigue from labor	Give analgesia as ordered if patient wants it; offer hot drink and nourishment; provide period of undisturbed rest and sleep in a quiet environment	Patient comfortable and has the fluids, nourishment, rest, and sleep she needs
	Alterations in nutrition: less than body requirements related to decreased intake during labor		
	Sleep pattern disturbance related to labor and birth		

Remain calm

Provide cleanliness

Control the birth of the baby's head

Calm.   Even though she must think and act quickly, the nurse must keep calm in order to instill confidence in the mother and obtain her cooperation, which may be vital to the safety and well-being of both mother and baby.

Cleanliness.   In precipitate delivery, events frequently occur so rapidly that cleanliness is sacrificed in order for the birth to be controlled. However, efforts should be made to use only clean supplies; and the place of the birth and the nurse's hands should also be clean. If the mother is in the hospital, it may be possible to transfer her quickly to the delivery room where she can be prepped and draped and the nurse can put on sterile gloves before the birth. Any measures taken to provide cleanliness will help prevent infection in the mother and baby.

Control birth of baby's head.   Controlling the birth of the baby's head to prevent its sudden expulsion is the most important thing for the nurse to do in a precipitate delivery (Fig. 11-18). This is done to prevent cerebral damage to the baby and lacerations to the mother. As soon as the head becomes visible at the vaginal opening, the nurse must focus her attention on it so that when it starts to crown she can exert gentle pressure on it to control its progress. At the same time, the mother is instructed to pant

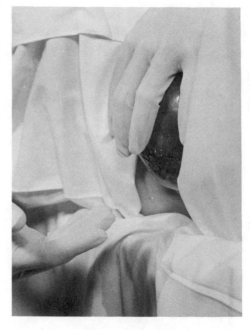

FIG. 11-18. *The hands are used to control the birth of the baby's head. The right hand is ready to receive the head and the left hand gives steady gentle pressure to prevent sudden expulsion.*

with her contractions to control the force with which the head is being expelled. If possible, the head should be delivered between contractions since this lessens the expulsive force and makes controlling it much easier. *The nurse must never hold back the baby's head to prevent birth.*

After the head is born, the nurse concentrates on clearing the baby's airway so that it can breathe. This is done by suctioning the mucus and fluid from its mouth and nose. If a bulb syringe is not available, a clean cloth can be used to wipe the mouth and nose. Then the nurse feels along the baby's neck to see if the cord is around the neck. If it is, she should try to slip it gently over the baby's head. If this cannot be done easily, she can try to slip it over the shoulder. If this is not possible, and she has sterile clamps and scissors, she should clamp the cord with two clamps and then cut between them. This will free the cord so the rest of the body can be delivered without undue strain on the cord.

External rotation usually occurs spontaneously after the head is out. Then the nurse can place a hand on either side of the head and lower it gently to deliver the anterior shoulder. The posterior shoulder is delivered by raising the head gently; the rest of the body slips out easily after the shoulders are delivered. A newborn baby is very slippery, and the nurse must hold it securely to prevent dropping it.

Immediately after birth the infant should be dried thoroughly and wrapped in a clean blanket. As soon as its breathing is well established, it can be placed on the mother's abdomen where she can see and touch it and where her body heat can help keep it warm. The cord should be left attached until sterile clamps and scissors are available. This is safer for the baby than using unsterile supplies.

The mother is observed for signs of placental separation. When these appear she is asked to bear down with the next contraction to expel the placenta. After the placenta is delivered, the uterus should be kept firmly contracted, by massaging it if necessary, to prevent excessive blood loss. Because the uterus may have a tendency to relax following a precipitous labor, the mother should be watched closely for hemorrhage.

CLINICAL REVIEW

ASSESSMENT. Mrs. M. is a 27-year-old gravida 3, para 2, who was admitted at term at 6:30 P.M. She stated that she had been having contractions at 7- to 10-minute intervals since 4 P.M. They lasted 30 seconds. She also stated that she had been having "a lot of false labor" and hoped that this was "the real thing." Her membranes were intact. Mrs. M.'s temperature, pulse, and respirations were normal and her blood pressure was 124/80 mm Hg. The fetal heart tones were 134 and regular. The nurse examined Mrs. M. and found that the baby's head was at +1 station, and the cervix was 4 cm dilated and 80% effaced. She reported her findings to the physician and he ordered a prep and enema, and Demerol 50 mg with Atarax 50 mg to be given intramuscularly when needed.

1. Do you think Mrs. M. is in false labor? Give reasons for your answer.

2. Why is the prep done? Why is an enema given?

3. As Mrs. M. was getting into bed after expelling the enema, her membranes ruptured. What is the first thing that you would do after this occurs? Why?

4. After her membranes ruptured, her contractions began coming every 4 minutes and lasted 45 to 55 seconds. They were moderately strong. Why is it important for Mrs. M. to relax during her contractions? How can you help her to relax?

5. When do you think Mrs. M. should be given the medication ordered by the physician? What safety measures should be taken at the time the medication is given? What observations should be made after it is given? Why? What observations would you report to the physician.

   At 7:45 P.M., Mrs. M. complained that she was shaking. The nurse noted that there was an increase in the bloody show and the amniotic fluid. She suspected that Mrs. M. was in transition, so she examined her. The head was at +2 station, the cervix was 8 to 9 cm dilated, and effacement was complete. The nurse notified the physician and transferred Mrs. M. to the delivery room. The physician gave her a pudendal block and did a midline episiotomy. At 8:05 P.M. Mrs. M. gave birth to a 7 lb 5 oz (3317 gm) boy in the LOA position. The nurse put medicine in the baby's eyes and placed an identifying bracelet on his right wrist and right ankle. A matching bracelet was placed on the mother's wrist. A thumbprint of the mother and footprints of the baby were taken. The baby was shown to his mother and then taken to the newborn nursery. At 8:08 P.M. the placenta was expelled.

6. Why is the medicine put in the baby's eyes?

7. Why is it important to put identification on the baby in the delivery room?

8. What care should Mrs. M. receive before she is transferred to the recovery room? Why?

BIBLIOGRAPHY

Jensen MD, Bobak IM: Maternity Care: The Nurse & The Family, 3rd ed, pp 436–502. St. Louis, CV Mosby Co, 1985

Reeder SR, Martin LL: Maternity Nursing, 16th ed, pp 457–524. Philadelphia, JB Lippincott Co, 1987

Normal Postpartum Period 6

normal body changes **12** during the puerperium

BEHAVIORAL When the goals of this chapter are reached, the student will
OBJECTIVES be able to:

○ *Define: puerperium, involution, lochia, afterpains.*

○ *Discuss breast engorgement.*

○ *Explain how colostrum differs from breast milk.*

○ *Explain how involution occurs and tell how long it takes.*

○ *Describe how the rate of involution is measured.*

○ *Name and describe the three types of lochia and tell when each usually appears.*

○ *Describe postpartum changes in the cervix, vagina, and perineum.*

○ *Tell when menstruation will probably return if a mother nurses her baby and when it will return it she does not nurse.*

○ *Describe the effects of birth on the urethra and bladder and tell how soon they return to normal.*

○ *Discuss the effects childbirth may have on sexual activity.*

○ *Describe the postpartum examination.*

✓The 6 weeks immediately after delivery are called the *puerperium,* or the *postpartum* period. During the puerperium changes occur in the body that restore it to approximately its prepregnant condition. The reproductive organs return to their normal size and position, although they are never again exactly as they were before pregnancy.

Most physicians have the mother come for an examination 6 weeks after delivery. At this time the mother's blood pressure is taken, a urinalysis is done, the breasts are examined, and a pelvic examination is performed. If corrective measures are necessary, arrangements are made at this time. The mother is encouraged to discuss with the physician any health problems she may have. The physician usually asks the mother to return for another checkup in 6 months.

CHANGES IN REPRODUCTIVE ORGANS

BREASTS

The breast changes that occur immediately after delivery are a continuation of the preparation for lactation that started early in pregnancy. The lactogenic hormone, prolactin, causes an increase in the blood supply of the breasts and in the activity of the breast glands. As a result, the breasts become distended, hard, and painful. This congested condition, called *engorgement,* develops about the third day after delivery and lasts 24 to 36 hours; it then subsides and is followed by lactation. During lactation the breasts are softer and comfortable.

The first substance that the newborn infant obtains from the mother's breasts is a thin, yellowish fluid called *colostrum.* Colostrum contains more protein and salts but less fat and carbohydrate than breast milk. Colostrum is secreted by the breasts until the third or fourth day after delivery, when it is replaced by breast milk.

Two essential processes are involved in lactation: secretion, or production, of milk and expulsion of milk. *Secretion* of milk depends on stimulation by the lactogenic hormone and on frequent and complete emptying of the breasts. The lactogenic hormone becomes active soon after the baby is born and continues to function during the time the baby is breast-fed. Emptying of the breasts occurs when the baby suckles. The *expulsion* of milk is controlled by the let-down reflex. This reflex is influenced favorably by physical factors such as comfort and restfulness, and unfavorably by pain and fatigue. It is also influenced by emotional factors—favorably by happiness and contentment, unfavorably by worry and tension.

UTERUS

The returning of the uterus to its normal size and position is called *involution* (Fig. 12-1). Involution begins immediately after the placenta is expelled and takes approximately 6 weeks to complete. The large vessels

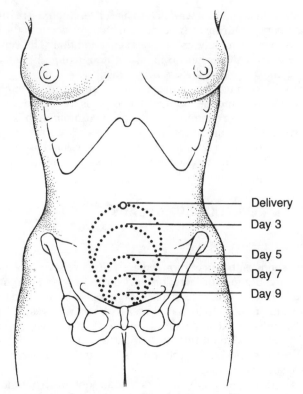

FIG. 12-1. *Involution of the uterus.*

at the placental site become compressed and thrombosed as the uterus contracts and decreases in size. Eventually these vessels are obliterated and new, smaller vessels develop. The muscle cells in the uterus decrease in size. Some of the protein material in the uterine wall is broken down and cast off in the urine. The decidua separates into two layers. The outer layer sloughs off and becomes a part of the vaginal discharge following delivery, while new endometrium develops from the inner layer.

Assessment of involution. The height of the fundus of the uterus indicates the rate at which involution is occurring; this is measured in fingerbreadths in relation to the umbilicus (Fig. 12-2). The bladder should be empty when the height is measured, since a full bladder raises the uterus one or more fingerbreadths. The rate of involution varies with individuals. Usually, however, the fundus is even with the umbilicus or one to two fingerbreadths below it soon after delivery. It may remain even with the umbilicus for one or two days after delivery; then it decreases in height by approximately one fingerbreadth each day. By the tenth day the uterus normally is so low it cannot be felt through the abdomen. Some physicians prescribe ergonovine (Ergotrate) for a day or two following delivery to hasten involution.

Lochia. The vaginal discharge following delivery is called *lochia* and contains blood from the placental site, particles of decidua, and mucus. Changes occur in the lochia as healing takes place at the site where the placenta was implanted. For the first two or three days postpartum, the lochia is red and bloody and is called *lochia rubra*. On the third or fourth day postpartum, the lochia decreases and is more serous. It is pink or brown and is called *lochia serosa*. On the ninth or tenth day the discharge is scant and appears yellowish-white. It is called *lochia alba*. Three weeks after delivery there is little or no discharge.

The amount of lochia varies, and is usually more profuse in multigravidas than in primigravidas. The amount of lochia usually increases when the mother ambulates for the first time after delivery, because ambulation promotes drainage of lochia that has accumulated in the vagina. Lochia has a characteristic odor that is not offensive. A foul odor indicates that an infection is present.

Afterpains. During the first few days postpartum, the mother may experience abdominal discomfort known as *afterpains*. Following delivery the uterus contracts down into a firm mass. A uterus that has good tone contracts and stays retracted; a uterus that does not have good tone

FIG. 12-2. *The nurse measures the height of the fundus.*

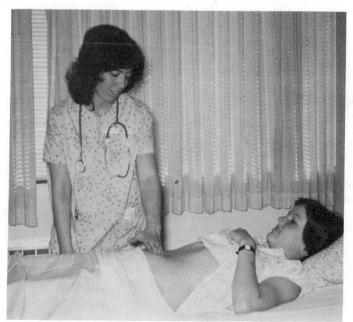

contracts and then relaxes. It is the contraction of the uterus following a brief period of relaxation that causes afterpains. Since the uterus loses some of its tone with each pregnancy, the multipara is more likely to have afterpains than the primipara. The mother who nurses her baby may have afterpains at the time she feeds the baby, because breast-feeding stimulates the uterus to contract.

CERVIX, VAGINA, AND PERINEUM

The number of muscle cells in the cervix increases after delivery. The internal os returns almost to its normal size while the external os may remain slightly dilated. Lacerations of the cervix that occurred during delivery heal; and the cervix gradually regains its tone. The vagina and perineum also regain their tone and the vagina decreases in size, although it never completely returns to its prepregnant condition.

RETURN OF MENSTRUATION

The time of the mother's first menstrual period after delivery depends somewhat on whether or not she nurses her baby. If she does not nurse her baby, she probably will have her first menstrual period within 8 weeks after delivery. If she does nurse her baby, she probably will not have a menstrual period until about 2 months after lactation ceases. Both nursing and nonnursing mothers can become pregnant before menstruation returns; thus, breast-feeding should not be regarded as a form of birth control.

OTHER CHANGES

VITAL SIGNS

Temperature. The woman's temperature, taken orally, should remain within normal limits during the puerperium. Although a slight rise in temperature may occur after delivery for no apparent reason, a temperature of 100.4 °F (38 °C) or higher on any two consecutive days postpartum, exclusive of the first 24 hours, is considered a symptom of infection. When a slight temperature elevation occurs, its significance can usually be determined by assessing the pulse rate: if the pulse rate is slow, the slight rise in temperature is usually not a symptom of infection.

It was once believed that a temperature elevation normally accompanied the onset of lactation. This was called *milk fever*. This is no longer considered true. Although a sharp rise in temperature may occur with extreme vascular and lymphatic engorgement of the breasts, this elevation does not last longer than 12 hours; if it persists for a longer period, infection must be suspected.

Pulse. The pulse rate may be slower than usual soon after delivery and may remain so for one or two days. A slow pulse rate, between 60 and 70 beats per minute, is considered a good sign, whereas a rapid pulse rate following delivery may be a symptom of shock or hemorrhage. A rapid pulse rate later in the puerperium may be a symptom of infection.

ABDOMINAL WALL AND SKIN

The abdominal muscles lose much of their tone during pregnancy. Regaining muscle tone is a gradual process. Good nutrition, adequate rest, and proper exercise help the muscles regain tone much faster.

The striae on the skin gradually become silvery in appearance but do not disappear completely.

↓ peristalsis RIT ↓ volume RIT birth.

CIRCULATORY, METABOLIC, AND URINARY SYSTEMS

The blood volume returns to normal within the first 2 weeks after delivery. The excess water that was in the blood or retained by the body tissues during pregnancy is excreted by the kidneys. This causes a marked increase in the daily output of urine (diuresis). Changes in metabolism at this time cause the mother to perspire profusely (diaphoresis), particularly at night. Through diuresis and diaphoresis the mother loses 4 to 5 lb (1.8 kg to 2.3 kg) of weight. *20'*

The mother may have difficulty urinating after delivery because the urethra is swollen or the area is sore. Also, the bladder may become distended with urine without the mother's feeling the urge to urinate. This is usually due to loss of bladder tone resulting from trauma during labor or to the anesthesia used for delivery. Bladder tone is usually restored within 24 to 48 hours.

DIGESTIVE SYSTEM

RIT metabolism, sweating, labor work.

Immediately after delivery the mother is usually thirsty, but may be too tired to desire food. After she has rested she usually has a hearty appetite.

To most mothers constipation is a problem. Constipation is due to relaxation of the abdominal wall and loss of intra-abdominal pressure, as well as sluggishness of the bowel caused by crowding of the enlarged uterus. The physician usually orders a laxative or an enema to take care of the problem during the first few days postpartum. With good nutrition, plenty of fluids, exercise, and return of bowel tone, this problem is corrected. *∴ IV, clear fluids & juices may be given. because digestion ↓; ↑ glucose needed*

EMOTIONAL ASPECTS

Immediately after the birth of her baby, the mother is excited. The long months of waiting are over. She and her husband are busy spreading the

emotional Tasks 1950's FP.
Reva Rubin : Tasks of PP women
24-48° - "taking in" phase (mom's babied)
"Taking Hold" phase: mom takes on respons.

grown'-up, taking care of another.)

278 sodomy
⊖ intercourse
⊖ tampons } 3-6 wks P.P.

news of the new arrival. She is showered with attention—congratulations, flowers, telephone calls. As the excitement decreases, the mother experiences a let-down feeling, and may become irritable or tearful. This feeling is thought to be related to the abrupt hormonal changes, fatigue, and discomfort that occur postpartum. So common is this feeling that it has been labeled *postpartum blues*. Usually, it occurs about the third day postpartum and is of short duration.

MARITAL RELATIONS

Marital relations—sexual activity and intimacy—are expressions of the caring and devotion each partner has for the other and are vital to the harmony and well-being of the married couple. Satisfaction or lack of satisfaction in marital relations affects every other aspect of married life.

To promote spontaneous, satisfying marital relations, the couple needs uninterrupted time together in private without fear of distractions. Before the birth of a child, the couple is usually able to arrange periods of uninterrupted privacy and can concentrate all their attention on each other. After the birth of a child, the attentions of the couple are concentrated more on the needs of the infant and less on each other. The wife may have less desire for sexual activity because of the pain of the episiotomy; the husband may be afraid of hurting his wife during sexual intercourse; both may be so exhausted from lack of sleep that they have little desire for sexual activity. The infant's crying may interrupt their sexual activity, and lack of privacy is likely to decrease spontaneity.

CLINICAL REVIEW

1. Why is it important for a mother to be rested and free from pain and worry when breast-feeding her infant?
2. How do the changes in the uterus that follow delivery differ from the changes that occurred as a result of pregnancy?
3. "Catheterize if unable to void" is included in most postpartum orders. Why is this sometimes necessary?
4. Why are laxatives or enemas often necessary during the first few days postpartum?

BIBLIOGRAPHY

Fischman SH, et al: Changes in sexual relationships in postpartum couples. J Obstet Gynecol Neonatal Nurs 15(1): 58–63, 1986
Jensen MD, Bobak IM: Maternity Care: The Nurse & The Family, 3rd ed, pp 737–745. St. Louis, CV Mosby, 1985
Reeder SR, Martin LL: Maternity Nursing, 16th ed, pp 569–579. Philadelphia, JB Lippincott, 1987

postpartal care
Reva Rubin

3 kinds lochia
rubra - red
serosa - pink-brown
alba - whitish

nursing care during the 13 puerperium

BEHAVIORAL OBJECTIVES When the goals of this chapter are reached, the student will be able to:

○ Discuss the probable feelings of the new parents immediately after birth.

○ Tell what nursing measures are indicated when chilliness and shaking occur after delivery.

○ Tell what observations are made during the first hour after delivery.

○ Explain the difference in the feel of the uterus when it is contracted and when it is relaxed.

○ Discuss the significance of the lochia during the first hour or two after delivery.

○ Explain why checking the perineum is part of the recovery care.

○ Describe the daily examination of the breasts postpartum and the findings the nurse should expect.

○ List two findings related to the episiotomy that should be reported to the physician.

○ Discuss ways in which the nurse can help the mother obtain rest and sleep.

○ List three or four measures taken to prevent infection in the postpartum patient.

○ Discuss the tasks confronting the new mother during the early postpartal period and tell how the nurse can help her work through these.

○ Discuss how the labor and delivery nurse can help the new mother to assimilate her labor and delivery experience.

○ Describe appropriate action on the part of the nurse should she discover a mother with the "blues."

○ List four or five points the nurse may need to teach the new mother regarding her own care.

○ List four or five points the nurse needs to keep in mind when teaching the mother in order to make the instruction meaningful and acceptable.

○ *Discuss the advantages and disadvantages of seven or eight methods of contraception.*

○ *Select a postpartum patient and develop an appropriate care plan for her.*

EARLY POSTPARTUM ASSESSMENT AND INTERVENTIONS

EMOTIONAL

The newly delivered mother is usually excited and happy. She is eager to see her husband and share the joy of the occasion with him. The father is just as eager to see his wife and to know that all is well. Both parents are bubbling with curiosity about the baby; they are eager to see it and to find out how much it weighs and how long it is. They want to count fingers and toes and see that the infant is normal in every way. They are curious to know the color of the eyes and whether the baby has hair. They want to study its features to see whether it looks like father, mother, sister, or brother. It is hard to believe that the waiting is finally over and the baby is really here. Both parents feel proud and satisfied with their accomplishment.

The time immediately following birth is crucial to the bonding process between parents and infant. The mother needs to be able to hold and caress the infant in order to promote and enhance her attachment with it and so that she can begin to realize that the baby is now a being apart from herself. The father also needs the interaction with his child so that he can begin bonding and appreciate the fact that the baby is really here. Fathers who attend expectant parent classes with their wives and who participate in labor and are present at the birth of their child form strong attachments to the child and are active in the subsequent care of it. The infant needs to be held and caressed by the parents so that it can begin attachment to them. Infants who are separated from their mothers immediately after birth and deprived of the opportunity to form attachments to them often experience *failure to thrive syndrome,* a condition in which there may be physical, emotional, and mental deterioration. It is the privilege and responsibility of the nurse to promote parent–infant bonding by making sure that they have time together immediately after birth, in the case of a healthy infant, and as soon as it can safely be arranged in the case of an ill infant.

PHYSICAL

After the mother has seen her husband and baby, she should be permitted to rest. Labor and delivery make heavy demands on her reserves of energy and, although she is happy and excited, she is probably also physically exhausted. The father can also be encouraged to go home and get some rest at this time.

The first hour after delivery, often called the fourth stage of labor, is a critical period for the mother; it is during this time that most postpartum hemorrhages occur. Mothers who have had general anesthesia may not have completely regained consciousness. To make sure that the mother receives the close observation needed immediately after delivery, many hospitals provide recovery rooms. The mother usually stays in the recovery room one or two hours (Fig. 13-1).

Immediately after delivery, the mother may feel chilly and may shake uncontrollably. The exact cause of this reaction is not known, although several factors are believed to contribute to it. It may result from rapid cooling of the body following the perspiring that accompanied the pushing during delivery. It may be due to the sudden loss of weight that occurs as the baby is born, or it may be due to nervousness and exhaustion. By keeping the mother warm, the nurse can help to prevent and relieve the chilliness and shaking. The mother should be covered with a warm blanket and, if she is not nauseated, she can be given a hot drink. It is important that she be told that it is normal to feel this way after delivery so that she does not think something is wrong.

The newly delivered mother is usually thirsty, and may also be hungry if food and fluids have been withheld during labor. She should be provided with water and encouraged to drink; this helps to replace fluids lost

FIG. 13-1. *The nurse checks the mother in the delivery room.*

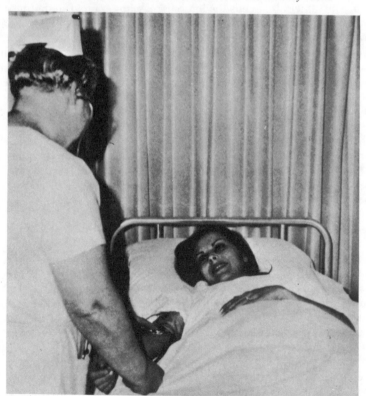

during labor and also promotes kidney function. After it is evident that the mother is able to tolerate liquids without becoming nauseated, she can be given solid foods if she so desires.

Nursing assessment

During the first hour after delivery, the mother's blood pressure, pulse, fundus, lochia, and perineum are checked at least every 15 minutes. If she has had general anesthesia, she is also observed for signs of returning consciousness and for nausea.

Vital signs. The blood pressure and pulse should stay within normal limits. A fall in blood pressure, accompanied by a rapid, thready pulse, is a sign of hemorrhage. A rise in blood pressure is a symptom of preeclampsia. The physician must be notified if these changes develop. The temperature is usually within normal limits, but it may be slightly elevated.

Uterus. The fundus of the uterus is checked for height and tone. The fundus is usually even with or one or two fingerbreadths below the umbilicus right after delivery. It may be one or two fingerbreadths above the umbilicus if the uterus has been overdistended with a very large baby, twins, or hydramnios. A full bladder can cause the uterus to relax and to rise two or more fingerbreadths above the umbilicus. When the bladder is full, the uterus may be displaced to one side instead of being centrally located.

The uterus should have good tone and be well contracted to prevent hemorrhage. A contracted uterus feels firm to the touch and should not be massaged, because unnecessary massage can tire the uterus and decrease its ability to remain contracted. A relaxed uterus is soft and boggy and may be difficult to feel. Massage may stimulate it to contract.

Lochia. The lochia is described as "heavy," "moderate," or "scant," depending on the amount present. Although there is more lochial discharge during the first hour or two after delivery than at any other time, the amount should be moderate even at this time. Heavy lochia is excessive bleeding that is frequently accompanied by clots. When the lochia is heavy, the cause must be found and corrected to prevent the mother from losing a dangerous amount of blood. When the lochia is scant, the nurse must be sure that the blood is not collecting inside the uterus instead of draining onto the perineal pads. An accumulation of blood within the uterus can prevent it from contracting, causing hemorrhage.

Perineum. The perineum is observed for unusual swelling and discoloration, which could be signs that a *hematoma* is developing. A hematoma is a collection of blood caused by bleeding into the tissues from a ruptured blood vessel. Occasionally a small vessel ruptures as the tissues are stretched during delivery, or a vessel is cut with the needle as the episiotomy is being repaired. When a vessel ruptures, the hematoma usually develops within the first few hours following delivery. Not all hematomas can be seen by inspecting the perineum, and therefore it is important that a mother's complaint of excruciating pain in her stitches or rectum be investigated. This complaint is often the first clue that a hematoma is developing and must be reported to the physician at once. Blood loss may be excessive unless the hematoma is detected early.

RECOVERY ROOM CARE
Every 15 minutes for the first hour, check:

VITAL SIGNS:

o Blood pressure should stay normal. Elevation may be a sign of preeclampsia; drop may be a sign of hemorrhage. Pulse may be slow. Rapid pulse may be a sign of hemorrhage. Temperature is taken before transferring patient to postpartum room.

FUNDUS: *ck c̄ bed flat*

o Tone should be firm. Boggy uterus should be massaged until firm to prevent hemorrhage.
o Height should be at umbilicus or one or two fingerbreadths above or below umbilicus.

LOCHIA:

o Should be moderate; occasionally will be scant. If scant, make sure it is not collecting inside uterus. If heavy, find out cause and treat.

PERINEUM:

o Unusual swelling and discoloration may be symptoms of hematoma.

WARMTH:

o Warm blanket and warm room are helpful to combat chilly feeling; also protects infant from cold stress.

BLADDER:

o Prevent distention. A full bladder can cause bleeding by preventing the uterus from contracting. It will displace uterus upward and to the side.

CLEANLINESS:

o Give perineal care and change pad as needed.
o Perform oral hygiene.
o Before transferring to postpartum room, give bath as per hospital routine.

EMOTIONAL:

o Provide privacy when checking patient and giving care.
o Provide for infant and husband to be with patient as desired.

ck for hemorrhage:
ck for contracted fundus (c̄ uterine atrophy)
Big clots are sign fundus is not contracted.
If fundus is midline & ↓ umbilicus,

Subsequent assessment and interventions

A bed bath may be included in the care given the mother in the recovery room. If it is not, the mother should be given the opportunity to freshen up by washing her face and hands. Oral hygiene is also important at this time. Perineal cleansing should be performed as needed to keep the mother comfortable.

If all is well after the first hour or two, the mother is transferred to the postpartum room. Observations of the height and tone of the fundus and of the amount of lochia are continued for the first 12 hours postpartum. If during this time the uterus remains contracted and the lochia is not excessive, hemorrhage is not likely to occur later.

After being transferred to the postpartum room the mother should be allowed a period of uninterrupted sleep and rest.

Ambulation.   Ordinarily the physician decides whether the mother is allowed out of bed within a few hours after delivery or whether she must stay in bed for a day or two. Many physicians encourage early ambulation, as circulatory complications and bladder problems can be prevented or minimized with early ambulation after delivery. In addition, the mother regains her strength more rapidly. Although early ambulation is good, it must not be overdone. The mother should be instructed to resume her activities gradually. She must also be instructed to have the nurse with her the first time or two that she gets up, to protect her from falling and hurting herself should she become faint (Fig. 13-2).

Bladder function.   Within 8 to 12 hours after delivery, most mothers are able to urinate without difficulty. Occasionally a mother does not feel the urge to urinate even though her bladder is full. It is the responsibility of the nurse to check the mother's bladder at frequent intervals and to make sure that it is emptied before it becomes overdistended. A distended bladder takes longer to regain tone and is easily infected.

The mother who is permitted out of bed can be assisted to the bathroom to urinate. In this normal place and position she is more likely to empty her bladder successfully than if she has to use a bedpan. The first voiding should be measured (Fig. 13-3, p. 287), and, after the voiding, the bladder should be felt to see if it is empty. The height and location of the fundus should also be checked to see if the bladder is empty. If the mother is unable to empty her bladder, catheterization may be necessary. To avoid the risk of infection resulting from repeated catheterizations, some doctors prefer that an indwelling catheter be inserted and left in place until bladder tone is restored. Usually within 24 to 48 hours after delivery, the bladder tone returns and the mother has no further problem urinating. Primiparas and mothers who experience a great deal of discomfort in the perineal area are most likely to have difficulty urinating.

[handwritten notes:]
Oxytocin IV, IM
* methergen PO, IV } ↑ BP
Ergetrate PO

CK MD order for methergen
DNG if BP

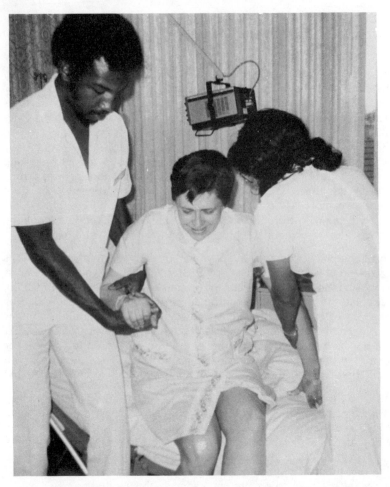

FIG. 13-2. *Two nurses assist the mother out of bed for the first time following delivery.*

DAILY POSTPARTUM CARE

The daily nursing care during the postpartum hospital stay consists of observations to detect early signs of complications and to determine the rate of involution; measures to promote the comfort and well-being of the mother and to protect her from infection; and instruction and support to help her adjust to her new responsibility.

PHYSICAL ASSESSMENT

Vital signs. The temperature, pulse, and respirations are measured every 4 hours during the day. If elevations occur, they are measured

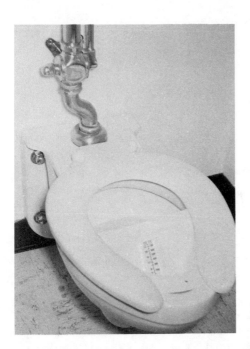

FIG. 13-3. *Pan used for collecting and measuring the first voiding.*

every 4 hours during the night also. A temperature of 100.4 °F (38 °C) or higher is generally considered an indication of infection except in the first 24 hours after delivery, when it probably is due to dehydration. A rapid pulse can also be a sign of infection, even though the temperature remains normal.

Each morning the nurse examines the mother to determine the condition of the breasts and nipples, the height of the fundus, the appearance of the lochia, and the condition of the stitches. Before beginning her examination, the nurse should provide privacy and explain to the mother what she intends to do and why. To protect the mother from infection, the nurse must wash her hands thoroughly and begin the examination with the breasts and nipples, then proceed downward, inspecting the stitches last. She must wash her hands again after completing the examination.

Breasts. The breasts are examined by gently feeling the outer sides to see if they are soft, firm, or engorged (Fig. 13-4). It is not necessary to feel the entire breast, since the outer aspects of the breasts, which are nearest the blood and lymph supply of the axillae, experience changes as soon as the rest of the breast. The breasts usually feel soft until the glands begin to enlarge in preparation for milk production, when they become firm. On the third or fourth day postpartum they may become engorged and painful. In 24 to 36 hours the engorgement subsides and the breasts become softer and comfortable.

• Depends on supply ě demar

q 1½ hr → 3hr. baby nursed because

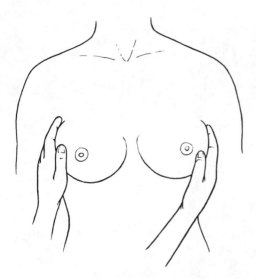

FIG. 13-4. *The breasts are examined by gently feeling the outer side of each breast.*

The nipples should be in good condition with no cracking or bleeding. Cracked nipples are uncomfortable to the mother and offer bacteria ready access to the breasts. When cracked nipples are discovered, the physician should be notified so that appropriate measures can be taken to prevent infection.

Fundus and lochia. With the bladder empty and the mother lying flat on her back, the relation of the fundus to the umbilicus is measured in fingerbreadths daily, to determine the rate of involution (see Fig. 12-1). The appearance of the lochia is determined by inspecting the perineal pad. (The normal rate of involution and the appearance of the lochia have been described in Chapter 12.) The placental site is usually completely healed within 3 weeks after delivery, after which there is no lochia.

Stitches. For inspection of the stitches, the mother is requested to turn onto her side and bring her upper leg forward (Fig. 13-5). In this position,

FIG. 13-5. *The stitches are inspected with the mother on her side and her upper leg forward.*

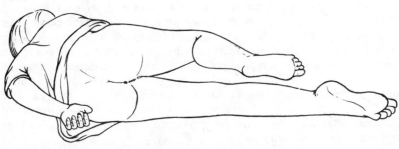

episiotomies are done sub cuticular and are dissolvable. only see a straight

with the perineal pad removed, the stitches can be inspected without touching the area. Separation of the episiotomy or purulent drainage around the stitches is reported to the physician.

INTERVENTIONS TO PROMOTE COMFORT AND WELL-BEING

Measures to promote the comfort and well-being of the mother include diet, a daily bath, breast care, perineal care, pain relief, provision for rest and sleep, bladder and bowel care, and measures to protect her from infection.

Diet. During the postpartum period, the mother usually has a hearty appetite. In most cases, mothers are given a menu and permitted to select their own diets. In addition to three regular meals a day, a mother may be given a between-meal snack in the afternoon and at bedtime. These snacks can be especially beneficial to the nursing mother because she needs additional calories, protein, minerals, and vitamins. The mother is encouraged to drink plenty of fluids during the postpartum period. An abundant fluid intake helps to replace fluids lost during labor and as a result of postpartum diuresis and diaphoresis. It is also important in maintaining bladder and bowel function. The diet following delivery may be supplemented with medicinal iron just as it was during pregnancy, if the physician feels the mother needs it.

Bathing. The first bath the mother receives following delivery is usually a bed bath. This care by the nurse enables the mother to regain her strength before resuming responsibility for her own care. In addition, it provides opportunity for her to talk to the nurse about labor, birth, and the baby and to ask questions about herself, the care of the baby, or about the unit routine. The nurse has an opportunity to get acquainted with the mother and to give her support and encouragement. She can also instruct the mother in the care of her breasts and stitches.

After the mother is ambulatory, she is usually permitted to take a shower. The first time she does this the nurse helps her to assemble the supplies she will need—clean gown, perineal pad, bag for disposal of soiled pad, soap in soap dish, shower cap, washcloth, and towel—and accompanies her to the shower. The nurse shows her how to regulate the water temperature and remains nearby so that she can hear the mother if she calls. If the mother gets along well the first time, it is usually not necessary for the nurse to stay with her for subsequent showers.

Breast care. The breast care a mother receives depends on whether or not she breast-feeds her baby. When a breast-feeding mother is given a bath or takes a shower, her breasts are washed first. Because the baby will put her nipple in its mouth to obtain food, it is important that the breasts and nipples be as clean as possible, and that organisms from other parts of the body not be brought to the breasts and nipples.

A broad-strap bra that gives good support without constricting the breasts should be worn. Nursing bras that open in front to make breasts and nipples easily accessible at feeding time are available. The nursing mother should have at least two bras so that, by washing one every day, she can put on a clean one after her bath each morning.

The breasts should be bathed with soap and water once a day. More frequent bathing removes the natural oils secreted by the glands of Montgomery, which lubricate the nipples and make them pliable. To supplement these natural oils, some physicians prescribe an ointment that helps prevent soreness and cracking. A small amount of this ointment is placed on the fingers and gently worked into the nipples after each feeding. Probably the most effective way to prevent soreness and cracking of the nipples is to be sure that the baby has all of the nipple and most of the areola in its mouth when nursing. Soreness of the nipples can also be avoided by not permitting the baby to nurse too long at each feeding before the milk comes in.

When the mother's breasts become very full or engorged, the nipple may become flattened, making it impossible for the baby to grasp. Before the baby is put to breast, the breasts may be pumped or some milk may be expressed manually so that the baby can get hold of the nipple. During the time that the breasts are uncomfortable due to engorgement, the physician may prescribe hot compresses for them, which improve circulation and relieve the discomfort. Medication for pain relief can also be given.

The breast care for the mother who is not nursing her baby includes measures to suppress lactation. The physician usually prescribes hormone preparations, such as stilbestrol or Deladumone, to suppress the action of prolactin. He may permit the mother to wear her own bra or he may order that a breast binder be worn. The breast binder compresses the milk glands, so that secretion of milk is suppressed by mechanical means.

During the time of engorgement, the physician may prescribe ice bags applied to the breasts of the nonnursing mother to relieve the discomfort temporarily and to discourage further engorgement by constricting the circulation and slowing metabolism. The mother can also be given medication for pain relief. The breasts of the nonnursing mother should not be pumped, because this stimulates the breasts to produce more milk.

Perineal care. Following delivery, the episiotomy should heal without causing too much discomfort to the mother and without becoming infected. The mother is more comfortable, healing is more rapid, and there is less danger of infection if the area is kept clean. The cleansing may be done with a washcloth and soap and water or it may be done with sterile cotton balls, forceps, and a sterile solution. Cleansing may be done by the nurse or, after she is properly instructed, by the mother. The person giving the care must first wash her hands thoroughly with soap and water. Cleansing should be done gently, and it is very important that it be from front to back, to prevent organisms from being carried from the anus to the stitches and vagina. For the same reason, when the pad is applied, it should be attached in front first and then in the back. Before touching the pad, the hands must be washed thoroughly with soap and water. Nei-

episiotomy coming apart may be a hematoma.

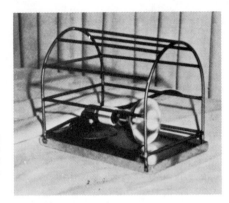

FIG. 13-6. *One type of heat lamp that may be used for applying dry heat to the perineum is covered by a frame which supports the bedclothing, allowing the mother to be covered during treatment.*

ther the nurse nor the mother should touch the side of the pad that is placed next to the body, to protect the mother from infection carried by the hands. In some hospitals gloves are being worn by nurses when giving perineal care as a precaution against autoimmune deficiency syndrome.

Many physicians prescribe dry or wet heat treatments for the stitches. Dry heat is applied by means of heat lamps (Fig. 13-6), and wet heat is applied by means of compresses or sitz baths (Fig. 13-7). Heat temporarily

FIG. 13-7. *Wet heat applied in the sitz tub promotes healing and relieves discomfort of the episiotomy. (A) Nurse prepares sitz tub. (B) A mother takes a sitz bath for relief of perineal discomfort.*

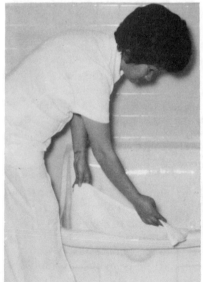

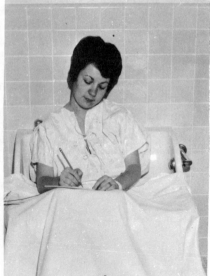

A   B

[handwritten: ice 1st, then heat]

[handwritten: 2 kinds heat: Dry, moist]

relieves the discomfort of the stitches and promotes healing. Sprays or ointments also may be prescribed for relief of discomfort, and medication for pain relief may be given.

Some women have hemorrhoids before they become pregnant. Others develop them during pregnancy as a result of pressure from the gravid uterus on the pelvic veins, and from straining at stool because of constipation. During the second stage of labor as the mother pushes, these hemorrhoids may become greatly enlarged. Swollen hemorrhoids may cause considerable discomfort to the mother during the early days of the puerperium. Measures used to relieve pain in the stitches, such as heat lamps, sitz baths, sprays, and ointments, may also help to relieve hemorrhoidal pain. Other measures that the doctor may prescribe include cold witch hazel compresses and rectal suppositories. As the circulation improves, the hemorrhoids gradually disappear or return to their pre-pregnant size.

Pain relief. During the first few days postpartum the mother may experience afterpains, pain in the area of the episiotomy, and pain due to breast engorgement. Anticipating these discomforts, the physician prescribes analgesics, such as aspirin plus codeine (Empirin with codeine) or propoxyphene (Darvon), to be given every 3 to 4 hours as needed. Within the limits set by the physician, the nurse uses her judgment in administering the analgesics. The mother should be encouraged to request this medication when she first begins to feel uncomfortable, because the sooner it is given the more effective it is. The breast-feeding mother can be given an analgesic just before the baby nurses so that she can complete the feeding without being bothered with afterpains. Afterpains can also be avoided if the mother who is receiving ergonovine (Ergotrate) is given medication for pain relief at the same time.

Rest. Periods of undisturbed rest and sleep are important to restore the mother's physical and emotional energies and to help her to make a satisfactory adjustment following delivery. Freedom from pain and worry contribute to her ability to rest and sleep. Therefore, the nurse should do all in her power to make the mother comfortable and to relieve her anxieties and tensions. Some maternity units have a certain time during the day during which unit activities are stopped and the mother is encouraged to rest. Limiting visitors to certain hours of the day is also helpful in providing rest for the mother. The physician usually prescribes a "sleeping pill" for bedtime. The nurse can help the mother to relax by rubbing her back and straightening her bed linens and can provide an atmosphere conducive to sleep by dimming or turning off lights and eliminating noise. The baby on formula can be fed in the nursery at night so that the mother's sleep is uninterrupted. The breast-fed baby can also be fed in the nursery at night until the mother's milk comes in.

Bladder and bowel care. After the first 12 to 24 hours postpartum, the problems that may have prevented a mother from being able to empty her bladder should have disappeared. Occasionally, however, a mother may have a bladder problem for 2 or 3 days; the nurse must be on the alert to detect this. Forcing fluids and preventing the bladder from becoming

[handwritten left margin: pains, uterus contractions]

[handwritten bottom: Dry heat bad for hemorrhoids.]

measure voiding 3x

overdistended can aid in regaining bladder tone and in preventing bladder infections. Giving the mother an analgesic 10 to 15 minutes before she attempts to empty her bladder may so relieve the soreness and discomfort in her stitches that she is able to relax and urinate without difficulty. When possible, the mother should be permitted to use the bathroom instead of the bedpan, since this is more natural and therefore more conducive to normal functioning.

The causes and treatment of constipation following delivery were discussed in Chapter 12. The woman who normally has a bowel movement each day may need to be reassured that failure to have a bowel movement for a day or so after delivery is normal and that regular bowel habits will return soon. Proper diet and abundant fluids, along with exercise and a regular time for elimination, promote the return of regular bowel habits.

Preventing infection. The nurse must be mindful of the ease with which the mother may become infected during the puerperium and must be constantly on guard to protect her from infection. She must wash her hands well before and after giving care or handling supplies and equipment used by the mother. Each mother should have her own supplies and equipment and these should be washed and sterilized before being used by another mother. The nurse should wear a clean uniform each day. Nurses or other personnel who have colds should not take care of the mother. A mother who develops an infection must be isolated, and the nurse who cares for her should not care for other mothers.

Exercise. The postpartum woman is generally motivated to exercise when she sees the flabby appearance of her abdomen. Depending on the type of labor and delivery she has had and how much energy she has, she can begin simple exercises a day or two after delivery. It is important that she start slowly and gradually increase as she can tolerate it (Fig. 13-8). She should stop before she becomes tired and avoid exercises that put strain on the episiotomy. More strenuous exercises are postponed until after the 6-week checkup.

Maternity units usually provide mimeographed sheets of exercises or exercise booklets for new mothers. These tell which exercises to start when and the steps in doing them. Pharmaceutical and formula companies also supply exercise booklets for new mothers.

Listed below are some exercises that may be started as soon after

FIG. 13-8. *The basic exercise for firming the abdominal muscles may begin on the first day postpartum. The patient inhales, exhales, pulls in the abdomen, holds for a count of five, and relaxes. Other exercises, such as pelvic rock, situps, and straight leg raising are developed from this position later in the postpartum.*

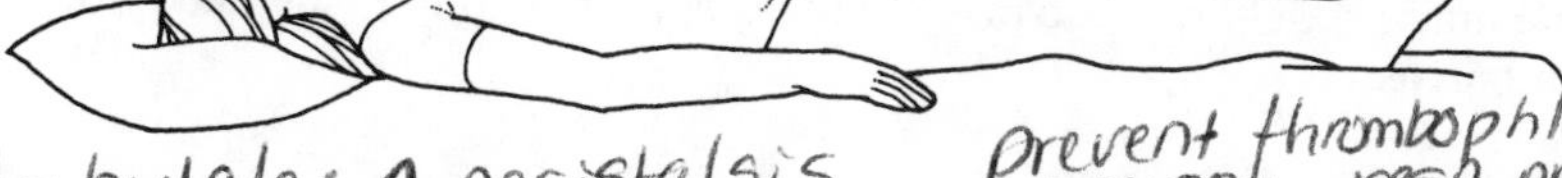

Ambulate: ↑ peristalsis helps voiding dystocia ??? prevent thrombophlebitis prevent resp. problems

delivery as the mother wishes. The first four increase muscle tone and relieve backache and tension; the fifth reduces congestion and discomfort in the perineal area, increases the ability of the muscles to control the openings of the urethra, vagina, and rectum, and improves support to the pelvic organs.

EXERCISES FOR EARLY POSTPARTUM PERIOD

- *Deep abdominal breathing:* Take in a deep breath, hold it briefly, then exhale slowly while contracting the abdominal wall at the same time. Do this four or five times.

- *Head raising:* Lie flat on back without pillow and with arms at sides. Raise head so that chin touches chest, at same time contract abdominal muscles. Repeat several times; repeat exercise several times daily.

- *Stretching from head to toe:* Lie flat and extend arms above head. Repeat several times.

- *Lower back exercise:* Lie flat on back with knees bent and feet flat on bed (or floor). Keep one knee bent and slowly lower other leg while pressing lower spine against bed. Keep spine completely flat against bed. Repeat, using other leg.

- *Kegel:* Gradually tighten muscles around vagina and anus, then gradually release them. This exercise can be done any time, any place, and as often as desired.

EMOTIONAL SUPPORT

The changes in the mother's body as it returns to the prepregnant state are accompanied by changes in her thinking and in behavior as she faces her new responsibilities. On the third or fourth day the mother may experience "postpartum blues."

The nurse can give the mother support and guidance as she learns her new role. She can reassure her by explaining what is happening. She can encourage her to talk about her feelings by being an interested and understanding listener. She can help the mother to develop confidence in her own abilities by showing approval of her efforts to assume her new responsibilities.

The nurse who discovers a mother crying should first determine whether the cause is due to physical or emotional factors that might be relieved by nursing measures. If the mother assures her that "nothing is wrong," and she does not "know why" she is crying but she "can't seem to stop," the nurse can be fairly certain that the mother has postpartum blues. The nurse can then explain that this is a normal reaction to all the excitement of having a baby and that it will pass. One mother may wish to have the nurse sit with her until she feels better, another may wish to be alone. The wishes of each mother should be respected. In any event, the nurse should provide privacy for the mother so that she need not be embarrassed.

Potential nursing diagnoses:

Knowledge deficit related to self-care (breasts, lochia, episiotomy, nutritional needs, and so forth)

Alterations in comfort: pain related to episiotomy, afterpains, breast engorgement, hemorrhoids

Sleep pattern disturbance related to labor, delivery, care of infant

Potential alteration in parenting related to inexperience or feelings of inadequacy

Anxiety related to appearance

POSTPARTUM TASKS

Just as the woman had certain tasks to accomplish during pregnancy, so also she has tasks to work through during the early postpartal period. These tasks relate to herself, her baby, and her husband.

Tasks pertaining to herself. The tasks relating to herself have to do with her labor and delivery experience, her body image, and her skills as a mother. The new mother needs to be able to deal with her feelings regarding her labor and delivery experience so that she can rid herself of any anxieties she may have regarding it. Unless she is able to assimilate her experience, any negative feelings that are unresolved may surface with increased anxiety in her next pregnancy. Perhaps one of the most effective ways of helping her work through this task is for the nurse who was with her during labor and delivery to visit her a day or so after the birth and let her discuss her experience. As the mother recounts her labor and the birth, the nurse can clarify details that are vague and help the mother align them in proper sequence; the mother should feel free to express her feelings about the experience and her perception of her performance. At this time she can also get answers to questions she may have about her labor and the birth. If the mother shows embarrassment over something that happened during labor or delivery, the nurse must be careful not to make remarks that, although intended to make the mother feel less embarrassed, may actually result in keeping her from further expressing her true feelings about her experience.

One of the biggest concerns of the new mother after delivery is her body image. If she expected the trim figure she had before becoming pregnant, it can be quite a shock to see her abdomen still looking pregnant. The nurse can assure her that with proper nutrition and exercise her figure will be restored. The nursing mother should be cautioned against dieting to regain her figure during lactation. If the episiotomy is a concern to the mother, the nurse can reassure her that this is a temporary discomfort and that the analgesic ointments, sprays, heat treatments, and so forth will help. When the nurse inspects the episiotomy each morning she can tell the mother how it looks and that it is healing properly; this is reassuring.

The multipara may feel quite confident in her mothering skills because of her previous experience, but she still needs to be commended for her care of this infant. The woman who has just given birth to her first child but who has had much experience with caring for younger brothers and sisters, or who has done a lot of babysitting of very young children, may also be confident in her ability to care for her infant; however, she too needs reassurance from the nurse that she is doing a good job. The woman who has just given birth to her first child and who has had no previous experience with babies is likely to be very dependent on the nurse to teach her what to do for her infant, how to do it, how to get acquainted with him, and what his cry means. The nurse needs to spend a lot of time with this mother and provide opportunity for her to actually do the care, after being shown, so that she can develop skill and confidence in her ability before going home. She probably will feel self-conscious and scared at first, but the nurse can encourage her with praise; it is extremely important that the nurse permit the mother to give the care even though she may be slow and awkward in the beginning.

Tasks pertaining to her infant. The task related to the infant has to do with fantasies the mother developed during pregnancy about the infant in utero and the realities of the baby she gave birth to. She may have imagined a baby of a different sex, size, coloring, or temperament from that of the actual child. To care for and respond to the real infant she must relinquish her fantasized infant. Claiming this infant as her own seems to be easier for the mother if he functions normally. Therefore, his ability to suck, burp, eat, cry, and have bowel movements is very important to the mother's ability to integrate him into reality.

Tasks pertaining to her husband. The task relating to her husband has to do with their relationship. The new mother is very sensitive to her husband's feelings about the labor and delivery experience, the baby, her appearance, his role as father, his expectations of her now as compared to what they were before the pregnancy, and how he sees her as the mother of their child. Working through this task involves defining their relationship in a new setting with each of them assuming new roles. The degree to which this task is accomplished affects her marital satisfaction and is indicative of her postpartal adjustment and adaptation.

The postpartum tasks come at a time when the mother is probably tired from labor and from lack of sleep, sore from the birth and the episiotomy, and emotionally vulnerable. The postpartum nurse can help the new mother to accomplish these tasks in a number of ways.

WAYS THE NURSE CAN HELP THE POSTPARTAL MOTHER ASSUME HER TASKS

1. Be aware of the tasks facing the new mother.
2. Be a good listener and provide opportunity for her to express her feelings freely without judging her.

3. Provide exercises and nutrition counseling that will help her regain her figure.
4. Arrange for her to have early and frequent, if not continuous, contact with her infant.
5. Find out what resources, such as family or friends, are available to the mother and encourage her to use them to help with household chores when she goes home.
6. Stress the importance of rest periods during the day so that the mother will not become exhausted from loss of sleep.
7. Instruct the mother in infant care skills and permit her to practice them before she goes home.
8. Reinforce the mother's self-confidence through honest praise when she does well in providing infant care.
9. Help the mother to realize that during the first weeks at home she should not expect to be able to do all the things (such as keeping a spotless house, entertaining, cooking, and so forth) that she did before the baby came.
10. Help the husband to have realistic expectations of what the new mother can do when she goes home.
11. Remind the couple of the importance of communicating with each other and working out an arrangement so that both share in the family responsibilities.
12. Remind them that occasionally they should find time when they can get away alone together for a few hours.
13. Provide them with the phone number of the postpartum unit so that they can call if they have questions; this is particularly helpful if a problem arises in the middle of the night.

POSTPARTUM TEACHING

The postpartum nurse has opportunities and responsibilities for meeting the mother's need for information about the care of herself and her baby. Soon after delivery, the mother should be taught the importance of drinking plenty of water in order to maintain bladder function. The nursing mother should be taught that her nutritional needs and those of her baby require that her diet contain an increased amount of calories, proteins, minerals, and vitamins. The importance of milk in her diet can be emphasized by explaining to her that 1½ quarts of milk a day will supply the additional protein and minerals and part of the additional vitamins needed.

For her safety, the mother is instructed to have a nurse with her the first few times she gets out of bed and the first time she takes a shower. She should also be reminded that although ambulation has many advantages over staying in bed, she should resume her activities gradually.

The breast-feeding mother is taught to wash her breasts first when taking a bath or shower. For the sake of cleanliness, she is also encouraged to wear a clean bra each day. The nurse can explain that only two bras are necessary if the mother washes the one she takes off each morning.

The mother should be shown how to apply the nipple cream prescribed by the physician.

The mother needs to know that a simple and safe way of cleaning the perineal area is to use soap and water and wash the vulva and perineum first, avoiding the rectum, then to rinse and dry the vulva and perineum. The rectum should then be washed, rinsed, and dried from the *back*. Once the washcloth has come into contact with the rectum, it must never be brought back up over the perineum and vulva, to prevent organisms from the rectum being carried to the stitches and vagina. The importance of washing the hands well with soap and water after handling the perineal pads should be stressed. The mother should also be taught not to touch the side of the pad that goes next to her body, and she must be instructed how to apply the spray or ointment prescribed by the physician for her stitches or hemorrhoids.

Individual or group instruction in the care of the newborn should be available to the new mother. By learning what care is needed and how to give it, the mother can be comfortable in meeting the needs of her infant. She should be taught how to meet her baby's need for food,

FIG. 13-9. *The mother is encouraged to bathe her baby with the assistance of the nurse.*

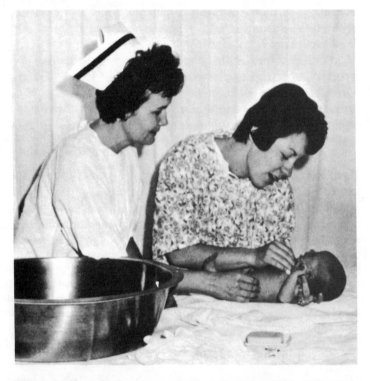

FIG. 14-9. *The mother is encouraged to bathe her baby with the assistance of the nurse.*

whether it is breast-fed or formula-fed, when and how to burp the baby, the importance of cuddling, and how to hold the baby so that it feels secure. She must know how to diaper and bathe the baby (Fig. 13-9). She needs to learn how her physician wants her to care for her baby's skin, navel, and circumcision. She should be taught how to protect her baby from infection. Instructions for the mother in the care of her baby are included in Chapter 15.

In all of her efforts to provide the mother with information, the nurse should remember to speak clearly and distinctly and to use terms that the mother can understand. Her teaching should be realistic and practical, as far as possible using supplies that are available to the mother at home. Some means, such as having the mother actually give her baby a bath under the nurse's supervision, should be used to see how well the mother understands what has been taught. Questions from the mother should be encouraged. The nurse must not only teach the mother what *she* feels is important for the mother to know but should also permit the mother to tell what she feels she needs to learn. The nurse should never force information and should try to develop a good relationship so that the mother will trust her and seek her help. The nurse must be aware of the physician's instructions to individual patients so that her teaching does not conflict with his.

The nursing-care plan for the postpartum patient, which summarizes the information presented in this chapter, is described in Table 13-1 (see pages 304–305).

POSTPARTUM TEACHING

DIET AND FLUIDS

○ If breast-feeding, provide additional calories and nutrients needed during lactation; do not diet while breast-feeding

○ If breast-feeding, avoid excess sweets and gas-forming foods that can affect baby

○ Drink six to eight glasses of fluids daily; important for lactation, circulation, elimination

AMBULATION

○ Nurse with her first time or two

○ Limited activity at first; gradually increase

○ Prevents many complications (bladder, circulatory, etc.)

AFTERPAINS

○ More likely in multipara, after taking oxytocic drugs (methergine, etc.), and when nursing baby

○ Medication to relieve may be excreted in breast milk but will not harm infant; take 15 to 20 minutes prior to breast-feeding so that she can be comfortable and more successful

BREAST CARE

o   Keep nipples clean and dry

o   Wear uplift bra; change daily

o   Use nipple cream or ointment to prevent sore nipples

o   For sore or cracked nipples, use heat lamp for 20 minutes twice daily; exposure to fresh air following breast-feeding beneficial

o   Report cracked nipples to doctor

BATHING

o   Shower first 2 weeks

o   Tub bath after 2 weeks if desired

LEGS

o   Avoid constricting items (garters, etc.)

o   Report tenderness, swelling, redness

PERINEUM

o   Keep clean; may use soap, water, and washcloth; discard washcloth after it comes in contact with anus; may use plastic squeeze bottle to rinse in bathroom; blot dry from front to back

o   Wash from front to back

o   Apply pad from front to back; avoid touching inside of pad; make pad snug so it does not slide from anus to vagina; change pad each time bathroom is used

o   Heat lamp or sitz bath for discomfort; cleanse perineum before using heat lamp so as not to dry lochia on skin and sutures

o   Analgesic ointments or sprays for discomfort; ointments keep sutures soft and pliable (relieve drawing sensation); ointment can be put on soft tissue, then tissue put next to sutures

o   Inflated plastic ring to sit on if sitting uncomfortable; to relieve tension on sutures when sitting, first sit down, then lift slightly, squeeze buttocks together, sit back down

o   Kegel exercises to restore muscle tone: gradually tighten muscles around anus that are used to prevent bowel movement and muscles around vagina and urethra, then gradually relax them; start few days postpartum and continue daily for rest of life

REST AND SLEEP

o   Essential to emotional and physical well-being

o   Control tendency to overdo

o   Morning and afternoon rest periods even if can't actually sleep

o   Should be comfortable and free from pain

URINARY

o First day or so postpartum an occasional patient will have to be catheterized because of swollen tissues or anesthesia

o Prevent bladder distention to avoid infection

o Output increased during first few days postpartum as fluids retained during pregnancy are excreted, also blood volume returns to prepregnant level

LOCHIA

o Increased amount upon arising in the morning or after resting in bed because of pooling in vagina

o Changes from bloody to pink to pale yellow

o Slight increase when she first goes home and increases her activity

o May need to wear pad 4 to 6 weeks

o Tampon may be worn after about 3 weeks if healing permits insertion without discomfort

o Report foul odor; may be sign of infection *if* pads are changed frequently and cleanliness is maintained

o Report persistent blood-tinged lochia; may be sign that involution is not occurring as expected or that a piece of placental tissue has been retained

HEMORRHOIDS

o Size and amount of discomfort decrease within few days postpartum as circulation to area improves

o Heat or cold applications can help: ice compresses, heat lamp, sitz baths

o Witch hazel compresses (Tucks)

o Analgesic ointment or sprays

o Rectal suppositories

ELIMINATION

o Take stool softener and/or laxative first few days postpartum to prevent constipation; enema or suppository second or third day postpartum if no bowel movement

o If breast-feeding, follow doctor's orders regarding laxatives; some are excreted in breast milk and can affect baby

o Practice good bowel habits: regular time of day, roughage in diet, plenty of fluids, exercise

NIGHT SWEATS

o Normal first week or so postpartum as body rids itself of fluids retained during pregnancy

EXERCISES

o Simple exercises may be started during first few days postpartum with gradual progression to more difficult; do slowly, few times at first, gradually increasing

o Avoid fatigue

o Lying on abdomen first few days postpartum helps uterus return to normal position

o Kegel restores tone to perineal muscles

MENSTRUATION

o If not breast-feeding, returns in about 8 weeks

o If breast-feeding, may not return until breast-feeding discontinued; sometimes it returns before

o Ovulation may occur before breast-feeding is discontinued, making pregnancy possible before return of menstruation

SEX

o Intercourse may be resumed by third or fourth week postpartum, depending on comfort and sexual desires

o Takes 3 to 6 weeks for episiotomy, placental site, and lacerations of cervix, vagina, or perineum to heal

o Fatigue, lack of sleep, new responsibilities, changes in home routine may decrease wife's sexual desires for first year after the birth

o Low hormone levels for first 6 months postpartum result in poor lubrication of vagina; may also cause vaginitis; use water-soluble gel to decrease tightness and dryness of vagina

o Proceed cautiously at first because of tenderness and discomfort of episiotomy

o Disruptions will occur (baby crying, etc.)

o Patience, understanding, open communication are needed to adjust to differing sexual desires

o Breast-feeding woman's breasts may be tender, reducing desire for breast stimulation; milk may leak or spurt from breasts as result of sexual stimulation (wearing bra with absorbent pad can help)

o Breast-feeding women normally experience sexual arousal in response to the infants' suckling

SAMPLE DISCHARGE INSTRUCTIONS

The following is a sample list of instructions the physician may give to the mother when he discharges her from the hospital:

1. No physical exertion for 2 weeks, except to care for yourself and the baby. REST frequently in bed. After 2 weeks let the amount of discharge and your

feelings be a guide to your activities. DO NOT take over full household duties for 3 to 4 weeks.

2. Tub baths, shower baths, and hair washing are permissible.

3. No douching for 6 weeks, unless otherwise directed.

4. No intercourse for 6 weeks.

5. No tampons, unless perineal pad is irritating.

6. Whether or not you are nursing your baby, wear a good supportive bra. If you are not nursing, ice bags and aspirin will alleviate much of the breast discomfort.

7. Avoid going up and down steps. If necessary to go upstairs, rest after taking a few steps.

8. You will probably continue to flow intermittently for 4 to 6 weeks.

9. Hemorrhoids should respond to hot sitz baths and ointment as prescribed. Occasionally, rectal suppositories are necessary. If a laxative is needed, take 1 oz of mineral oil.

10. If your episiotomy stitches are painful, daily hot sitz baths and application of the medicated ointment will relieve the discomfort.

11. Driving a car should not be attempted for 2 weeks. Riding as a passenger in a car is possible at any time.

12. Finish taking any prenatal vitamins that you may have at home. These may be refilled and taken if you so desire.

13. A girdle may be worn.

14. Exercises should not be attempted until 3 weeks after delivery, because of undue strain on the episiotomy.

15. Please call immediately following your arrival home and make an appointment for your 6-week postpartum examination. At this time, your blood pressure, hemoglobin, and urine will be checked and a gynecological examination done.

DANGER SIGNS TO REPORT

Danger signs the woman should report to the doctor if they develop after she goes home from the hospital:

o Persistent bright red vaginal bleeding or an increase in vaginal bleeding with passage of clots

o Temperature of 100.4 °F (38 °C) or higher on two consecutive readings, taken at least 4 hours apart

o Foul odor of the vaginal discharge

o Pain, tenderness, and redness in thighs or calves of the legs

o Unusual pain in the episiotomy or purulent discharge from it

o Cracked nipples or hard, reddened, painful breasts

(*Text continues on p. 306*)

TABLE 13-1 NURSING-CARE PLAN FOR POSTPARTUM PATIENT

ASSESSMENTS	POTENTIAL NURSING DIAGNOSES	INTERVENTIONS	EXPECTED OUTCOME
Observe, listen to, and question patient regarding understanding of self-care	Knowledge deficit related to self-care (breasts, lochia, episiotomy, nutritional needs, etc.)	Teach patient self-care	Patient demonstrates understanding of self-care
Take vital signs q. 4 hr for 24 hr, then b.i.d., or as ordered; examine breasts and nipples daily	Potential for injury, infection related to postpartum status, cracked nipples or milk stasis, etc.	Record vital signs on appropriate forms; report abnormal findings; teach patient how to breast-feed to prevent nipple soreness; report cracked nipples; treat breast engorgement	No infection; nipples remain intact without cracking or unusual soreness; signs of infection detected early
Check rate of involution daily; inspect episiotomy and perineum daily; note color, amount, and odor of lochia daily	Potential for injury and complications related to subinvolution, hemorrhage, hematoma formation	Record height and tone of fundus on appropriate form; report separation of episiotomy; report increase in discoloration and swelling of perineum; record color and amount of lochia on appropriate form; report abnormal findings; report foul odor of lochia	Involution occurs normally without complications; signs of complications detected early; healing occurs without complications
Check bladder and urinary output	Potential alteration in patterns of urinary elimination related to trauma of labor and birth	Assist to bathroom; measure amount voided; palpate bladder after voiding; catheterize for residual if necessary	Patient empties bladder completely
Determine bowel elimination	Potential alteration in bowel elimination: constipation related to decreased peristalsis, dehydration, perineal pain	Encourage fluids; include roughage in diet; give stool softeners or laxatives as ordered; give analgesic prior to attempted elimination	Patient has bowel movement

Anticipate need for assistance with ambulation	Potential for injury, syncope related to anesthesia, medication, blood loss, weakness	Assist patient out of bed first time or two after delivery; assist to show first time and stay with patient	Patient ambulates without injury
Anticipate need for rest and sleep	Sleep pattern disturbance related to labor, delivery, or care of infant	Provide periods of uninterrupted rest and sleep	Patient receives sleep and rest she needs
Anticipate discomfort	Alterations in comfort related to episiotomy, afterpains, engorged breasts, hemorrhoids	Give analgesia as ordered; apply analgesic sprays or foams to episiotomy, hemorrhoids; teach her how to use sprays, foams, ointments; apply heat or cold to engorged breasts as indicated; teach patient to support breasts with good bra	Discomfort relieved
Observe parenting skills and interactions with infant	Knowledge deficit related to care of infant, normal infant behavior, feeding Potential alteration in parenting related to inexperience or feelings of inadequacy	Provide opportunity for mother and infant to be together; teach mother how to care for infant; demonstrate care; arrange for return demonstration; answer questions; praise her; give her postpartum unit telephone number so she can call if questions arise at home	Patient demonstrates understanding of care of infant; holds, feeds, bathes infant with confidence; knows where to get help if needed
Discuss sexual activity and contraception with couple	Knowledge deficit related to sexual feelings after childbirth, when sexual activity can be resumed after childbirth, and how to make it less painful for the wife	Explain postpartum sexual feelings and their cause; instruct regarding when intercourse can be resumed; explain how to prevent dryness and tightness of vagina; answer questions	Couple verbalizes understanding of sexual feelings after childbirth, when sexual activity can be resumed, and how to make it less painful for the wife

FAMILY-CENTERED CARE

ROOMING-IN FACILITIES

Family-centered maternity care is directed toward maintaining the family as a unit during the mother's and baby's hospital stay. Efforts toward achieving this type of care have been made in several ways, most commonly by providing facilities whereby the baby can "room-in" with the mother. In strict rooming-in, the baby must stay once it has been brought to the mother. The mother is permitted no visitors other than her husband. In permissive rooming-in, the mother may have her baby with her as much or as little as she desires and is encouraged to send the baby to the nursery at bedtime so that she can get a good night's sleep. In this arrangement the baby can also be taken to the nursery during visiting hours so that the mother can have visitors. Where permissive rooming-in is practiced, many of the emotional and psychological needs of both parents and infant can be met.

In a rooming-in situation, both parents can learn to care for the baby under the guidance and supervision of the nurse. The baby is usually on "demand feeding," which means that it is fed when hungry rather than on a rigid hospital schedule. Many hospitals provide the father with a guest tray so that he can eat with his wife. He is usually permitted to be with his wife and baby anytime. He wears a special gown while with his wife and baby; both parents are instructed to wash their hands well before handling the baby (Figs. 13-10 and 13-11).

Where rooming-in is not possible because of lack of space or for other reasons, family-centered care has been attempted by having the same nurse take care of mother and baby. She is then better informed about the baby and is better prepared to answer the mother's questions than if she were taking care of the mother only. She is also better acquainted with the mother and more aware of her needs than if she were caring only for the baby.

SIBLING VISITATION

A recent innovation in maternity care that contributes to family unity by promoting early acceptance of the new baby by other children in the family is *sibling visitation*. This arrangement consists of visits to the hospital to see mother and baby by brothers and sisters of the new baby.

For many years, state health department regulations stipulated that children under the age of 14 or 16 years could not visit patients in hospitals. These regulations were designed to prevent the spread of infection, particularly communicable diseases common to children, which a child may be carrying before symptoms appear. These diseases can be disastrous when contracted by those who are already ill or who are recovering from surgery, or by newborn infants with limited defenses against disease.

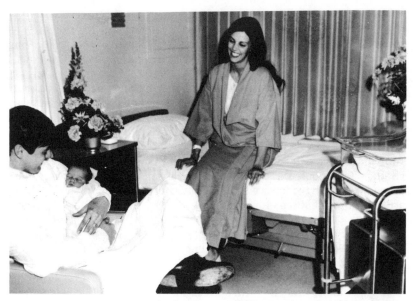

FIG. 13-10. *Where rooming-in facilities are available, parents and child can become acquainted before the baby is taken home.*

FIG. 13-11. *Rooming-in also helps the parents gain confidence in their ability to care for the baby.*

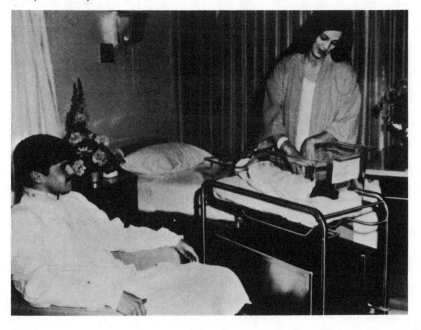

It was also thought that these regulations were necessary to protect the children from the diseases of hospitalized patients. Furthermore, it was recognized that children who are not properly supervised can, by being noisy and unruly, cause tension and discomfort in hospitalized patients.

Maternity department regulations were even more restrictive. Visitors were limited to the husband and grandparents. Some maternity patients were not permitted to leave the maternity unit during their hospital stay for fear they might become infected and transmit infection to their babies.

With advances in epidemiology, which have reduced considerably the incidence and severity of the communicable diseases of childhood, and with increasing demands by the public for more leniency in hospital visiting regulations, there has been a relaxing of some of these rules. Some hospitals have lowered the age limit for child visitors, while others are permitting children of all ages to visit patients in medical and surgical units.

A few maternity departments have begun experimenting with less rigid rules. Some have extended visiting privileges on the maternity unit to anyone except children. Others permit the mothers to meet visitors, including children, in the hospital lobby. Still other hospitals are permitting sibling visitation. The other children in the family can visit their mother and can see, touch, and hold the new baby (Fig. 13-12).

When young children are separated from their mother for a period of time, as when a mother is hospitalized for childbirth, they may feel abandoned. This can cause deep emotional trauma. One of the purposes of sibling visitation is to prevent this feeling of abandonment, and thus reduce the anxiety of children, by breaking up the period of separation with contacts with their mother. Another hoped-for benefit of sibling visitation is early acceptance of the new family member with a minimum of jealousy and rivalry.

Mothers may also benefit from sibling visitation. A mother who has never been separated from her child before may find her hospital stay almost unbearable without physical contact with her child. Another mother may have had to leave her child with a baby-sitter who was not familiar with the child and the family's habits. Her husband or the sitter may inform her that the child is not eating well and is spending a great deal of time crying for her. Sibling visitation is usually welcomed by these mothers, who can thus be reassured of the well-being of their child.

Not all members feel that sibling visitation is a good idea. Some feel it is too emotionally upsetting to the child and to themselves when the visit is over and the child cries because it is time to leave. They feel that the adjustments to repeated separations are more difficult than the adjustment to one initial separation. No doubt the age and disposition of the child as well as the degree of emotional dependence on the mother and the emotional maturity of the mother are factors that influence the actual value of sibling visitation.

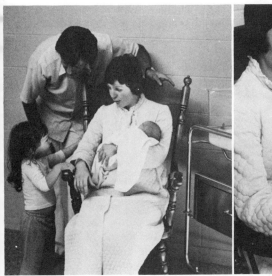

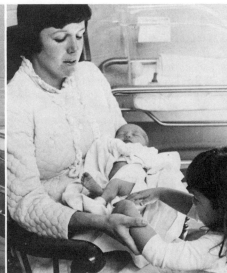

"Is that our baby?"

"Can I touch her?"

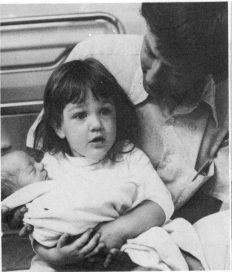

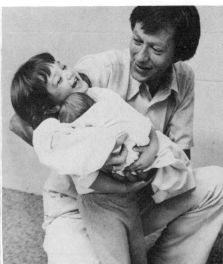

"I can hold her."

"Let's keep her!"

FIG. 13-12. *Stephanie goes to the hospital with her father to see her mother and meet her new baby sister, Kristie.*

Some maternity departments that offer sibling visitation have found that the children are more interested in eating and running up and down the hallways and making noise than in visiting with the mother and baby. Because the parents often do nothing to curb this behavior, sibling visitation may be more disruptive than helpful. When the true purpose of sibling visitation is realized, however, it can be a satisfying experience for all involved.

BREAST-FEEDING AND WORKING MOTHERS

Some mothers who work want to continue breast-feeding after they return to the job. Depending on the type of work they do and the facilities available, they may be able to do this. If there are facilities for refrigerating the milk after it is expressed manually or by breast pump, the milk can be saved for feeding the baby the next day while the mother is at work. To save the milk, the mother needs to take a sterile bottle with her in which to collect it. Sometimes it is possible for the mother to go home for lunch or for the infant to be brought to her at lunchtime for feeding. Whether she is able to breast-feed her infant on the job or must empty her breasts manually or by pump, she needs privacy and a relaxed, supportive atmosphere so that the let-down reflex can function to make the milk available.

If refrigeration and other desirable conditions are not available, a working mother must adjust the feeding schedule so that she feeds the infant just before leaving for work and immediately upon return. This may cause considerable discomfort for her for the first couple of weeks, but gradually the supply of milk produced during the day decreases and the discomfort lessens. However, there is risk of infection from stasis of milk in this arrangement.

Sometimes working mothers find their milk supply decreases when they return to work. This may be due to many factors, including inadequate rest, tension, insufficient fluids, and an inadequate caloric intake.

CLINICAL REVIEW

ASSESSMENT. Mrs. S. gave birth to her first child, a 7 lb 8 oz (3402 g) girl, at 6:24 A.M. She had caudal anesthesia and a midline episiotomy. Outlet forceps were used. After the placenta was delivered, Mrs. S. was given 1 ml of oxytocin intramuscularly. At 6:55 A.M. she was transferred to the recovery room. Her blood pressure was 126/80 mm Hg, her pulse was 88 beats per minute, and her fundus was two fingerbreadths below the umbilicus and firm. Mrs. S. plans to breast-feed her baby.

1. What do you think are Mrs. S's greatest needs immediately after delivery?

2. Four hours postpartum, Mrs. S. attempted to urinate but was unable to do so. How could the nurse explain to her why she could not urinate? What nursing measures may be helpful in enabling her to urinate?
3. What instruction should Mrs. S. be given regarding:
   a. Ambulation
   b. Diet
   c. Breast care
   d. Care of her episiotomy
   e. Care of her baby

BIBLIOGRAPHY

Anthony CP, Thibodeau GA: Textbook of Anatomy and Physiology, 10th ed, pp 634–636. St. Louis, CV Mosby, 1979

Broome ME: Breastfeeding and the working mother. J Obstet Gynecol Neonatal Nurs 10(3):201–202, 1981

Fischman SH, et al: Changes in sexual relationships in postpartum couples. J Obstet Gynecol Neonatal Nurs 15(1):58–63, 1986

Jensen MD, Bobak IM: Maternity Care: The Nurse & The Family, 3rd ed, pp 756–774. St. Louis, CV Mosby, 1985

Mercer RT: The nurse and maternal tasks of early postpartum. Am J Maternal-Child Nurs 6:341, 1981

Reeder SR, Martin LL: Maternity Nursing, 16th ed, pp 580–618.

The Normal Infant 7
at Birth

the normal newborn 14 at birth

BEHAVIORAL When the goals of this chapter are reached, the student will
OBJECTIVES be able to:

Define: caput succedaneum, cephalhematoma, phimosis, circumcision, milia, icterus neonatorum, Moro reflex.

Give the average length and weight of the normal newborn.

Describe the anterior and posterior fontanelles and tell when they usually close.

Discuss the newborn's ability to see and hear.

Discuss the chemical and physical factors that influence initiation of respirations in the infant at birth.

Describe the breathing of the newborn and tell what factors play a part in initiating it at birth. Discuss fetal breathing movements, including their possible use in the future for assessing fetal well-being.

Tell the normal pulse rate and blood pressure of the newborn. *120 - 160* *√BP*

Explain how the infant is prepared to obtain nourishment. *rooking & sucking reflex*

Tell what type of vomiting should be reported to the physician. *projectile*

Tell which types of food substances the infant can digest at birth and which types cannot be digested as easily.

Describe the types and number of stools of the newborn.

Explain the cause of pseudomenstruation. *hormones from mom*

Name and describe seven or eight reflexes normally present in the infant at birth.

Back or side = sleeping position

EXTERNAL APPEARANCE AND CHARACTERISTICS

GENERAL APPEARANCE

Normally, the length of the newborn at birth varies from 18 to 22 inches *AV* (45 to 55 cm) and the weight ranges from 5.5 to 10 lb (2495 to 4536 g). The *7-7* skin of white infants is pink or reddish; that of black newborns and others of nonwhite ancestry is often pink or reddish at birth, but within a few minutes or hours it becomes darker than that of white infants but not as dark as that of adults of their race. The skin may be covered with a white, cheesy substance called *vernix caseosa*, which protected it while the fetus was in the amniotic fluid. Areas of fine downy hair called *lanugo* may be present on the body, particularly on the back and shoulders. Fingernails, toenails, eyebrows, and eyelashes are present, and there may be hair on the head. The cry is loud and lusty, and the infant is very active, although movements are uncoordinated. The baby usually assumes the position occupied before birth—the legs and arms are flexed and the hands are close to the face. The infant is likely to suck on the fist, fingers, or anything else that comes in contact with the lips.

SPECIFIC CHARACTERISTICS

Head. The head is the largest part of the newborn's body, the average circumference ranging from 13.5 to 14 inches (34 to 35 cm). The bones of the skull are separated from each other by membranous spaces called sutures (Fig. 14-1). Because these bones are soft and have not grown

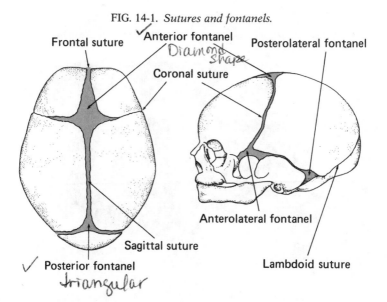

FIG. 14-1. *Sutures and fontanels.*

together, they overlap and the head is able to mold to the birth canal. If much molding occurs during labor and birth, the shape of the head may be long instead of round; however, the head loses its elongated appearance within a few hours after birth. An elongated appearance of the head may also be due to *caput succedaneum*, particularly if the mother has a long labor (Fig. 14-2). Caput succedaneum is swelling caused by prolonged pressure on the head by a partially dilated cervix; it usually subsides within 24 to 48 hours after birth. Treatment is not necessary.

Pressure from the birth canal or from forceps sometimes causes a blood vessel in the periosteum of a skull bone to rupture, and bleeding then occurs between the periosteum and the bone. This is known as a *cephalhematoma*. A cephalhematoma is seen as a bump on one or both sides of the baby's scalp (Fig. 14-3). It may not be noticeable until a few hours after birth because the bleeding is usually slow. Several weeks may be necessary for a cephalhematoma to disappear, depending on its size. No treatment is necessary.

At the junction of the bones in the front of the baby's scalp there is a diamond-shaped space, or "soft spot," called the *anterior fontanel.* At the junction of the bones in the back of the head there is a smaller, triangular space called the *posterior fontanel* (see Fig. 14-1). As the bones of the head grow together these spaces close. The posterior fontanel usually closes by the time the child is 3 months old, and the anterior fontanel usually closes by the 18th month.

The newborn's face is small in comparison with the rest of the head. Because the lower jaw is small, the chin is small. The nose is flat except for the tip, which is prominent. At birth the eyes appear blue or slate-gray. They attain their permanent color by the age of 3 months. Although a

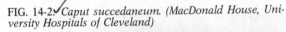

FIG. 14-2. *Caput succedaneum. (MacDonald House, University Hospitals of Cleveland)*

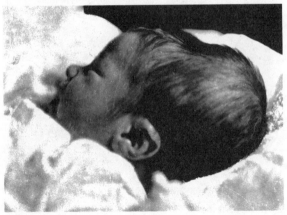

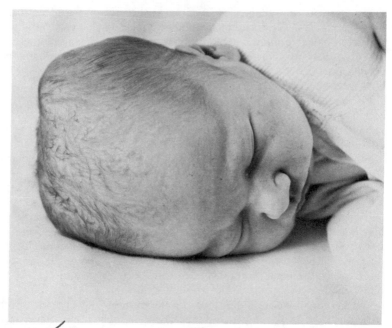

FIG. 14-3. *Cephalhematoma. (MacDonald House, University Hospitals of Cleveland)*

newborn infant has only limited visual ability, it can distinguish between light and dark and does not like bright lights. The infant is unable to focus the eyes and may seem to be cross-eyed when trying to do so, because muscle coordination is lacking. Tears are not usually produced when the newborn cries, because the lacrimal glands do not function for several weeks following birth. The ears of the newborn are flattened against the head. Normally hearing is present and improves as the ear is cleared of vernix and amniotic fluid.

Neck and chest. The newborn's neck is so short that the head seems to rest on the shoulders. The chest is a little smaller than the head and is round. Within the first few days after birth the breasts of either the female or male infant may become engorged due to hormones produced by the placenta during pregnancy. If left alone, the engorgement subsides within a few days and does not reappear.

Abdomen. Because of the size of the abdominal organs and the lack of tone in the abdominal muscles, the abdomen of the newborn appears large and flabby. The umbilical cord protrudes from the navel until 6 to 10 days after birth, when it drops off. There may be spotting of blood from the navel until it heals, which usually takes about a week.

Genital area. The labia of the female infant and the scrotum of the male infant may appear large at birth. The foreskin of the penis may

lose a point on APGAR

be adherent to the glans. The opening at the end of the foreskin may be so small that the foreskin cannot be pulled back over the glans, a condition called *phimosis*, which interferes with cleansing of the penis. The physician may correct this condition by stretching the opening with an instrument or by *circumcision*, the surgical removal of the foreskin of the penis (Fig. 14-4). Circumcision may also be done for religious or cultural reasons.

Extremities. The arms and legs of the newborn are short and are usually flexed, with the hands close to the face and the soles of the feet almost touching each other. The hands and feet usually feel cool to the touch and appear bluish in color for a few hours after birth because of poor peripheral circulation.

Skin. The newborn infant's skin is often so dry that breaks occur in it, particularly around the ankles. The skin of some newborns is so tender and sensitive that even minor irritation causes it to develop large, red, hivelike areas called *erythematous blotches* (Fig. 14-5). On the skin of the nose and the forehead may be found tiny white spots called *milia*. Small, deep pink areas may be present on the eyelids, just above the nose or on the nape of the neck. These areas of thin skin, sometimes called "stork bites," usually disappear within a few months.

Often there are dark bluish areas on the buttocks, lower back, or other parts of the body of nonwhite infants. These are called "mongolian spots," although they are not associated with mongolism. These spots disappear spontaneously during the first year.

FIG. 14-4. *The baby is prepared for circumcision. Note the tray containing necessary supplies for the doctor.*

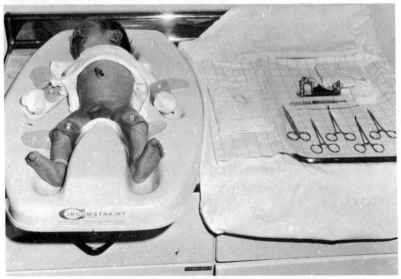

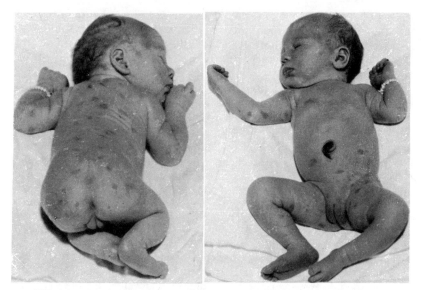

FIG. 14-5. *Erythematous blotches on the newborn due to sensitive skin.*

INTERNAL DEVELOPMENT AND ACTIVITY

RESPIRATORY SYSTEM

Before birth the lungs are collapsed; the baby receives oxygen and gets rid of carbon dioxide through the umbilical cord. As soon as breathing begins, the lungs begin to expand and to function.

Although the infant does not take in air through its lungs before birth, movements of the lungs simulating breathing have been noted in 55% to 90% of cases. These movements are sporadic, irregular, and vary in depth and rate. The rate ranges from 30 to 70 times per minute. They have been detected by ultrasound as early as the 11th week of gestation and appear to be affected by hypoglycemia and mild hypoxia, which decrease them, and by an increase in carbon dioxide, which increases them. These movements become abnormal during labor when the pH and PO_2 are decreased, so that in time they may be used to assess the well-being of the fetus. LOOK for sternal retraction, acrocyanosis (not impro

Exactly what causes the infant to start breathing is not definitely known, but several factors, including chemical and physical changes, are believed to be involved. An important chemical change is the increased amount of carbon dioxide in the infant's circulation, which results from a decreased supply of oxygen caused by pressure on the cord during birth or by clamping of the cord. An increased amount of carbon dioxide for a *brief* time stimulates respirations; the same amount for a *prolonged* period has the opposite effect and depresses respirations.

One of the important physical changes is the change in temperature the infant experiences upon emerging from the warm uterus into the cool room air. Another physical change is the skin stimulation that occurs as the baby comes in contact with the birth canal and the hands of the obstetrician.

Within 1 or 2 minutes after birth, circulation through the umbilical cord stops. This is timed to coincide with the expansion and functioning of the baby's lungs. Since the cord is no longer needed, it is clamped and cut.

The newborn infant breathes through the nose. The abdomen rises and falls with breathing while the chest remains almost still. For this reason, breathing is said to be abdominal rather than chest. Breathing is irregular and quiet; normally there are 35 to 50 breaths a minute.

CIRCULATORY SYSTEM

The newborn is pinkish purple because of the lowered oxygen concentration of the blood. After breathing is established, the skin color quickly changes to pink. However, the hands and feet as well as the area around the mouth may be blue for a few hours because of poor circulation to them.

The normal pulse rate of the newborn ranges from 120 to 150 beats per minute. However, the rate may be influenced by the infant's activity, so that it may be less than 120 during sleep and more than 150 during periods of crying. To obtain an accurate pulse rate, the nurse should count the *apical* pulse while the infant is quiet.

The newborn infant's blood pressure is usually low, ranging around 80/46 mm Hg at birth and increasing to about 100/50 mm Hg by the time it is 10 days old.

Because oxygen concentration is lower before birth than after birth, the red blood cell count of the newborn is high, ranging from 5 to 7 million. Soon after birth, destruction of the excess red blood cells occurs, producing more bilirubin than can be taken care of by the immature liver. The excess bilirubin spills out into the tissues and makes the skin look slightly yellow, a condition known as *physiologic jaundice* or *icterus neonatorum.* Physiologic jaundice usually appears on the second or third day after birth and begins to disappear 4 or 5 days later. The iron that is released from the breakdown of the red blood cells is stored in the body for future use.

chgs from Rt. side → lt. side (↑ pressure)

TEMPERATURE-REGULATING MECHANISM

The temperature of the baby is probably the same as the mother's at birth. It usually drops 2 to 5 °F immediately after birth, but returns to normal within 8 hours. Because the heat-regulating mechanism is not

hypothalamus

mature at birth, the infant's temperature is unstable and responds to the temperature of the environment.

GASTROINTESTINAL SYSTEM

At birth the normal newborn is specially equipped to obtain food by sucking. The ridges in the roof of the mouth help the infant grasp and hold the nipple, and fat pads inside each cheek, called sucking pads, prevent them from being pulled in while sucking. The sucking muscles are strong. The taste buds are present and capable of functioning at birth.

The newborn's stomach is capable of holding approximately 2 oz (57 ml). However, it is possible for the infant to take more than this amount at a feeding, because the stomach is able to stretch and because some of the feeding empties into the duodenum before the feeding is completed.

The cardiac sphincter of the newborn's stomach is not completely developed at birth; therefore, the infant may regurgitate (spit up) some of the feeding. Spitting up may also occur if the infant is given too much at a feeding or is not burped during and after the feeding. Vomiting may occur during the first hours following birth as a result of discharges swallowed during birth. *Forceful (projectile) vomiting should be reported to the physician.*

The caloric requirements of the infant are small during the first 2 or 3 days of life but increase as growth and activity increase. Proteins and carbohydrates are digested easily, but fats cannot be digested as well because the supply of the enzyme lipase, which is necessary for fat absorption, is deficient at first.

Before birth the fetus drinks amniotic fluid but normally does not have a bowel movement. The first stool is usually passed within 8 to 10 hours after birth. *The physician must be notified if the baby does not have a stool within 24 hours following birth,* since an abnormality may be the cause. The first stool is a thick, dark, sticky material called *meconium.* After the infant has taken milk for a day or so, the stools are thinner and are greenish yellow; these are called *transitional,* because they are changing from meconium to milk stools. Transitional stools are followed by yellow stools. The consistency and odor of the yellow stools depend on whether the infant is breast-fed or formula-fed. The number of stools an infant has each day varies, with two to six being common.

At birth the average weight of the newborn is 7.25 lb (3289 g), with boys weighing a little more than girls. The size of the baby seems to be genetically influenced by the size of the parents, large parents having large babies and small parents having small babies. Often each succeeding baby born to the same mother is a little larger than the previous infant.

During the first few days after birth the newborn infant loses as much as 5% to 10% of the birth weight. This normal loss of weight is referred to as *physiologic weight loss,* and it occurs because the newborn's output exceeds intake. During the first few days the food and fluid intake is very low; at the same time the infant loses weight by excreting excess fluid from the tissues and by having bowel movements. About the third or fourth day after birth, intake increases, and the infant stops losing weight and starts to gain. Although weight fluctuates from day to day, the birth weight is usually regained within 10 to 14 days.

GENITOURINARY SYSTEM

The female infant may have a small bloody vaginal discharge 2 or 3 days after birth. This is a result of hormone action on the lining of her uterus before birth and is known as *pseudomenstruation* (*pseudo* = false). It does not recur.

Before birth the kidneys function and the fetus urinates. At birth the bladder is an abdominal organ because the pelvis is too small to hold it. The newborn voids at birth or within 12 to 24 hours afterward. Occasionally a reddish or rusty color may be seen on the diaper of the newborn following a voiding. The color is due to uric acid excreted in the urine.

NERVOUS SYSTEM

Although the nervous system of the newborn is immature, certain reflexes, which are indications of normal development and functioning at this time, should be present. These include the rooting, sucking, swallow-

FIG. 14-6. *Rooting reflex.*

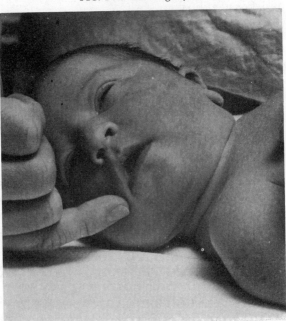

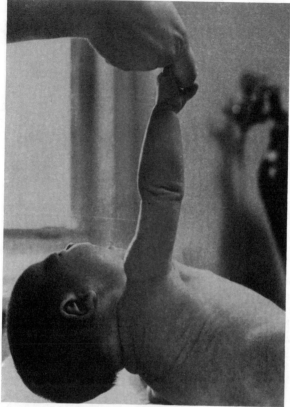

FIG. 14-7. *Grasp reflex.*

ing, gag, cough, sneeze, grasp, startle, and tonic neck reflexes. Absence of these reflexes may be an indication of immaturity or brain damage.

When the cheek is stroked gently, the newborn's head turns in that direction in search of food; this is the *rooting* reflex (Fig. 14-6). Sucking movements begin when anything touches the lips—the *sucking* reflex. The *swallowing* reflex involves the ability to swallow fluid placed far back on the tongue. The *gag* reflex is stimulated when the mouth is too full to permit swallowing. The *cough* and *sneeze* reflexes enable the infant to remove small obstructions, such as mucus or lint, from the nose or throat. When an object is placed in the hands, the newborn takes hold of it momentarily, using the *grasp* reflex (Fig. 14-7). A loud noise or sudden movement of the crib when the infant is lying quietly elicits the *Moro* or *startle* reflex: the infant draws up the legs and brings the arms upward and forward (Fig. 14-8). The *tonic neck reflex* is a positional response of the infant's arms and legs when placed on the back with the head turned to one side. In this position, the arm and leg on the side toward which the

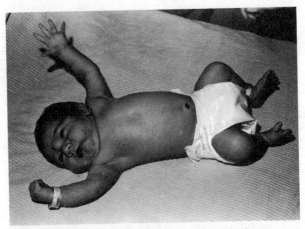

FIG. 14-8. *Moro reflex. (Courtesy of Mead Johnson)*

infant is facing become partially or completely extended while the arm and leg on the opposite side are flexed (Fig. 14-9). This reflex is a result of the immaturity of the infant's nervous system; as the nervous system matures, the reflex disappears.

The newborn spends about 20 of the 24 hours a day sleeping. There is a great deal of movement during sleep, and the infant awakens easily.

FIG. 14-9. *Tonic neck reflex. (Courtesy of Mead Johnson)*

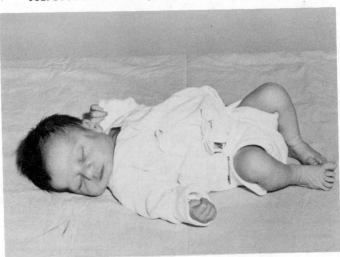

CLINICAL REVIEW

ASSESSMENT. Mrs. P. is 18 years old. She was in labor for 19 hours before she gave birth to her first baby. She had general anesthesia and a low forceps delivery. The baby, an 8 lb 5 oz (3770 g) boy, cried lustily as soon as he was born. He became pink right away except for his hands and feet, which remained blue. His head was quite elongated because he had a caput succedaneum.

1. Mr. P. saw his son for the first time through the nursery window. He asked the nurse why the baby's head had such an odd shape. What should the nurse answer?

2. After Mrs. P. recovered from her anesthetic, her son was brought to her so that she could hold and inspect him. When he was unwrapped, Mrs. P. asked the nurse what would happen to the cord that was still attached to the baby's navel. She also asked the nurse why the baby's hands and feet were blue. What should the nurse tell her?

3. When asked if she wanted the baby circumcised, Mrs. P. replied that she did not know what was meant by circumcision. How could the nurse explain this to her?

4. Two days after the baby was born, the nurse went into Mrs. P.'s room after the pediatrician had visited her. Mrs. P. confided to the nurse that she was worried about the baby and thought she should put him on a formula instead of continuing to breast-feed him, because the pediatrician had told her that the baby weighed 7 lb 14 oz (3572 g) today. How could the nurse relieve Mrs. P.'s concern?

5. Mrs. P. also told the nurse that she had noticed that the baby's eyes were crossed but she had forgotten to tell the pediatrician. What explanation could the nurse give Mrs. P. for this?

6. Four days after the baby was born, Mrs. P. told the nurse she thought there was something wrong with him because his skin was yellow. How could the nurse explain this to her?

BIBLIOGRAPHY

Jensen MD, Bobak IM: Maternity Care: The Nurse & The Family, 3rd ed, pp 583–602. St. Louis, CV Mosby, 1985

Pritchard JA, MacDonald PC, Gant NF: Williams Obstetrics 17th ed, pp 379–387. New York, Appleton-Century-Crofts, 1985

Reeder SR, Martin LL: Maternity Nursing, 16th ed, pp 617–653. Philadelphia, JB Lippincott, 1987

nursing care of the 15 newborn

BEHAVIORAL When the goals of this chapter are reached, the student will
OBJECTIVES be able to:

○ *Define: neonatal period, Apgar scoring system, demand feeding.*

○ *Explain why the physician may delay clamping the cord until it stops pulsating.*

○ *Tell why it is necessary to clamp the umbilical cord.*

○ *Discuss cold stress and its effects on the newborn.*

○ *List three or four ways the delivery nurse can prevent heat loss in the newborn.*

○ *Discuss ways in which parent-infant bonding can be promoted.*

○ *Tell what precautions are taken if the newborn is placed in an incubator for warmth.*

○ *Describe the procedure for the first bath the infant receives.*

○ *Discuss the observations the nursery nurse makes of the newborn regarding cord, mucus, breathing, stools, and voidings.*

○ *Demonstrate the proper way to suction the infant with a bulb syringe.*

○ *List six or seven measures that are taken to protect the newborn from infection.*

○ *Teach a new mother how to bathe her infant.*

○ *Describe the clothing worn by the infant in the nursery and tell how this clothing is treated.*

○ *Describe the care of the infant after circumcision.*

○ *Teach a new mother how to prepare formula using both the aseptic and the terminal methods of sterilization.*

○ *Tell what measures are taken to minimize bacterial growth in formula.*

○ *Instruct and assist a new mother in formula-feeding her baby.*

○ *Name four or five measures the nurse can take to promote comfort of the infant.*

NEONATAL PERIOD

The neonatal or newborn period is the 4 weeks immediately following birth. During this time the newborn adjusts to life outside the uterus. During this time, also, more infants die than at any other period in early childhood. The nursing care the newborn receives during the hospital stay is important to later adjustment and can be a major factor in reducing the number of infant deaths. Likewise, the care the newborn receives from the parents at this time and the bonding or lack of bonding that develops between them can be significant to the establishment of a positive or negative relationship and can affect the child's future relationships. The support and assistance the new parents receive from the nursing staff in their efforts to care for the infant can also be crucial to them as they adapt to their new parenting roles.

IMMEDIATE CARE AFTER BIRTH

DELIVERY ROOM CARE

The care of the newborn in the delivery room is directed toward promoting its physical safety and comfort and emotional well-being. As soon as the infant is born, he may be placed on the mother's abdomen so that there is direct skin-to-skin contact with her, or he may be placed in an incubator or a heated crib, or he may be placed in a container of warm water with his head supported above the water. If he is placed on the mother's abdomen or·in the crib, he should be dried with a soft, warm blanket and then covered with a warm blanket to prevent cold stress; the mother's body will provide warmth where his body touches hers but a warm blanket should be placed over him to keep the rest of him warm. If the father is present and wants to hold the infant, this can be arranged.

Clearing the airway. For physical safety, the airway must be clear so that the infant can breathe without obstruction. As soon as the head is born, the nose, mouth, and throat are suctioned to remove fluid and mucus before the first breath is taken, so that these materials are not aspirated. When birth is complete, the head is held lower than the body so that the mucus can drain into the mouth and nose, from which it is easily removed. Clearing the airway also promotes emotional well-being, since an infant who must struggle to breathe because of an airway obstruction becomes very frightened.

After clearing the airway, the physician inspects the baby for any obvious abnormalities. A thorough physical examination is done later in the nursery.

Clamping the cord. The infant's blood volume can be increased 50 to 100 ml by waiting until the cord stops pulsating before clamping it.

The cord usually stops pulsating within a minute after birth. Clamping is necessary to prevent hemorrhaging from the cord blood vessels.

Assessment. The Apgar scoring system is a method of assessing the physical condition of the baby. This assessment is done in some hospitals at 60 seconds and 5 minutes after birth and in others at 60 seconds and again at 2, 5, and 10 minutes after birth. The heart rate, respiratory effort, muscle tone, reflex irritability, and color of the baby are scored 0, 1, or 2, according to the degree to which they are present (Table 15-1). The total score is the sum of the scores for each item; 10 is the highest score and 0 the lowest score possible. Usually the nurse assesses the baby's condition using the Apgar method, although in some instances the physician may do so.

Preventing cold stress. An important function of the delivery nurse caring for the newborn infant is to prevent cold stress. Cold stress results from excess heat loss. The cold-stressed infant is more susceptible to other problems such as apnea, hypoglycemia, acidosis, and respiratory distress syndrome. Newborn infants lose heat rapidly through evaporation, conduction, convection, and radiation unless appropriate preventive measures are taken.

Heat loss by evaporation occurs when a wet infant is born in an air-conditioned delivery room. Drying the infant immediately and thoroughly, including the head, can help prevent heat loss by evaporation. Heat loss by conduction occurs through direct contact with cold objects. Thus it is important to place the infant, wrapped in a prewarmed blanket, in a heated crib. Heat loss by convection occurs through the flow of air; thus an infant born in a room with a temperature of 72 °F (22 °C) is more likely to lose body heat by convection than an infant born in a room with a higher temperature. Radiant heat loss occurs when an infant is placed near a cold surface such as an outside window. Even the sides of a cold crib can cause radiant heat loss if the infant is not properly covered. To be properly covered, the entire body except the face should be wrapped snugly in a warm, soft blanket.

When cold stress is present, the oxygen needs of the infant increase, causing an increase in the respiratory rate. Unless the situation is corrected so that oxygen needs and respirations are decreased, the infant may become fatigued and develop apnea. Also, when cold stress is present,

TABLE 15-1 APGAR SCORING CHART

SIGN	0	1	2
Heart rate	Absent	Slow (below 100)	Over 100
Respiratory effort	Absent	Slow, irregular	Good, crying
Muscle tone	Flaccid	Some flexion of extremities	Active motion
Reflex irritability	No response	Grimace	Cry
Color	Blue, pale	Body pink, extremities blue	Completely pink

metabolism of glucose and fat increases, so the infant may use up reserves of glucose and develop hypoglycemia. Untreated hypoglycemia may result in brain damage. Since more fat is burned in an effort to keep warm, the store of brown fat may become depleted. Brown fat is a special fat located in the upper thorax, axillae, and beneath the skin in the upper part of the back of the newborn. Its purpose is to generate heat during cold stress. When an excessive amount of fat is burned, fatty acids accumulate in the blood, producing acidosis. If uncorrected, acidosis can lead to death. In addition, heat loss leads to a reduction in the amount of surfactant, a material that lines the air sacs in the lungs and is essential to the expansion of the lungs. An insufficient amount of surfactant results in collapse of the lungs and respiratory distress syndrome. Thus, the importance of maintaining the body temperature of the newborn is obvious.

To prevent heat loss, the delivery nurse instills the eye medication and carries out the identification procedure with minimum exposure of the infant. Before the infant is taken to the nursery, the parents are provided an opportunity to hold their new child. During this time, cold stress is avoided by keeping the infant wrapped warmly. Remember, it is just as important to avoid overheating the infant as it is to prevent cold stress.

NEWBORN BEHAVIOR

Normally the infant starts to breathe and cry within a few seconds after birth. Within 1 minute respirations are well established, the infant cries lustily, the arms and legs move vigorously, and the color is pink except for the hands and feet. This is the traditional response of the infant at birth.

This initial behavior can sometimes be modified by controlling the environment in which birth occurs and by the manner in which the infant is handled. When the noise and lights in the delivery room are diminished before birth, and when infants are held gently and spoken to softly as the airway is suctioned and immediately after, they lie quietly and look around. They appear relaxed and content, and although they do not cry and beat the air with their arms and legs, they breathe normally, and their color changes to pink as quickly as if they did cry. This type of environment and manner, which minimize the factors that appear to be frightening to newborns, are thought to promote both physical and emotional comfort. Parents who expect crying may have to be reassured that all is well even though the infant is quiet.

PROMOTING PARENT-INFANT ATTACHMENT

Maternal–infant bonding and paternal–infant bonding are subjects of current research in maternity care. Bonding involves the development of strong attachments between parents and infant. When bonding has occurred, parents have a deep love for the infant and willingly accept responsibility for its care, putting its needs and interests above theirs. The child, in turn, develops a preference for the parents and a feeling of belonging. Bonding helps cement family ties and promotes family stability and solidarity. In addition, it may have long-lasting effects on the physical and mental health of the child and on the child's ability to develop later relationships with others.

Interaction between parents and child is essential to bonding. The sooner the interaction is begun, the sooner bonding is established. The first hour after birth seems to be the ideal time to begin the bonding because, at this time, the infant is wakeful and alert and the parents are thrilled and excited about their new baby. Since the senses (sight, touch, smell, hearing) are the means by which bonding occurs, the parents should be given the opportunity to hold, touch, caress, kiss, and talk to their infant. Visual interaction is one of the most powerful ways of establishing bonding; it is therefore important that the parent and infant be positioned so that their eyes meet fully on the same vertical plane. (This is referred to as the *en face* position.) When eye-to-eye contact is established, the infant may stare at the parent and follow the movement of the parent's face if it is moved slowly. Also, if the room is quiet, the infant may turn

FIG. 15-1. *An infant responds to an animated smiling face.*

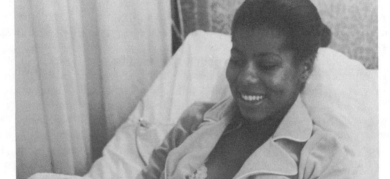

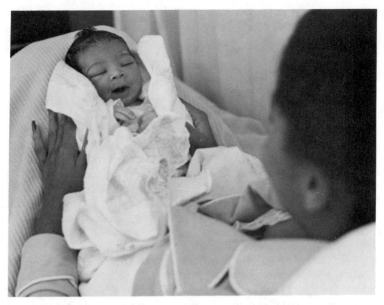

FIG. 15-2. *The infant begins to move his mouth as the mother smiles and talks.*

toward the sound of the parent's voice. These responses may be brief, but parents can be encouraged to watch for them because they make the interaction more meaningful. When the parents become aware that the infant is responding to them, they are better able to recognize that their child is an individual with personality, even at this early age (Figs. 15-1 and 15-2). They are usually eager then to discover other responses by the infant; thus the bonding process is encouraged. When both parents share in the discovery of their infant's ability to interact with them, harmony and family unity are promoted.

Breast-feeding is also important to maternal-infant bonding and should be possible during the first hour after birth if it is the way the infant is to be fed.

Throughout the hospital stay the mother and infant should be able to choose the time they spend together. This means that the infant can be fed when it is awake and hungry or desiring to suck. It also means that the mother can choose to be with the infant other than at feeding times if she wishes. By choosing to be with the infant when she is free of pain and discomfort, the quality of her contacts with it can be improved. The father should have the same freedom of contact with the infant when he is able to visit.

The nurse can promote parent–infant bonding by providing opportunity for interaction between parents and infant, by praising parents for their caretaking efforts, by providing information when parents request it, and by helping the mother to have periods of uninterrupted rest and freedom from pain and discomfort.

CARE IN THE FIRST HOURS

Initial care in the nursery includes weighing, maintaining body temperature, bathing, measuring, and observing the newborn closely.

Weighing.   The normal newborn is usually weighed soon after birth, either in the delivery room or in the nursery, and every day or every other day thereafter. The scale should be located in a warm part of the room away from outside windows and out of drafts from doors and air vents. Before the infant is weighed, a soft piece of paper or a towel that has been sterilized and prewarmed can be placed on the scale as a protection from infection and from heat loss due to contact with the cold scale. The scale can be adjusted to compensate for the paper or towel so that an accurate weight is obtained. While babies are being weighed, the nurse keeps her hand over them so that she can hold onto them if they become active. Because the infant must be undressed for weighing, weighing should be completed as quickly as possible to avoid chilling (Fig. 15-3).

Temperature maintenance.   The rectal or axillary temperature is taken when the infant arrives in the nursery and every 2 hours for the next 8 hours. Then it is taken at least twice a day during the hospital stay. If the temperature is lower than normal, external heat may be provided by a radiant heat warmer (Fig. 15-4) or by an incubator. If these means are used, the infant's temperature and the incubator temperature must be measured every hour to make sure the desired effects are obtained and to avoid overheating. Because the heat-regulating mechanism of infants is immature, their temperature is unstable and is readily affected by external heat.

Bathing.   To allow the newborn's temperature to stabilize, bathing may be delayed for 3 or 4 hours after birth. In the meantime, the temperature is taken at 2-hour intervals. If possible, a radiant heat warmer should be used to reduce heat loss during the bath; if this is not possible, the room temperature should be increased. The bath should be given in the warmest part of the nursery and away from outside windows; drafts from doors and air vents must also be avoided. Heat loss can be minimized by keeping the baby wrapped except for the part that is being bathed. After each part is bathed, it is dried thoroughly and covered. Warm water and a mild soap can be used. Cotton balls are generally used because they create less friction than washcloths on the newborn's sensitive skin. While the baby is being bathed, the nurse inspects him or her for abnormalities. After the bath, the infant should be dressed in prewarmed clothing and wrapped in a prewarmed blanket.

Measuring.   At the time the bath is given, the infant is measured. Measurements usually consist of the length of the infant and the circumfer-

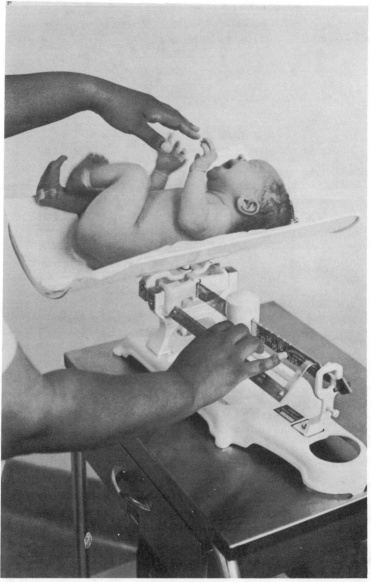

FIG. 15-3. *When weighing the newborn, the nurse keeps one hand ready to take hold if the infant becomes active. Note the paper on the scale to prevent the infant from coming in contact with the scale.*

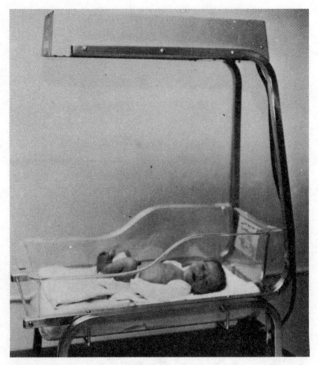

FIG. 15-4. *External heat can be supplied to the newborn by means of a radiant heat warmer.*

ence of the head and chest. With the infant lying with the legs extended, the length is measured from the top of the head to the sole of the foot (Figs. 15-5 and 15-6). The normal newborn is 18 to 22 inches (45 to 55 cm) long, the average being 20 inches (50 cm). The circumference of the head averages between 13 to 14 inches (34 to 35 cm), and the circumference of the chest is a little less.

Nursing observations. The infant is observed closely during the first hours following birth. The cord is inspected frequently, and if bleeding occurs, another clamp or a tie can be applied. The newborn is observed for mucus, which can cause choking. During the first hours the baby is positioned on one side, which is favorable to the drainage of mucus. Tilting the crib so that the head is lower than the body also promotes drainage of mucus. A bulb syringe can be kept in the crib so that it is readily available for suctioning when needed. To avoid forcing air or fluid from the bulb syringe into the throat and lungs, the syringe should be squeezed before it is put into the baby's mouth or nose.

The respirations are also watched closely to see that they are normal and that the infant is having no difficulty breathing. The color is observed for cyanosis, paleness (pallor), and jaundice. Interference with breathing

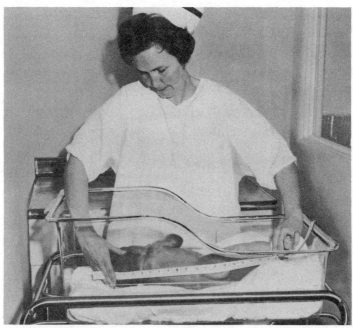

FIG. 15-5. *The length of the newborn is obtained by measuring from the top of the head to the sole of the foot with the leg extended.*

FIG. 15-6. *Measuring the circumference of the head. A nonstretchable tape is placed just above the eyebrows and over the most prominent part of the occiput.*

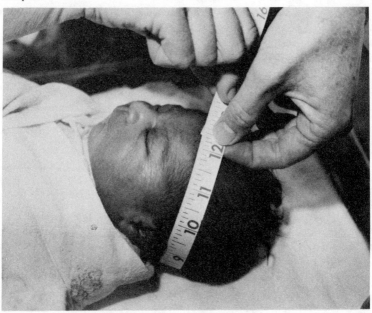

and certain heart conditions may cause the infant to become cyanotic. *Pallor or jaundice within the first few hours after birth may be an indication of a pathologic condition and must be reported to the physician.* The baby's general behavior is also noted. Babies who appear listless and lethargic may have to be stimulated to cry.

The nurse observes and records the time of the infant's first voiding and first bowel movement, which usually occur within 8 to 12 hours after birth. *If the infant does not urinate or does not have a bowel movement within 24 hours after birth, the physician must be notified, since it could indicate a problem.* One way to tag the crib of an infant who needs to be observed for the first voiding or first stool is to tape colored cards (yellow for voiding and green for stool) on the crib. The time of the first voiding is noted on the chart, and the yellow card is removed from the crib. Similarly, the first bowel movement is noted on the chart, and the green card is removed.

CIRCUMCISION

For many years circumcision of newborn baby boys was done almost routinely. Now, however, parents are beginning to question the necessity for this procedure, and fewer circumcisions are being done. The decision about circumcision is the responsibility of the parents. Written consent by one or both parents is necessary before circumcision can be done. Circumcision may be done in the delivery room or it may be done a day or two after birth. The trend is toward doing it a day or two later. Ritual circumcision, a religious ceremony for Jewish infants, is usually done when the infant is 8 days old.

A circumcised baby must be watched closely for bleeding for several hours (Fig. 15-7). *If bleeding occurs, the physician should be notified.* When a circumcision is done, a red card can be taped to the crib as a reminder that the infant has been circumcised and must be watched for bleeding; it can be removed when there is no longer any danger. Immediately and for 12 to 18 hours following the circumcision, a generous amount of petrolatum jelly on a square of gauze can be applied to the penis to prevent the diaper from sticking to it. The wound usually heals in 3 or 4 days. Until then, the penis is bathed gently with a moist cotton ball at bathtime. No other care is usually necessary.

DAILY NURSING CARE

The daily care that newborn infants receive during their hospital stay is designed to meet the need to be free of infection, physical needs, and emotional needs.

Preventing infection.   The nurse must be constantly aware of newborns' susceptibility to infection and must be on guard to protect them

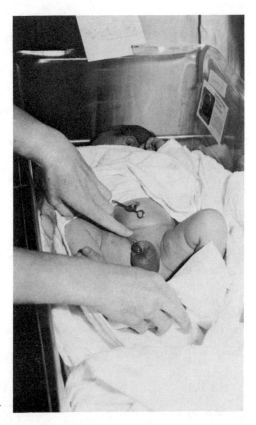

FIG. 15-7. *Postcircumcision inspection.*

from it in the nursery. Measures that should be taken by nurses to prevent infection include:

Wearing a clean scrub gown each day before going into the nursery

Washing hands and arms up to the elbows before beginning nursery duties and washing again after caring for each baby or touching any nursery equipment

Giving special attention to the fingernails, keeping them short and free of polish, because long fingernails and cracked polish can harbor pathogenic organisms

In addition to these measures, the number of people who go in and out of the nursery is limited to the personnel involved in the care of the infants. Anyone with an infection is barred from the nursery, and any baby suspected of having an infection is isolated. Babies not born in the hospital are not admitted to the regular nursery.

To further guard against infection, each baby is provided with his or her own supplies and equipment, which are kept in the drawer of the crib.

The cribs are spaced at least 2 feet apart and the rows of the cribs are spaced at least 3 feet apart. Ideally, only five or six babies are placed in each nursery, and no new babies are added until all five or six go home. This limits the exposure of an infant to other babies and reduces the hazard of infection.

Another way to prevent infection in newborns is to wrap them in a square of muslin at each feeding time and take them to their mothers in their cribs. If they are kept wrapped until the feeding is completed, they do not come in contact with the mothers' bed linens, from which they could possibly become infected. Taking them to their mothers in their cribs lessens exposure to infection through close contact with other infants, as would occur if a common carrier were used. After the feeding, the infants are unwrapped, lifted into their cribs, and returned to the nursery. The wrappers are placed with the soiled linen and are washed and autoclaved before being reused.

Care of the skin. During the bath, the baby's skin is inspected for moist, irritated areas, pustules, and blisters, which may be indications of infection. If these are found, the baby is isolated and the physician notified.

Until the cord drops off and the navel has healed, the newborn is given a sponge bath. After the navel has healed, a tub bath may be given. If the baby has been circumcised, a tub bath is not given until the wound has healed. Bathing every other day is usually adequate during the first month, although the face and genitalia should be washed daily, and more often if necessary. Shampooing two or three times a week is usually sufficient.

The bath at home should be given at a time when the mother is not hurried, so that she can devote all of her attention to the infant. It should not be given soon after a feeding, because handling may cause the infant to vomit. The room should be free of drafts and comfortably warm, not hot. The working area should be of comfortable height and have adequate space for the bathtub, baby, and supplies. The mother should remove her rings, watch, and other jewelry that might scratch the infant. The baby should never be left alone on the table or in the tub. If the telephone or the doorbell rings, the mother should either put the infant back in the crib or take the infant with her to answer it. A washcloth or diaper can be put on the bottom of the tub to prevent the infant from slipping. The newborn may cry and give every indication of disliking the bath. However, if the mother uses a soothing voice, holds the infant gently but securely, avoids extremes in temperature of the bath water, and is unhurried in her movements, the child will soon learn to enjoy being bathed.

BATH SUPPLIES FOR BABY

- Bathtub
- Mild soap

- Pad
- Soft towel and washcloth
- Cotton balls
- Warm water
- Alcohol
- Cotton-tipped applicators
- Bag or other container for waste
- Clean shirt and diaper and outer clothing as desired

BATHING AND DRESSING THE BABY

1. Wash your hands and arms well with soap and water, giving special attention to fingernails.

2. Assemble supplies and arrange in convenient order.

3. Put 2 or 3 inches of warm water into bathtub. Test water with elbow. It should be neither hot nor cool.

4. Place infant on pad on table.

5. Moisten cotton ball. Holding infant's head firmly, wash eyes with cotton ball, wiping from inner canthus outward. Use a separate cotton ball for each eye.

6. Dip thumb and forefinger into water and then twist end of cotton ball between them. Again holding head firmly to prevent sudden movement by infant, clean the nose by rotating twisted end of cotton ball in nostril. Clean other nostril in same manner, using different cotton ball. Cotton balls should not be dipped into water, because if they are too wet some water might get into nose and frighten infant.

7. Wrap washcloth around hand and dip into water. Squeeze out excess water and wash infant's face and ears. Do not use soap. Pat dry with soft towel.

8. With infant's head supported in left hand, place infant's left hip against your left hip, permitting the infant to be held securely with one hand and arm while the other hand is free; this is "football hold."

9. Make lather with right hand and wash baby's head using circular motion. Wash creases behind ears. Avoid getting soap in eyes and water in ears. Rinse head and creases well, using washcloth and clean water. Pat dry.

10. Place infant flat on pad. Remove infant's clothes. Keep hand between pin and baby when unpinning diaper to prevent pricking. If diaper is soiled, moisten cotton ball and cleanse genitalia before continuing bath.

11. Lather both hands with soap. Beginning with neck, soap entire body, front and back. To get into neck crease, lift shoulders so that head drops back slightly. If hands get dry, dip into water and continue soaping body, giving attention to creases. To get into creases of hands and between fingers, put your thumb into baby's fist, then let go. Baby will automatically open hand, making it easy to wash hands and fingers.

12. Until the navel and circumcision wounds are healed, rinse body with washcloth and clean water. After healing, the baby can be rinsed in the tub. Be

sure all soap is removed from creases, which otherwise can become quite sore.

13. Pat dry with towel, giving special attention to creases.

14. *Female babies:* Separate labia. Using moistened cotton ball, wipe each side of area from front to back. Use separate cotton ball for each side. Pat dry. *Male babies:* To bathe genitalia of circumcised baby until the wound heals, gently clean the penis with a moistened cotton ball. After healing no special care is usually necessary. The physician instructs the mother how to care for the uncircumcised male baby.

15. Dip a cotton-tipped applicator into the alcohol and clean the navel. After the navel heals, this step is omitted.

16. Apply powder or oil if the physician approves and the mother wishes. Some physicians object to the use of oil, because it may cause a rash by clogging the pores of the skin. When powder is used, it should be sprinkled into the mother's hands rather than directly onto the baby so that the baby does not inhale it. Powder and oil should not be applied together, because this causes caking of the powder.

17. Dress the infant, beginning with the diaper. Keep a finger between the pin and the infant. Point the pins to the side. When putting the shirt on, gather the sleeve so that the infant's hand can be grasped and brought through, thus preventing fingers from getting caught and being bent backward.

18. When dressed, the infant can be fed or placed in the crib.

After the bath an ointment may be applied to the dry areas of the infant's skin if the physician permits. A thin layer of petrolatum jelly applied to the buttocks after the bath and after each bowel movement helps prevent irritation and sore buttocks by keeping the stool from sticking to the skin.

Care of the cord. Care of the cord consists of keeping it dry and preventing infection and irritation. Usually it is dry enough for the clamps to be removed within 24 hours after birth. To keep the cord dry and thereby promote healing, the baby is not given a tub bath until the cord is off and the navel has healed. The cord heals faster if left exposed to the air. To prevent infection of the cord and to keep it dry, alcohol is usually applied at least twice a day (Fig. 15-8). Diapers and other clothing must be prevented from rubbing and causing irritation to the cord.

Clothing. The clothing worn by the infant in the nursery is limited to a diaper and cotton shirt, which is easy to launder. The diaper may also be of cotton or it may be of paper, which is used once and then discarded. Soiled cotton diapers are collected in a covered receptacle until they are sent to the laundry. To prevent infection, all nursery linen should be washed separately from other hospital linen and should be autoclaved before it is reused.

Comfort measures. The nurse can promote the physical comfort of infants by:

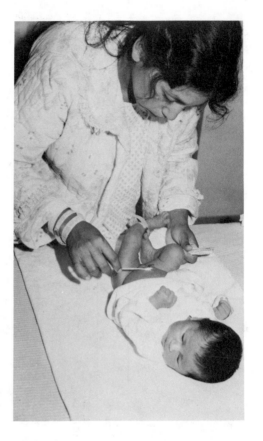

FIG. 15-8. *The mother should be taught to give cord care to her infant.*

Feeding them when they are hungry

Changing their diapers when soiled

Changing their position frequently

Preventing the crib linens from becoming crumpled under them

She can also make sure that their clothing is not too tight and that the room temperature is such that they are neither too cool nor too warm.

Emotional care.   Rooming-in (Chapter 13) is an effective way of meeting the emotional and psychological needs of newborns, for they can then have the tender attention of their mothers as they desire. Where rooming-in is not possible, the emotional needs of infants can be met by such means as "demand feeding" and permitting their mothers to hold and cuddle them at times other than feeding time. New mothers can be taught to hold their babies firmly, with the head well-supported, so that the baby feels secure.

The nursing-care plan for a newborn infant is presented in Table 15-2.
(*Text continues on p. 348*)

TABLE 15-2 NURSING-CARE PLAN FOR NEWBORN INFANT

ASSESSMENTS	POTENTIAL NURSING DIAGNOSES	INTERVENTIONS	EXPECTED OUTCOME
Observe breathing	Ineffective breathing pattern related to obstructed airway	Position on side; suction as necessary; tilt head of crib as necessary to promote drainage; keep bulb syringe in crib	Breathes normally
Take temperature; observe color	Potential alteration in body temperature related to birth and newborn status	Place in warmer; record temperature on appropriate form; record temperature of warmer frequently; bathe when temperature is stable; avoid drafts when bathing; wrap warmly after bath	Infant warm, temperature stable
	Impaired gas exchange related to cold stress		Cold stress avoided; color normal
Note physical appearance and status; vital signs; determine gestational age; note neurologic development; observe behavioral pattern: sleep and activity, responsiveness	Potential for infection related to newborn status and lack of normal skin flora; potential impairment of skin integrity related to lack of normal flora and peeling and cracking of skin	Weigh and record; measure and record length and head circumference; wash hands before and after caring for infant; use individual technique; cleanse cord with anti-infective agent according to hospital policy	Infant adjusts to extrauterine life without problems; no infection; intact skin; infant responds to stimulation; alternates sleep and activity
Inspect cord and circumcision (male infants)	Potential for injury and bleeding related to circumcision and cord	Reclamp cord if bleeding occurs; report bleeding from cord or circumcision	No bleeding

Determine well-being of infant	Alterations in comfort: pain related to wet diaper, position, hunger, circumcision	Change diaper as necessary; change position frequently; feed when hungry; hold and cuddle infant; apply vaseline to circumcision to keep diaper from sticking to it	Comfortable
Observe for first and subsequent stools and urinations	Alteration in bowel elimination related to imperforate anus	Record color, consistency, and amount of all stools; report if no stool in first 24 hr	Has meconium within first 24 hr
	Alteration in patterns of urinary elimination related to insufficient fluid intake	Record number of wet diapers; report if no urination in first 24 hours; report if number of wet diapers decreases	Urinates within first 24 hr and 6 to 10 times every 24 hr
Observe parent-infant interaction	Potential alteration in parenting related to inexperience and feelings of inadequacy	Provide opportunity for parents to hold and get acquainted with infant; assist parents as necessary; stay in background when not needed	Parents comfortable with infant and confident caring for him; positive interaction

FEEDING

Feedings for the healthy infant are more successful if they are given when he is hungry. Some newborn infants are hungry within a few minutes after birth; others may not be hungry for several hours. The hungry infant who is to be breast-fed can be put to breast in the delivery room or recovery room. The infant who is to be bottle-fed can also be fed at this time if he is hungry; his first feeding is usually sterile water. Sterile water is less likely than formula to cause lung problems if he should vomit because of mucus in his stomach and aspirate part of the feeding.

Feeding the infant when he is hungry is called "demand feeding." Demand feeding reduces the difficulty of trying to keep the infant awake and eating at feeding time when he would rather sleep. It also prevents a hungry, crying infant from having to wait until a rigid feeding schedule permits him to eat. A demand feeding schedule meets the infant's needs and makes feeding time more rewarding for the new mother since the infant takes the feeding better. The infant should also be permitted to decide how much he wishes to eat at a feeding; when he has eaten all he wants he should not be forced to take more.

The demand feeding schedule can vary considerably during the first few days after birth. Sometimes the infant may eat every 2 hours and sometimes he may go 6 or 8 hours between feedings. The amount he takes at a feeding also fluctuates at this time. Usually after the first week or so, a relatively consistent feeding schedule of every 3 to 4 hours is established, although occasionally he may want to eat more often.

Whether babies are breast-fed or formula-fed, mothers are taught to burp them before, during, and after the feeding. After a feeding, babies are placed on their side so that any of the feeding they regurgitate will run out of the mouth, and they will not choke.

Breast-feeding. The mother who wishes to breast-feed should be given encouragement and all the help she needs. When it is time to feed the baby, the mother is reminded to wash her hands and get into a comfortable position. She is instructed to put all the nipple and as much of the areola as possible in the baby's mouth to prevent her nipples from becoming sore and also to enable the baby to express milk while sucking by pressing on the sinuses containing the milk (Fig. 15-9).

The physician usually instructs the mother about the length of time the baby should nurse at each feeding. Until her milk comes in, the baby nurses only about 5 to 7 minutes on each breast—long enough to stimulate milk secretion but not long enough to make the nipple sore. After the milk is in, the baby nurses longer on each breast. The contentment and satisfaction of the baby, accompanied by weight gain, are indications that the breast-fed infant is getting sufficient milk. During the hospital stay, however, the breast-fed infant may be weighed before and after a feeding to find out how much milk has been obtained.

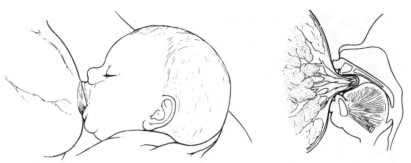

FIG. 15-9. *Note the proper position of the infant's mouth on the breast for feeding.*

Breast-feeding is more successful and less frustrating to mother and baby if the baby is brought to the mother when hungry. For this reason many breast-fed infants are placed on "demand feeding." When sleeping, they are not disturbed.

Formula-feeding.   For the formula-fed infant there is a variety of milk substances. Evaporated milk, water, and a carbohydrate preparation, such as Karo syrup, are ingredients commonly used in preparing formula. The doctor prescribes the amount of each ingredient to be used for the formula.

Formulas are available already prepared and in bottles ready to use. Prepared formula is more expensive than the evaporated milk formula the mother prepares, but it may be more convenient in some instances. Formula, like breast milk, usually contains 20 calories per ounce.

The mother who formula-feeds her baby is encouraged to hold the baby while feeding. She should tilt the bottle so that the milk fills the nipple, to prevent the baby from sucking in air (Fig. 15-10).

Teaching the mother to prepare the formula.   The nurse should make certain that the new mother who plans to formula-feed her baby understands the recipe for the formula prescribed by the doctor, and also knows how to prepare it. The mother who breast-feeds her infant should also know how to prepare formula, because it may be necessary at some time to feed the infant formula.

The recipe prescribed by the infant's doctor may read: 1:2 E.M. 1 T dark Karo. The "1:2 E.M." means one part evaporated milk to two parts of water, so that if 24 oz of formula is desired, she would use 8 oz of milk and 16 oz of water. The "1 T dark Karo" indicates the amount (one tablespoon) and type (dark Karo syrup) of sweetener to be added. The amount of formula prepared depends on how often and how much the infant eats. A newborn may eat as often as every 3 to 4 hours and may take from 1 to 3 oz at a feeding. It is usually advisable to plan on feeding every 4 hours and providing 4 oz at a feeding. Within a few weeks the baby will sleep through the night, thus eliminating at least one feeding;

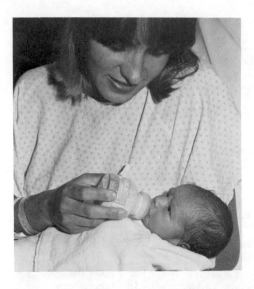

FIG. 15-10. *When bottle-feeding her infant, the mother tilts the bottle in such a way that the nipple is filled with milk.*

however, at the same time, the baby will be eating more at each feeding. The amount of formula offered should usually be more than the infant is expected to take; thus, the infant is always assured of getting enough. Also, because the infant will soon be taking more formula than at first, the nurse should suggest that the mother use 8-oz bottles from the start. This is more economical than buying smaller bottles.

There are two common methods of preparing formula: the aseptic method and the terminal method. In the aseptic method, all the supplies (bottles, nipples, etc.) are washed and *sterilized* by boiling for 5 minutes. The water for the formula is boiled, and the evaporated milk and sweetener (sugar, syrup, or special sweetener) are measured and added to it. An equal amount of formula is then poured into each of the bottles. Nipples are put on the bottles, and nipple covers or caps are put on the nipples. The formula is refrigerated until feeding time. This method is convenient when only one or two bottles of formula are needed. Considerable care must be taken, however, to avoid contamination while preparing the formula and putting the nipples on the bottles. After the first few weeks, it is not necessary to sterilize the formula if safe milk and pure water are used to prepare it. However, the supplies used in preparing it, including the bottles and nipples, should be scrupulously clean.

Cleanliness is very important in preparing formula, because bacterial growth in the formula can cause illness in the infant. To lessen the danger of bacterial growth, the formula must be refrigerated following sterilization; unused portions of a feeding should be discarded. The nipple on the formula bottle should be kept covered until ready for a feeding, and should not be handled before or during the feeding.

SUPPLIES FOR PREPARING FORMULA BY TERMINAL METHOD

- Six 8-oz bottles
- Six nipples
- Six nipple covers or caps
- Pitcher for mixing formula
- Measuring cup
- Measuring spoon
- Mixing spoon
- Can opener
- Bottle brush
- Alarm clock or timer
- Sterilizer with rack (boiler or pail may be used)
- Hot water
- Soap
- Recipe for fomula
- Can of evaporated milk
- Sugar, syrup, or special sweetener
- Warm water

HOW TO FEED THE BABY

1. Wash hands thoroughly.
2. Remove bottle of formula from refrigerator and remove nipple cover.
3. Place bottle of formula in pan of hot water to warm.
4. Change baby's diapers if wet or soiled.
5. Wash hands.
6. Test formula to see if warm by shaking a few drops on inside of wrist. It should be neither hot nor cold.
7. Wrap baby in receiving blanket.
8. Hold baby in arms with head supported at bend of your arm.
9. Feed. Make sure neck of bottle and nipple are full of milk to prevent baby from sucking in air.
10. Burp infant by leaning infant's head against your shoulder while patting back gently, or by sitting infant upright in lap, leaning head slightly forward over hand, and patting back gently with other hand.
11. Following feeding, place infant on side so that infant is less likely to aspirate vomitus if regurgitation occurs.
12. Rinse bottle and nipple with cold water to remove formula, thus making cleansing easier.

PREPARING FORMULA BY TERMINAL METHOD

1. Wash hands thoroughly with soap and water, cleansing well under fingernails.
2. Assemble supplies.
3. Wash bottles and nipples inside and out, using brush and hot, soapy water. Rinse thoroughly under hot running water and let drain dry. Wash spoons, measuring cup, pitcher, can opener, and can of evaporated milk with hot soapy water. Rinse with hot water and let drain dry.
4. Measure desired amount of warm tap water in measuring cup. Pour into pitcher. (Warm water dissolves sugar, syrup, or other sweetener more rapidly than cold water.)
5. Measure desired amount of sugar, syrup, or special sweetener into measuring spoon. Add to warm water in pitcher and stir until dissolved.
6. Measure desired amount of evaporated milk. Add to water and sugar mixture. Stir.
7. Pour equal amounts of formula into bottles.
8. Put nipples on bottles. Cover nipples with nipple covers or caps. If nipple caps are used, they should be loose to prevent a build-up of pressure inside bottles, which causes breakage.
9. Place bottles in rack in sterilizer. (If a boiler or pail is used without a rack, a washcloth should be placed in the bottom to prevent bottles from direct contact with boiler or pail. This is necessary to prevent breakage due to excessive heat on bottle bottoms.)
10. Add 2 inches of water to sterilizer (or boiler or pail).
11. Put lid on sterilizer. Place sterilizer on stove to boil.
12. When water in sterilizer begins to boil, set clock or timer for 25 minutes.
13. Keep water at a low boil for exactly 25 minutes, then remove sterilizer from stove. Wait until sides of sterilizer are cool enough to be handled before lifting the lid. This is important in preventing scum formation which could clog the nipples.
14. Remove bottles from sterilizer. Tighten caps. Place bottles in refrigerator.

INSTRUCTION IN BABY CARE

FEEDING

- Feed when hungry; may be every 2 to 3 hours at first.
- Infants differ in sucking behavior; some take feeding immediately, others are slower. It is better to adjust feeding period to infant than infant to feeding period
- Arrange for privacy, if desired.
- Mother should be in comfortable position and free from pain (tension and pain interfere with success). For first few days after birth, mother may take pain medicine 15 to 20 minutes before a feeding, so that she can be free to concentrate on the feeding in comfort.

- ○ First week after birth is learning time for mother and infant.
- ○ *Breast-feeding:*
  - Wash hands thoroughly after changing infant's diaper.
  - Position infant on same level as breast to avoid pull on nipple.
  - Touch nipple to baby's cheek. When he turns toward it, put nipple into his mouth.
  - Put all of nipple and as much of brown area (areola) as possible in mouth to allow compression of lacteal sinuses as well as sucking, and to prevent pain and possible nipple damage.
  - If infant has problem grasping nipple:
    —manually express some milk so that he can get hold, or use nipple shield, but discontinue as soon as nipple can be grasped by infant;
    —breast pump can be used to draw out nipple if it is flat; mother can place a finger on either side of nipple and brown area and shape it to shape of infant's mouth, making it easier for infant to grasp it.
  - Make sure nipple is on top of tongue.
  - Use forefinger to hold breast tissue away from infant's nose so he can breathe while nursing.
  - Vary infant's position when feeding to prevent sore nipples.
  - Limit feeding to 5 to 7 minutes on each breast to start. After milk comes in, gradually increase time to 10 to 15 minutes on first breast and for as long as infant wants to nurse on the second.
  - Alternate breast the infant starts with each time. A safety pin on bra strap on side to start next time works well as reminder.
  - Break suction before removing infant from breast by placing clean little finger into corner of his mouth or by pulling chin down. Remove nipple before he can grasp it again; breaking suction prevents pain and injury to nipple.
  - Burp infant before beginning feeding, again when changing breasts, and at end of feeding.
- ○ *Weaning:*
  - Start when mother or baby is ready. Many mothers breast-feed for 6 to 9 months, others anywhere from 2 weeks to a year or longer.
  - Do gradually.
  - May wean to cup or bottle, depending on age of infant.
- ○ *Bottle-feeding: (See Formula Preparation, above):*
  - Wash hands thoroughly after changing infant's diaper.
  - If formula is refrigerated, place in pan of warm water to take chill off. Formula may be room temperature or moderately cold. Serve at same temperature each time.
  - Hold infant in comfortable, semireclining position so swallowed air stays at top of stomach.
  - Person feeding infant should be comfortable and unhurried.

- Holes in nipple should be large enough to permit milk to drop freely but not to run out in a stream when bottle is tipped downward. If hole is too small, heat needle to red heat and plunge quickly into hole. Sterilize nipple so treated before using.
- While feeding keep formula in neck of bottle to minimize air swallowed.
o To dispel air bubble, hold infant upright to allow air to rise to top of stomach, then gently pat back.
  - Infant will not take exactly the same amount each time. When he is satisfied, do not urge him to take more.
  - Spitting up milk and some vomiting after feeding is normal for newborns and decreases as they get older. Gentle handling, burping, and keeping head higher than body after feeding will help prevent this.
  - Hiccupping after feeding is normal. No treatment is necessary, but water may be given.
  - Formula should meet nutritional needs for infant's age and size. Changes can be made according to growth and satisfaction of hunger.

DIAPERS

o Change before and after each feeding and at other times as needed.
o Diapers should fit snugly but not hamper movement.
o If safety pins are used, keep hand between them and baby while pinning and removing them.
o Prevent diaper rash by:
  - boiling diapers 3 to 5 minutes to kill bacteria;
  - thoroughly rinsing after washing with detergent;
  - changing diapers when wet;
  - minimizing use of plastic or rubber diaper covers.

WEIGHT

o Infant loses 5% to 10% of birth weight during first few days after birth.
o Regains birth weight in 10 to 14 days.
o Gains about 4 to 6 oz per week during first 5 months, then 2 to 4 oz per week.
o Doubles birth weight by 6 months of age; triples it by 1 year.
o Weight may stay the same for few days at a time, then increase again.

HANDLING

o Support infant under head and buttocks when holding. Hold firmly to make baby feel secure.
o Babies are active and make unexpected moves. They are slippery when wet and can wiggle out of hand.
o To lift infant from supine position, place one hand under head and neck; with other hand take hold of ankles with index finger separating ankles. You can also lift by placing one hand under neck and head and the other under the buttocks.

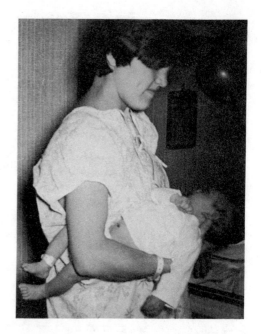

FIG. 15-11. *Using the football hold to carry the infant. Head and shoulders are supported with one hand while infant's hips rest against mother's hips. This frees one of the mother's hands.*

○ Football hold frees one hand while baby is held firmly with the other: place hand under baby's head, wrist under shoulder, hold rest of baby against hip with same arm (Fig. 15-11).

BATHING (See Bathing and Dressing the Baby)

○ No tub bath until cord is off and umbilicus is healed.

○ Warm room, no drafts.

○ Use mild soap and warm water. Water that feels warm to bather's elbow is right temperature. If thermometer is used, temperature should be 98 to 100 °F (37 to 38 °C).

○ Assemble all supplies and equipment before getting baby.

○ Proceed from cleanest areas to least clean.

○ *Never leave infant alone, not even for a minute.*

SKIN

○ Newborn's may be dry and cracked; cracks disappear in few days. Oils may clog pores and cause rash; water-soluble lotion may be helpful.

○ Newborn's skin is thin, delicate, tender, and easily irritated.

○ Infant does not perspire for about a month. Rash may develop if overheated. In warm weather dress lightly and keep room temperature cooler.

○ To prevent diaper rash:

  • keep buttocks clean and dry;

  • may use petroleum jelly or A and D ointment;

- if rash, expose to air and light several times a day; heat lamp for 30 minutes a day (25 to 40 watt bulb, keep lamp at least 1 foot from buttocks; keep diaper under infant during heat treatment) (Fig. 15-12).

CORD

o No tub bath until cord is off and umbilicus healed.

o Do not try to remove cord until it is completely separated.

o May apply alcohol to base of cord until it comes off.

o Report redness at base or foul discharge.

o Usually comes off 5 to 8 days after birth, but may be 12 to 14 days.

o Bloody discharge from umbilicus is normal for few days after cord comes off.

SLEEP

o Newborn sleeps 20 to 23 hours a day at first, but this varies with the individual.

o Infant wakens and cries when hungry.

o Sleep may be deep or light. In deep sleep, eyes are closed with no eye movements under lid, breathing is regular. Light sleep is characterized by rapid eye movements with the lids closed, irregular breathing, and random movements, including sucking movements.

o Change infant's position when awake.

o Make sure clothing and covering are lightweight, warm, and free of wrinkles.

o Position infant on either side or on abdomen to prevent aspiration if he should regurgitate.

CRY

o Fretful cry accompanied by green stools or gas indicates indigestion.

o Fretful cry with fists in mouth, flexed, tense extremities indicates hunger.

o Loud, insistent cry with drawing up and kicking of legs indicates colic.

CIRCUMCISION

o Day of circumcision:
  - observe penis closely for bleeding;
  - apply sterile petroleum dressing at each diaper change;
  - hold both feet when changing diaper so he does not kick against area.

o Cottonballs moistened with warm tap water are used to cleanse until healed.

o If Plastibell is used, petroleum dressing is not necessary.

STOOLS

o Change during first 5 to 6 days from tarry black to greenish black, to greenish brown, to brownish yellow, to greenish yellow, to soft yellow if bottle-fed or to golden yellow if breast-fed.

- Four to six stools per day by about fifth day; gradually decreases to one or two per day.
- Stools of bottle-fed infant have smooth, pasty consistency and foul odor.
- Stools of breast infant have mushy consistency and are influenced by mother's diet
- Report watery, green stools with much mucus accompanied by much flatus; may be symptom of digestive or intestinal problem.

TEMPERATURE

- Not necessary to take unless infant seems unusually warm or appears ill.
- Rectal temperature (preferred by many physicians): lubricate thermometer, insert about 1 inch into rectum, hold in place for 3 minutes; keep diaper under infant because of likelihood of stimulating bowel movement with thermometer. Wipe thermometer with toilet tissue and read; then wash thermometer with cold water and soap, rinse, dry, and put away.
- Axillary temperature: place thermometer under infant's arm and hold for 3 minutes by placing infant's arm firmly against it. Remove and read; wash, rinse, dry, and put away (Fig. 15-13).
- Be sure to shake thermometer so that mercury is below 96 °F (35 °C) before taking temperature.

FIG. 15-12. *Heat treatment for buttock rash. Lamp should be kept at least one foot from buttocks during treatment.*

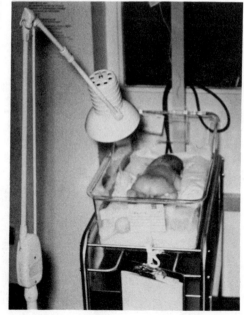

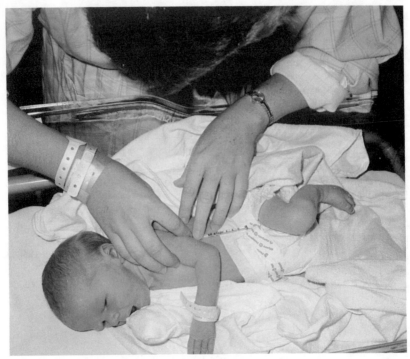

FIG. 15-13. *Taking axillary temperature.*

CLINICAL REVIEW

ASSESSMENT. Mrs. W. gave birth to her first child, a girl, at 10:19 A.M. The baby breathed spontaneously and cried lustily immediately after being born. She was very active and within 1 minute after birth she was pink, except for her hands and feet, which were blue. She was wrapped in a sterile blanket and kept warm while eye medication was instilled and identification applied to her and her mother. Then, after being shown to her mother, who was awake, she was taken to the receiving nursery.

1. What do you think Baby W.'s Apgar score should be?
2. Baby W. was weighed as soon as she was taken to the nursery. She weighed 6 lb 10 oz (3005 g). What precautions should be taken while she is being weighed?
3. Baby W. was observed closely during the first hours after birth. During this time the nurse noticed that she had a lot of mucus. What can the nurse do to help Baby W. get rid of the mucus?
4. Baby W. was to be breast-fed. At feeding time she was wrapped and taken to her mother in her crib. After Mrs. W. washed her hands and got into a comfortable position, her baby was lifted from the crib and

placed in her arms. What suggestions can the nurse give Mrs. W. to help her to be successful in breast-feeding her baby? Why might Mrs. W. be requested not to unwrap the baby while she is feeding her?

5. What can the nurse do to help meet the emotional needs of Baby W.?

BIBLIOGRAPHY

Anderson GC: The mother and her infant: Mutual caregivers. J Obstet Gynecol Neonatal Nurs 6:50, 1977

Cannon RB: The development of maternal touch during early mother-infant interaction. J Obstet Gynecol Neonatal Nurs 6:28, 1977

Dahl N, Frazier SA: Series I. The First Six Hours of Life. Neonatal Thermoregulation. Module 1, The National Foundation/March of Dimes, 1976

Erickson MC: Trends in assessing the newborn and his parents. Am J Maternal-Child Nurs 3:99, 1978

Gottlieb L: Maternal attachment in primiparas. J Obstet Gynecol Neonatal Nurs 7:39, 1978

Klaus MH, Kennell JH: Maternal-Infant Bonding. St. Louis, CV Mosby, 1976

Leonard SW: How first-time fathers feel toward their newborns. Am J Maternal-Child Nurs 1:361, 1976

Lincoln GA: Neonatal circumcision: Is it needed? J Obstet Gynecol Neonatal Nurs 15:463–466, 1986

Reeder SR, Martin LL: Maternity Nursing, 16th ed, pp 654–674. Philadelphia, JB Lippincott, 1987

Reiber VD: Is the nurturing role natural to fathers? Am J Maternal-Child Nurs 1:366, 1976

Management
of Health 8
Problems

health problems during 16 pregnancy

BEHAVIORAL When the goals of this chapter are reached, the student will
OBJECTIVES be able to:

○ *List the three leading causes of maternal mortality.*

○ *Discuss the symptoms of preeclampsia and eclampsia, and list symptoms that may indicate that the (preeclamptic) patient is about to have a convulsion.*

○ *List two safety precautions the nurse caring for a patient with pregnancy-induced hypertension should take.*

○ *List three or four causes of spontaneous abortion.*

○ *Name and define the five classifications of spontaneous abortion.*

○ *Discuss action that may be taken in an attempt to prevent threatened abortion.*

○ *Discuss nursing considerations related to abortion.*

○ *Discuss the follow-up care for hydatidiform mole.*

○ *Describe the symptoms of sudden rupture of the tube in ectopic pregnancy.*

○ *Describe the three types of placenta previa and give the characteristic symptom.*

○ *Explain the types of bleeding that may occur in abruptio placentae.*

○ *Discuss the responsibilities of the nurse caring for a patient with bleeding.*

○ *Discuss the concerns the mother in premature labor may have and the role of the nurse in alleviating them.*

○ *Describe the treatment and nursing care of the patient with hyperemesis gravidarum.*

○ *Describe Rh_o (D) immune globulin and explain how, to whom, and when it is given.*

○ *List three or four effects that diabetes may have on pregnancy.*

○ *Describe the precautions the pregnant woman with heart disease should take.*

○ *Mention two or three infectious diseases and discuss the effects they may have on pregnancy.*

○ *Discuss acquired immunodeficiency syndrome, its cause, who is at risk for it, and how it can be prevented.*

The expectant mother is susceptible to all the diseases and conditions of the nonpregnant state. In addition, health problems that are directly related to the pregnancy may threaten the health and life of either the mother or baby or both. When a woman dies as a direct result of a complication of childbearing, her death is classified as a maternal mortality. The three leading causes of maternal mortality are:

1 Pregnancy-induced hypertension
2 Hemorrhage
3 Puerperal infection

(Hemorrhage and infection occurring after delivery are discussed more fully in Chapter 19.)

PREGNANCY-INDUCED HYPERTENSION

The medical condition known as toxemia is now called pregnancy-induced hypertension (PIH), although it is still referred to as toxemia in some areas. PIH was initially called toxemia because it was believed that a toxin (poison) in the pregnant woman's blood was responsible for the symptoms. However, no toxin has ever been found. This condition, characterized by hypertension, occurs only during pregnancy, labor, or the puerperium (period following delivery). Although the symptoms and effects of PIH have been known for years, the cause is still unknown.

Approximately 6% of all pregnant women develop PIH. It occurs most often in young primigravidas, and it usually occurs after the 24th week of pregnancy. PIH is the leading cause of maternal death; in addition, it causes approximately 30,000 stillbirths and neonatal deaths each year. (A stillbirth is an infant born dead. Neonatal deaths are infant deaths occurring during the first 4 weeks after birth.) PIH can be prevented through careful antepartal care. Since PIH does not usually occur until after the 24th week of pregnancy, it is important that the mother be seen at frequent intervals during the last 2 or 3 months of pregnancy. The early detection and prompt treatment of signs and symptoms of toxemia can almost always prevent deaths from this disease. PIH is classified as preeclampsia or eclampsia, depending on the symptoms (Fig. 16-1).

PREECLAMPSIA

The symptoms of preeclampsia are:

Elevated blood pressure (hypertension). Normally, the blood pressure does not become elevated during pregnancy. A rise of 30 mm Hg or more in the systolic pressure or 15 mm Hg or more in the diastolic pressure above the normal levels for a pregnant woman is considered to be a symptom of PIH. This means that a mother whose blood pressure normally is 110/80 mm Hg is considered to have a symptom of PIH if she

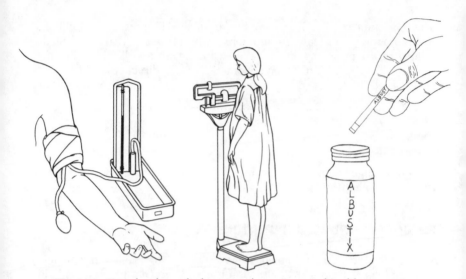

FIG. 16-1. *Tests for the early detection of pregnancy-induced-hypertension.*

has a blood pressure of 140/80, or 110/95, or 140/95 mm Hg, or higher. A blood pressure of 140/90 mm Hg for any pregnant woman is considered a sign of PIH unless she was known to have high blood pressure before she became pregnant. (Use of the rollover test to detect patients likely to develop hypertension late in pregnancy is discussed in Chapter 8).

Edema. The body tissues retain fluids to a greater extent during pregnancy than in the nonpregnant state, but in PIH this retention of fluids is increased even more. Retention of fluids may not be apparent at first, but it is suspected if the mother has a sudden, excessive weight gain. As the fluid in the tissues increases, it appears as swelling in the face, hands, or feet. Edema of the face may be first noticed as puffiness of the eyelids, while edema of the hands becomes apparent as the fingers become swollen. A ring that becomes uncomfortably tight may be the first indication of swelling that the mother notices.

Late in pregnancy, it is normal for the feet and ankles to become edematous by the end of the day. However, this swelling usually disappears after a good night's rest. If it does not disappear, it is an indication of PIH.

Albuminuria. The presence of albumin in the urine on two or more successive days is considered a symptom of PIH. Albumin may be present in varying amounts from a trace to 4+.

In severe preeclampsia one or more of the following is present:

The blood pressure is 160/110 mm Hg or higher, even though the mother is on bed rest.

The urine shows 3+ or 4+ albumin.

The edema is so extensive that pulmonary edema is present.

The urinary output is 400 ml or less in 24 hours.

ECLAMPSIA

The symptoms of eclampsia are the same as those of preeclampsia, but convulsions and coma are also present. Eclampsia occurs about once in every 500 to 800 deliveries. Eclampsia may occur during the antepartum period, during labor and delivery, or during the postpartum period (period immediately after delivery). Postpartum eclampsia occurs most often within the first 24 hours after delivery. The death rate in eclampsia is 10% to 15%.

TREATMENT

The treatment of preeclampsia depends on the severity of the symptoms. If there is only a slight elevation of blood pressure, and if this is the only symptom present, the physician may permit the mother to remain at home, having limited activity and spending most of her time in bed. When her blood pressure returns to normal, and if no other symptoms develop, she may resume her normal activities. However, the physician may want to see her at more frequent intervals so that he can detect the reappearance of symptoms early and institute appropriate treatment.

If more symptoms of PIH are present, or if the symptoms are more severe, the physician will probably hospitalize the mother. He will then prescribe treatment that may include the following:

Complete bed rest
Daily weight check
Fluid intake and output record
Blood pressure recorded every 4 hours
A balanced diet
Daily quantitative analysis of urine for albumin and microscopic analysis for casts
Sedatives
Antihypertensive drugs

Complete bed rest helps to lower the blood pressure by slowing metabolism. The patient's weight is a good indicator of the amount of fluid she is eliminating from her tissues. The record of her fluid intake and output informs the doctor of the balance between these two factors and helps him determine the efficiency of her kidneys. The blood pressure record and the findings of the urinalysis tell to what extent the mother is responding to treatment. The purpose of a well-balanced diet is obvious: the mother and fetus need an adequate supply of nutrients to meet the maintenance and growth needs of pregnancy.

Sedatives may be ordered to repress hyperactive reflexes and to forestall convulsions, especially if severe preeclampsia develops. Magnesium sulfate is most often used in these circumstances, but other sedatives may occasionally be used. Antihypertensive drugs such as hydralazine (Apresoline) may also be used in extreme cases as a temporary measure to reduce blood pressure and decrease the possibility of cerebrovascular accidents. However, the use of antihypertensive agents is somewhat controversial because of their possible adverse effects on the fetus, and their prolonged use is generally not recommended.

In the past, the physician probably would have recommended a restriction of salt intake, because salt tends to promote retention of fluid in the tissues. This practice is no longer considered valid, because it has been found that a drastic reduction in the salt intake reduces the circulating blood volume. This is particularly undesirable during pregnancy, when damage to both mother and fetus can result.

Certain problems may cause treatment of the mother with preeclampsia at home to be unsuccessful. The mother with mild preeclampsia usually does not feel ill, and it may be difficult for her to follow the physician's recommendation to stay in bed. In families with several small children, the mother may not be able to get the bedrest she needs.

Potential nursing diagnoses:

Knowledge deficit related to PIH and how it can affect her and the unborn child

Knowledge deficit related to the importance of following the physician's orders

Ineffective individual coping related to ability to carry on activities of daily living

Anxiety related to interruption of daily routines

Anxiety related to her health and that of her unborn child

Anxiety related to concern over care of her family while she is incapacitated

Potential for injury related to convulsions

Nursing interventions.   Often the nurse can help to obtain the cooperation of the mother by explaining the reason for the care and the importance of it. The mother with small children may be helped to obtain the rest she needs by having someone look after the children for a few hours each day. If this creates a problem financially, the services of a social worker may be needed to help find a solution. The mother must also be told to report to the doctor if she has headaches, visual disturbances, or swelling of the fingers or eyelids. The nurse who cares for the hospitalized mother with preeclampsia must carry out the physician's orders carefully. Because the mother needs rest and quiet, the nurse should do all that she can to relieve the mother of any worries that she may have.

A mother who is hospitalized with PIH should always be in a bed equipped with side rails, because of the possibility of convulsions and also because she is likely to be given sedatives. The side rails should be up to prevent her from getting out of bed. The mother is observed closely for signs indicating that she is about to have a convulsion, such as headache, epigastric pain, nausea and vomiting, and visual disturbances. The physician should be notified at once if a mother complains of any of these.

A tray or cart containing padded tongue depressors and emergency drugs should always be kept in the room of a mother with PIH. Should the mother convulse, the nurse should try to prevent her from biting her tongue by placing the padded tongue depressor between her teeth and should also try to prevent her from falling out of bed or otherwise hurting herself. Meanwhile, because the patient should never be left alone, the nurse should have called for assistance by using the call signal. The nurse should note the type of convulsion and how long it lasts.

The nurse should listen to the fetal heart tones at least four times a day and observe the mother for signs of labor. A mother who is sedated may be in labor without knowing it.

In cases of severe PIH, termination of the pregnancy may be necessary in order to save the life of the mother and the baby, sometimes causing the baby to be born prematurely. In such instances, the nursery must be alerted so that preparations can be made to care for the baby. Babies born of mothers with PIH may be sick and should be observed closely. They are given the same care that a premature infant is given, whether or not they are premature. After delivery, the symptoms of PIH gradually disappear. The mother must be observed closely for several days postpartum, however, since convulsions may occur after delivery as well as before.

PROBLEMS INVOLVING BLEEDING

The most frequent causes of hemorrhage during the first half of pregnancy are abortions and ectopic pregnancies. During the latter part of pregnancy, the most frequent causes are placenta previa and abruptio placentae.

ABORTION

Pregnancies that terminate before the age of viability are called abortions. The age of viability is considered to be 24 weeks' gestation, since the infant born at this time has some chance of survival if given expert care. Abortions are either spontaneous or induced.

Spontaneous abortion

A *spontaneous abortion* (miscarriage) is the termination of pregnancy without mechanical or medical intervention (*i.e.*, it occurs naturally). Approximately 10% of all pregnancies end in spontaneous abortion. Approximately 75% of spontaneous abortions occur before the 12th week of gestation.

Sometimes a woman may have three or more consecutive spontaneous abortions. This condition is known as *habitual* abortion.

Spontaneous abortions are often caused by defects in the sperm or ovum or defects in the intrauterine environment. They may also be due to maternal diseases, such as pneumonia and pyelitis; deficiencies of certain hormones, such as progesterone and thyroid; or an incompetent cervix. In many instances the cause of the abortion cannot be determined.

A spontaneous abortion is classified as:

Threatened
Inevitable
Incomplete
Complete
Missed

In a *threatened* abortion there is bleeding, sometimes accompanied by cramps or backache. In an *inevitable* abortion, the bleeding and cramps are accompanied by rupture of the membranes and dilatation of the cervix. In an *incomplete* abortion, part of the products of conception (the fetus) is expelled and part (the placenta) is retained. In a *complete* abortion, all the products of conception are expelled. In a *missed* abortion, the fetus dies but is retained for 2 months or longer before being expelled. In missed abortions the uterus stops growing and may become smaller due to absorption of the amniotic fluid and to maceration of the fetus.

Attempts are made to prevent threatened abortions by placing the mother on bed rest for 48 hours. The physician may also prescribe hormones to control the bleeding and muscle-relaxing drugs to relieve the cramps. If these measures are not effective within 48 hours, it is very likely that the mother will lose the fetus. If abortion does occur, the treatment depends on the situation.

In incomplete abortions, hemorrhage may be profuse, since the placenta may be partly separated and partly attached. Hemorrhage occurs because the uterus cannot contract and clamp off the bleeding vessels beneath the separated part of the placenta while part of the placenta is still attached to the uterus. A surgical operation called dilation and curettage (D & C) may be performed. In this operation, the cervix is dilated and curettage (scraping) of the uterus is done to remove the retained placenta and thus control the bleeding. When hemorrhage occurs, blood transfusions are prescribed. Antibiotics are prescribed if the mother develops an infection.

Abortions caused by an incompetent cervix may be prevented by a surgical procedure in which the cervix is reinforced with a purse-string suture. An incompetent cervix is one that starts to dilate when the fetus becomes large enough to place weight on it, usually between the fourth and sixth months of pregnancy. The purse-string suture may be removed when the mother goes into labor at term, or it may be left in place and a cesarean section done.

Diethylstilbestrol (DES) is a synthetic estrogen substance that was once frequently prescribed for women with threatened abortion. This practice has been largely discontinued because of the potential cancer-producing effect it may have on female offspring when taken by the mother during pregnancy, especially during the first 12 weeks of pregnancy.

Induced abortion

An *induced* abortion is the intentional termination of pregnancy before the age of viability (defined as 24 to 26 weeks' gestation). Induced abortions are *voluntary*, that is, the termination of the pregnancy is at the request of the pregnant woman.

Since the 1973 Supreme Court ruling, the decision for abortion during the first trimester has been left to the woman and her physician. After the first trimester, states have power to regulate the procedures and, after the age of viability, to prohibit abortion except when the mother's life or health is jeopardized.

Induced abortions may therefore be considered in 2 further categories. A *legal* abortion is the termination of pregnancy using medical means in an accredited medical facility. It is performed by qualified medical personnel. The liberalizing of the abortion laws has resulted in an increase in the number of legal abortions that are being done and in different methods of accomplishing them.

A *criminal* abortion is the deliberate termination of pregnancy without benefit of a qualified practitioner and/or in defiance of local laws. The danger to the mother's life from hemorrhage and infection is great because of the conditions under which criminal abortions are conducted.

In spite of the Supreme Court ruling, abortion is still a controversial issue. Each person is entitled to her or his own opinion and should respect the rights of others to theirs. Nursing and medical personnel who have moral or religious convictions about abortion should make their views known well in advance so that arrangements can be made for other personnel to provide care when this procedure is to be performed. Understanding, supportive care is needed by the woman having an abortion, and only personnel qualified and willing to provide such care should be involved in the procedure.

Before voluntary abortion is performed, the woman should be counseled regarding the risks involved, the possibility of continuing the pregnancy and placing the infant for adoption, and the use of contraceptive methods. Abortion is not a substitute for contraceptive methods. Women contemplating abortion should be counseled to do so during the first trimester because it is easier and safer then.

Methods for induced abortion

The method used for terminating pregnancy depends on the gestational age. During the first trimester, a D&C or suction curettage is usually performed. Either procedure can be done under local anesthesia or light general anesthesia as an outpatient procedure. The patient comes to the hospital or special facility the morning of the surgery, has the operation, is observed for bleeding for 2 or 3 hours after the procedure, and then, if no complications develop, is allowed to go home.

Suction curettage is a simple procedure in which a suction curette attached to an electrical pump is inserted into the uterus after the cervix has been dilated sufficiently with dilators (Fig. 16-2). Within seconds the uterine contents are aspirated into a container. These are labeled and sent to the pathology laboratory.

The dried stems of a seaweed *Laminaria digitata,* are sometimes used to dilate the cervix so that the uterus can be easily evacuated by curettage. The stems are prepared and packaged by size. After the length of the

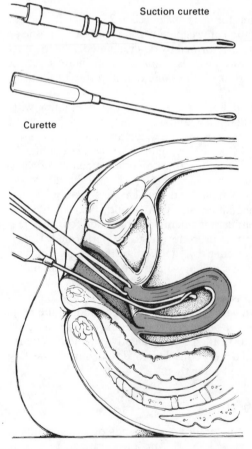

Suction curette

Curette

FIG. 16-2. *Curettage or vacuum aspiration for first trimester abortion.*

cervical canal has been determined, an appropriate-sized *Laminaria* stem is inserted so that the tip passes just beyond the internal os. The *Laminaria* stem absorbs fluid from the surrounding tissue and swells. As it swells it gradually dilates the cervix. Within a few hours the cervix is dilated sufficiently to permit passage of a curette and removal of the products of conception. Use of *Laminaria* stems is considered of value in preventing cervical lacerations.

After the first trimester, nonsurgical abortion may be performed by introducing a hypertonic saline solution or prostaglandins into the amniotic sac. These procedures are usually not done until after the 14th week of gestation, when a sufficient amount of amniotic fluid is produced to permit withdrawal of fluid before the solution or drug is injected. This is necessary to confirm proper placement of the needle.

When *saline injection* is to be done, the woman empties her bladder; then the abdomen is cleansed and a local anesthetic is injected at the site. A needle of proper length is inserted through the abdominal and uterine walls into the amniotic sac. Some amniotic fluid is withdrawn and a small amount of hypertonic saline is injected. If there is no adverse reaction, the remainder of the saline (usually 150 ml to 250 ml) is injected slowly. After several hours the patient goes into labor and the products of conception are expelled. The fetus is usually dead when delivered.

If labor does not occur, the saline injection can be repeated. If the second attempt fails, surgical removal by *hysterotomy* may be necessary. Hysterotomy is like a cesarean section except that the abdominal and uterine incisions are much smaller. Because of the danger of rupture of the scar during labor, patients who have had a hysterotomy and who subsequently become pregnant are delivered by cesarean section.

METHODS USED FOR INDUCED ABORTIONS

FIRST TRIMESTER

o D & C
o Suction curettage
o *Laminaria*

AFTER FIRST TRIMESTER

o Injection of hypertonic saline solution
o Prostaglandins
o Hysterotomy

RISKS ENCOUNTERED WITH ABORTIONS

o Hemorrhage
o Uterine perforation

- Cervical lacerations
- Infection
- Sterility
- Maternal death from: saline in maternal circulation; cardiac failure; septic shock; peritonitis; hemorrhage; disseminated intravascular coagulation; water intoxication
- Ruptured uterus

Saline injection for abortion is contraindicated in women who have:

A history of previous surgery involving the myometrium

Severe hypertension

Cardiac or renal disease

Severe anemia

Deaths due to entry of the hypertonic saline into the maternal circulation, cardiac failure, septic shock, peritonitis, hemorrhage, disseminated intravascular coagulation, and water intoxication have occurred following saline injection abortion.

Prostaglandins are chemical substances that occur naturally in the body and are capable of producing powerful contractions of smooth muscles. They may be administered intravaginally, intramuscularly, or intra-amniotically to empty the uterus.

When prostaglandins are to be injected intra-amniotically, the patient empties her bladder; then the abdomen is cleansed and a local anesthetic is injected at the site. A needle of proper length is inserted through the abdominal and uterine walls into the amniotic sac. A small amount of amniotic fluid is withdrawn to confirm proper location of the needle; then 5 ml of prostaglandins is injected slowly. If after 1 or 2 minutes there is no adverse reaction and amniotic fluid can still be aspirated, the remainder of the 40-mg dose is injected. A repeat dose of 20 mg may be given in 24 hours if abortion has not occurred. Nausea, vomiting, and diarrhea may occur with use of prostaglandins since they stimulate the smooth muscle of the gastrointestinal tract as well as the uterus.

Intramuscular injection of prostaglandins is sometimes used during the second trimester. This method is advantageous when the fetus has been dead for a long time and there is little or no amniotic fluid present.

Problems that may be encountered with the use of prostaglandins include nausea, vomiting, diarrhea, fever, delay in evacuation of the products of conception, hemorrhage, infection, and cervical lacerations, and fistula formation.

An intravenous infusion of an oxytocin solution may be administered to hasten the process when either saline injection or prostaglandins are used to induce abortion. This is a more concentrated solution of oxytocin than is used to induce labor at term. An oxytocin infusion is often administered after abortion to minimize bleeding.

Nursing assessment. The nurse caring for a woman having an abortion needs to recognize that abortion is an emotionally charged situation that involves not only the loss of the pregnancy but also potential risks to the life, health, and future reproductive capability of the woman. Many feelings are experienced when abortion is imminent: fear and guilt, whether the abortion is voluntary or spontaneous; failure and despair, if children are desired but repeated abortion has occurred; relief, if for some reason a child is not desired at this time (this is often followed by feelings of guilt and depression). The woman's partner may also experience deep feelings when abortion occurs. If the pregnancy has been greatly desired because children are wanted, the couple may experience a deep loss at the unexpected termination of the pregnancy before their hopes for a child have been realized. The nurse then must recognize the couple's need to go through the grieving process in order to cope and make a satisfactory recovery.

Potential nursing diagnoses:

Anxiety related to her own survival and the loss of the child

Potential for injury related to blood loss and Rh sensitization

Knowledge deficit related to abortion (causes, recurrences, etc.)

Disturbance in self-concept related to misplaced blame and responsibility for spontaneous abortion

Anxiety related to ability for future childbearing

Potential for dysfunctional grieving related to loss of a desired child

Anxiety related to abortion procedures

Nursing interventions. There may not be opportunity for the nurse and patient to become acquainted when spontaneous abortion is in progress or when voluntary abortion is scheduled. Therefore, the relationship of trust must be established in a situation that is moving rapidly and that is demanding of the nurse's time, knowledge, and skills. The nurse can project her caring and understanding through the tone of her voice, her touch, and her manner. This can be tremendously important to the woman.

In threatened abortion and inevitable abortion the nurse watches for signs, such as an increase in bleeding and cramping, that indicate that the cervix is dilating and that the products of conception may soon be expelled. In second trimester abortion, labor may be quite painful. The nurse can help lessen the pain by administering the analgesia prescribed by the physician, by rubbing the woman's back, and by staying with her and assisting her with breathing techniques to aid relaxation. Because surgical intervention is always a possibility, oral food and fluids are withheld until the uterus is emptied. Good oral hygiene should be maintained and the patient's lips should be kept moist if labor is prolonged. Privacy should be provided and opportunity given the woman to express her feelings about the abortion if she desires to do so.

In cases of missed abortion or induced abortion in which *Laminaria,*

prostaglandins, saline injections, oxytocin infusions, or surgical procedures are to be used, the nurse or physician should first explain to the
woman what is to be done and why, and what she can expect to happen. Some hospitals require written consent of the patient before these
procedures are performed. Obtaining this consent is usually the responsibility of the nurse. The nurse assembles the supplies, prepares the patient,
assists the physician, and, if general anesthesia is not used, provides continuous support to the woman during the procedure. After the procedure,
the nurse observes for hemorrhage and adverse reactions.

In spontaneous abortions, events may progress so rapidly that the
physician may not be present when the abortion occurs. The nurse then
must maintain a calm, confident manner while collecting the products of
conception in an appropriate receptacle. She should not leave the patient
alone at this time but, as soon as the immediate crisis is over and she has
determined whether or not the fetus and all of the placenta have been
expelled, she can leave the patient long enough to notify the physician. If
the abortion is incomplete, the physician will need to empty the uterus to
prevent excessive blood loss. This is done by curettage. The necessity for
this procedure should be explained to the woman, along with assurances
that she will be given medication for pain as necessary. The expelled
products of conception are placed in a container, labeled, and sent to
the pathology laboratory.

After the abortion the nurse carries out the physician's orders, which
may include administering an oxytocin infusion to minimize blood loss
and an injection of Rh_0 (D) immune globulin if the patient is Rh negative
(see below). The woman is given a bath, and perineal pads are applied.
Unless she is nauseated she can be given oral fluids. She is observed for
hemorrhage for 2 or 3 hours; then she may be discharged. If the physician
wants her to remain in the hospital overnight, she can be transferred to
a nonobstetrical unit.

HYDATIDIFORM MOLE

Hydatidiform mole is a benign neoplasm of the chorion in which the
chorionic villi become a mass of transparent vesicles filled with clear,
viscid fluid (Fig. 16-3). These vesicles resemble clusters of grapes. A fetus
is usually not present; however, when only some of the villi are involved,
there may also be a fetus.

A hydatidiform mole occurs about once in 2,000 pregnancies. The
pregnancy may appear normal at first, but then the uterus enlarges too
rapidly for the length of the gestation. Severe vomiting, bleeding, and PIH
may occur. The bleeding may vary from a small amount of dark brown
spotting to profuse hemorrhage. Some of the vesicles may be discharged
with the bleeding.

Treatment consists of removing the mole from the uterus. This may

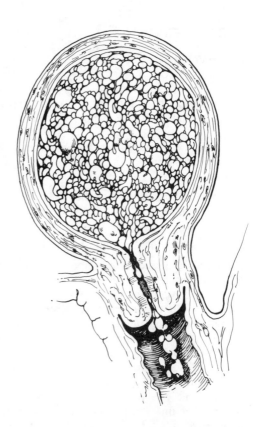

√ FIG. 16-3. *Hydatidiform mole.*

occur as a spontaneous abortion, or it may be achieved by stimulating the uterus with oxytocin or by dilating of the cervix and evacuating the uterus. In some instances, a hysterotomy or a hysterectomy may be performed.

The follow-up care includes tests to detect choriocarcinoma, a malignant growth that may develop after a hydatidiform mole. Blood serum is examined at frequent intervals to determine the amount of chorionic gonadotropin, a hormone produced in large amounts by hydatidiform moles and by choriocarcinoma. Normally the amount of chorionic gonadotropin in the serum steadily decreases following the removal of the mole; if the hormone level remains high over a prolonged period or increases, choriocarcinoma may be suspected. Because pregnancy also causes the production of chorionic gonadotropin, the woman may be advised against becoming pregnant until the follow-up studies for choriocarcinoma are negative. Chest x-ray studies may also be done periodically to find out if a malignancy from the uterus has metastasized to the lungs.

ECTOPIC PREGNANCY

Any pregnancy that occurs outside the uterine cavity is called an ectopic pregnancy. About 95% of ectopic gestations are located in the fallopian tubes. The others occur in the ovaries, horn of the uterus, cervix, and abdominal cavity. Ectopic pregnancies happen about once in every 100 to 200 deliveries. They occur more often in nonwhite women than in white women.

Ectopic pregnancies are caused by conditions that hinder or prevent the fertilized ovum from passing into the uterine cavity. Such conditions include:

Congenital abnormalities of the fallopian tubes
Kinking of the tubes due to adhesions resulting from infection
Chronic inflammation of the tubes
Tumors outside of the tube pressing on the tube

In ectopic pregnancy, the symptoms of pregnancy are present. As a result of hormone activity, amenorrhea is present and the uterus enlarges. As the pregnancy progresses, the area of the tube where the ovum has implanted becomes distended, causing the tube to rupture, usually by the 12th week of gestation. Rupture may be sudden or it may be a gradual tearing open of the tube. When it is sudden, the woman experiences a sudden, sharp, stabbing pain on the side of her abdomen and possibly extending to her shoulders. Because of the hemorrhage she appears very pale and may go into shock quickly; her abdomen is extremely tender, her blood pressure falls, and her pulse becomes very rapid. When the tube ruptures, hemorrhage into the peritoneal cavity occurs. There may or may not be vaginal bleeding. Prompt diagnosis and treatment are necessary to save the woman's life.

Gradual rupture of the tube results in mild symptoms. The woman feels continual pain in her abdomen. The bleeding is gradual and may not reach hemorrhagic proportions so that shock, a drop in blood pressure, and a rapid pulse may not be present.

✓ TESTS TO DIAGNOSE ECTOPIC PREGNANCY

○ **Beta-human chorionic gonadotropin (β-hCG).** Usually done on serum to determine hormone levels indicative of pregnancy.

○ **Ultrasound.** Performed to detect if a pregnancy is present in the uterus or a mass (swelling) on the tube or ovary that could be an ectopic pregnancy. It also shows if there is fluid in the cul-de-sac (area between the posterior wall of the uterus and the rectum. Bleeding from a ruptured ectopic pregnancy often collects in this space). It is possible to have an intrauterine pregnancy and an ectopic pregnancy at the same time.

○ **Culdocentesis.** A needle attached to a syringe is inserted into the cul-de-sac to aspirate any fluid there. Aspiration of more than 3 ml of unclotted blood is considered a positive sign of ectopic pregnancy if the pregnancy test is positive and ultrasound shows no intrauterine pregnancy. (Blood in the cul-de-sac may also be due to a hemorrhagic corpus luteum.)

o **Laparoscopy**. Performed to see if a tube has ruptured or if there is other evidence of ectopic pregnancy.

The treatment of ectopic pregnancy consists of surgical removal of the ruptured tube (salpingectomy) and blood transfusions to replace the blood loss. If the tube has not ruptured, the doctor may do a linear salpingostomy. In this procedure the anterior portion of the tube above the pregnancy is incised and the products of conception and the trophoblastic tissue are gently suctioned out. There is usually a good chance of successful pregnancy after this type of surgery. After an ectopic pregnancy the Rh-negative woman should be offered Rhogam.

Nursing assessment. The nurse looks for symptoms of hemorrhage and impending shock when assessing a woman suspected of having an ectopic pregnancy. (The nursing-care plan is outlined in Table 16-1.) These symptoms include pallor, a rapid, thready pulse, a drop in blood pressure, rapid respirations, air hunger, and cold, clammy skin. There may or may not be obvious vaginal bleeding. The nurse also notes the severity and location of pain: colicky pain on the affected side may be present in ruptured ectopic pregnancy. If these symptoms are present, immediate action must be taken to save the woman's life.

When the symptoms are less severe and the condition less life-threatening, the nurse needs to complete the data base. Information helpful to the physician in diagnosing an ectopic pregnancy includes the date of the patient's last menstrual period, past treatment for pelvic inflammatory disease, use of an intrauterine device (IUD) for contraception, history of a previous ectopic pregnancy, or history of previous voluntary or spontaneous abortions. These can all be factors in causing an ectopic pregnancy. The nurse also needs to find out the woman's religious affiliation because this may influence whether or not she wants the products of conception baptized and whether she will accept blood transfusions. The woman's Rh status should be determined so that she can be offered Rhogam if she is Rh negative.

PLACENTA PREVIA

In placenta previa the placenta is located near the internal os of the cervix instead of in the upper portion of the anterior or posterior wall of the uterus (Fig. 16-4). Placenta previa may be designated as central, partial, or marginal, depending on its relationship to the os. In a *central* placenta previa, also called complete or total placenta previa, the placenta completely covers the internal os. In *partial* placenta previa, the placenta covers part of the os. In *marginal* placenta previa, also called low implantation of the

TABLE 16-1 NURSING-CARE PLAN FOR ECTOPIC PREGNANCY

POTENTIAL NURSING DIAGNOSES	INTERVENTIONS	EXPECTED OUTCOME
	IMMEDIATE	
Knowledge deficit related to her condition and what is happening	Explain what is happening and what is being done; reassure patient	Understands condition and what is happening
Alterations in comfort: pain related to ectopic pregnancy	Give medication as ordered	Pain relieved
Potential for injury, weakness, shock related to blood loss	Record amount of blood loss; pad count; record vital signs every ½ hr; notify physician of excessive bleeding or abnormal vital signs; give blood transfusions as ordered; prepare for surgery	Blood loss controlled and corrected
	POSTOPERATIVE	
Knowledge deficit related to condition, causes, and chances of recurrence	Explain condition and causes; answer questions; explain chance of recurrence about 10%	Expresses understanding of condition, possible causes, and chances of recurrences
Potential for dysfunctional grieving related to loss of pregnancy	Allow patient to grieve; listen to her; arrange for clergy to visit if she wishes; allow family to stay with her if possible	Works through grief
Anxiety related to future fertility	Be honest; if this is first pregnancy, there is at least 50% chance she can have at least one normal pregnancy	Anxiety is relieved

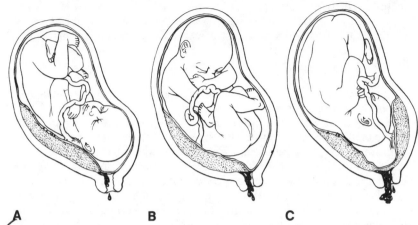

A   B   C

FIG. 16-4. *Placenta previa. (A) Marginal placenta previa. (B) Partial placenta previa. (C) Central (complete) placenta previa.*

placenta, the placenta is located near the os but does not cover any part of it.

Placenta previa is the most common cause of bleeding in the later months of pregnancy. It occurs approximately once in every 200 deliveries. It occurs most often when a mother has several pregnancies close together but rarely occurs in primigravidas.

Painless bleeding after the seventh month of pregnancy is the characteristic symptom of placenta previa. The bleeding is due to the separation from the uterus of the part of the placenta that is near or covering the internal os. As this separation occurs, the large vessels that were beneath that part of the placenta are left open. The amount of bleeding depends on how much of the placenta separates. The separation is due to the changes that normally occur in the cervix in preparation for labor.

Ultrasound scanning is considered the simplest, safest, and most accurate method of locating the placenta during pregnancy. With this method, it has been discovered that a low-lying placenta is present in 45% of pregnancies sometime during the second trimester. These placentas usually migrate upward toward the fundus later in pregnancy. When a low-lying placenta is detected, it is recommended that repeat ultrasound examinations be performed at 6- to 8-week intervals until the placenta has moved away from the cervix or the woman has delivered.

The physician decides whether the mother must be delivered immediately or whether to wait to see if the bleeding will stop. If the baby is small and the bleeding is not excessive, the physician may want to wait as long as is safely possible to give the baby more time to grow. He also decides whether to deliver the baby vaginally or by cesarean section. He prescribes blood transfusions and antibiotics as indicated. After delivery, the mother with placenta previa must be watched closely for hemorrhage, because the lower part of the uterus does not contract as well as the upper part to clamp off the open vessels where the placenta was implanted.

ABRUPTIO PLACENTAE

Abruptio placentae is the premature separation of a normally implanted placenta (Fig. 16-5). It occurs approximately once in every 250 deliveries; the cause is not known. All or only part of the placenta may separate.

Bleeding occurs at the site of the separation. If the separation occurs at the center of the placenta, the blood collects between the placenta and the wall of the uterus. In such instances, the blood does not pass out through the vagina; this is known as concealed bleeding. As the blood accumulates behind the placenta, the uterus becomes rigid and the abdomen becomes very tender and painful. There may be fetal distress or death, depending on the amount of bleeding.

If the separation occurs at the edges of the placenta—as it does in about 80% of cases—vaginal bleeding is present. In severe cases of abruptio placentae there may be hemorrhage into the muscles of the uterine wall. This interferes with the ability of the muscles to contract after delivery. Therefore, mothers who have abruptio placentae must be observed very closely for hemorrhage after delivery.

✓ GROUPS WITH AN INCREASED INCIDENCE OF ABRUPTIO PLACENTAE

- ○ Hypertensive women
- ○ Women in the lower socioeconomic group
- ○ Multigravidas, particularly gravidity over 5
- ○ Women with a history of reproductive loss (abortion, premature labor, prenatal hemorrhage, stillbirth, or neonatal death)
- ○ Women who have had a previous premature separation of the placenta

Abruptio placentae is most likely to occur among women with hypertension, those in the lower socioeconomic group, multigravidas (particularly gravidity greater than 5), those with a history of reproductive loss (abortion, premature labor, prenatal hemorrhage, stillbirth, or neonatal death), and those who have had a previous premature separation of the placenta. It is a leading cause of maternal death. In addition, about 15% of all perinatal deaths can be attributed to it. Approximately one third of the infants of women with this condition die, either from preterm birth or from intrauterine hypoxia. Of those that survive, some experience neurologic damage.

With abruptio placentae, as with placenta previa, the physician decides whether the mother must be delivered immediately or whether to wait.

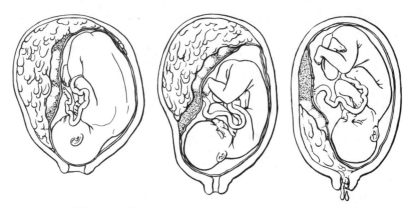

FIG. 16-5. *Abruptio placentae at various separation sites.*

This decision is based on the size of the fetus as well as the condition of the mother and the amount of bleeding present. Delivery by cesarean section may be necessary.

In the treatment of abruptio placentae, the physician usually prescribes blood transfusions to replace the blood loss. He may also prescribe antibiotics because excessive blood loss makes the mother very susceptible to infection.

DISSEMINATED INTRAVASCULAR COAGULATION

Disseminated intravascular coagulation (DIC) is a serious condition in which a coagulation defect prevents the blood from clotting. As a result, massive internal and external bleeding occurs. Although it is not known just where or how the blood clotting mechanism goes awry, certain stimuli can cause it to do so. These include bacterial debris or endotoxins, chemical and physical agents, anoxia, hemolytic processes, immune reactions, damage to the endothelium, and thrombocytopenia. DIC may occur in cases of abruptio placentae (most often), septic abortion, missed abortion when the fetus is retained for 5 weeks or longer, saline abortion, hydatidiform mole, ruptured uterus, amniotic fluid embolism, preeclampsia-eclampsia, and hemorrhagic shock. Immediate and effective treatment is absolutely essential to prevent death in this emergency.

Treatment consists of (1) transfusions of whole blood to maintain a hematocrit of 30% and intravenous infusions of Ringer's lactate to maintain a urinary output of 30 to 60 ml/hr; (2) transfusions of other blood components to supply additional clotting factors as necessary; (3) appropriate measures to correct the obstetric problem, such as delivery (vaginal or cesarean section) to remove the partially separated placenta, evacuation of the dead fetus in missed abortion, or evacuation of the infected fetal parts in septic abortion; (4) close observation of the patient's response to treatment with careful attention to the development of any secondary problems, such as kidney failure. This is a grave condition, and the prognosis depends on early diagnosis, prompt treatment, and restoration of the normal blood clotting process.

The nurse caring for a maternity patient with any obstetric problem should observe her closely to detect unusual bleeding. Excessive or persistent bleeding from slight injury, such as venipuncture, intramuscular or subcutaneous injection, nicks from shaving the perineum or abdomen, or insertion of a urinary catheter, as well as bleeding from the gums or nose, should be reported immediately to the physician, since this may be the first indication of a coagulation problem.

CERVICAL POLYPS

A polyp is a tumorlike growth with a pedicle or stem usually on a mucous membrane. Polyps situated at the external os of the cervix tend to bleed during the early part of pregnancy. Until the cause is diagnosed, this bleeding may be mistaken for threatened abortion. Bleeding from other lesions of the cervix may also occur in early pregnancy, especially after intercourse. However, lower abdominal pain and persistent low backache, which are present in threatened abortion, usually do not accompany bleeding from these causes.

MYOMAS

A myoma is a tumor of the muscle. Large myomas located beneath the endometrial surface of the uterine cavity may cause infertility by preventing implantation of the fertilized ovum. Myomas in the cervix or in the lower uterine segment may obstruct labor. Since myomas increase in size as pregnancy progresses, the uterus enlarges more rapidly than expected for the period of gestation. Following delivery, myomas decrease in size. Hemorrhagic infarction of a myoma occasionally occurs during pregnancy, causing pain and tenderness in the area, spotting, and sometimes a low-grade fever. Treatment consists of analgesia. A woman who has had surgical removal of a myoma of the uterus (myomectomy) before she became pregnant is usually delivered by cesarean section to prevent rupture of the scar during labor.

CARE OF PATIENTS WITH BLEEDING PROBLEMS

Nursing assessment. The nurse estimates the amount of bleeding that occurred before the mother arrived at the hospital by inspecting her clothing and the perineal pads and asking her to describe the bleeding she had. While the mother is in the hospital, the nurse keeps a close watch on the amount of bleeding that occurs. The number of pads used and the amount of saturation are noted and recorded on the chart. Excessive bleeding is reported to the doctor immediately.

The mother is observed for signs of shock, which include a lowering of the blood pressure and a weak, rapid pulse. If the gestation has reached 5 months or longer, the fetal heart tones are listened to at frequent intervals as ordered by the doctor. Slowing of the rate, irregularity, or absence of fetal heart tones should be reported to the doctor.

When bleeding is suspected or is present, the nurse never examines the mother to find out the dilatation of the cervix. Such an examination could cause severe hemorrhage.

The nurse must realize that emergency delivery by cesarean section may be necessary if bleeding becomes excessive; therefore, she must have everything in readiness for such an emergency. When pregnancy must be terminated before it has reached term, the nursery should be notified so that preparation can be made to care for the premature infant.

Potential nursing diagnoses:

Anxiety related to the bleeding

Fear related to her well-being and that of the baby

Anxiety related to care of her family while she is hospitalized

Anxiety related to finances

Knowledge deficit related to her condition

Alteration in comfort: pain related to internal bleeding

Nursing Interventions:

Maintain a calm attitude so as not to increase the mother's apprehension.

Be an understanding listener and encourage the mother to talk and express her feelings.

Be sensitive to the woman's feelings.

Estimate the amount of bleeding that occurred before the mother was admitted. Keep a pad count after she is admitted (the number of pads saturated in a given period of time). In some hospitals the pads are weighed to obtain a more accurate record of the amount of bleeding. If this is done, they should be weighed immediately after being removed, before they dry.

Watch for signs of shock. Take vital signs every 30 to 60 minutes until they stabilize, then every 2 to 4 hours.

Watch for signs of fetal distress. Listen to fetal heart tones each time mother's vital signs are taken. Fetal monitor can be used if available.

Be prepared by emergency delivery.

If care of her family is of concern and finances are worrying her, ask the hospital social worker to see her.

Explain her condition to her in terms she can understand. Be honest in discussing the possible outcome but positive in the availability of expert care for her and the baby.

Administer medication for pain relief in smallest doses possible if it is prescribed. The physician may not order analgesia because of the risk to the infant. Breathing techniques used for labor may be helpful. Reassurance through a positive attitude and permitting her spouse or support person to stay with her are also helpful. Explain why medication is not given.

✓INFECTIONS

TORCH

TORCH is the acronym for some of the most common infections that may be transmitted to the infant during the prenatal, intrapartum, and postpartum periods. It stands for:

T—Toxoplasmosis
O—Other: hepatitis B, syphilis, varicella, chlamydial infections
R—Rubella
C—Cytomegalovirus infections
H—Herpes simplex

TOXOPLASMOSIS

Toxoplasmosis is caused by a parasite, *Toxoplasma gondii.* The parasites are carried by cats, who get them from infected mice. People who take care of cat litter can get them through exposure to the contaminated feces of the cat. The parasites can be transferred from an infected mother through the placenta to the fetus.

✓Antibodies to *Toxoplasma gondii* can be detected through routine prenatal blood screening and through testing cord blood or a blood sample from the newborn at birth.

Although some infants of mothers with toxoplasmosis may not be affected, the risk to others may be life-threatening. Infants with toxoplasmosis may be born prematurely and may have intrauterine growth retardation, seizure disorders, hepatosplenomegaly, congenital defects such as chorioretinitis, microcephaly, or hydrocephalus, and cerebral calcifications.

The recommended treatment at the present time consists of pyrimethamine and sulfadiazine. Treatment during pregnancy is controversial since pyrimethamine, if given early in pregnancy, can cause abnormalities in the embryo. Sulfadiazine, which has a greater albumin-binding affinity than bilirubin, may result in such high bilirubin levels after birth that exchange blood transfusions may be necessary. Treatment of the newborn with these drugs is accompanied by folinic acid administration three times a week to prevent anemia. Although progression of the disease can be controlled with treatment, abnormalities and neurologic damage present when treatment is begun are not affected by the treatment.

CYTOMEGALIC INCLUSION DISEASE (CYTOMEGALOVIRUS INFECTION)

Cytomegalic inclusion disease (CID) results from infection by cytomegalovirus. Many adults have antibodies to this virus, and those who do not may manifest no clinical symptoms even though they have the virus. Therefore, it may be difficult to detect cytomegalovirus infection in a pregnant woman. However, detection may be very important to the welfare of the infant, since cytomegalovirus readily crosses the placental barrier and can infect the fetus, causing devastating results. Growth retardation, microcephaly, hydrocephalus, chorioretinitis with microphthalmia and blindness, mental retardation and other kinds of cerebral dysfunctions, as well as visceral and skeletal malformations are some of the problems caused by cytomegalovirus. Infected infants are usually born preterm and are small for gestational age. Soon after birth they may develop jaundice, petechiae, enlarged spleen and liver, dyspnea, and convulsions. Since there is no specific treatment against this virus, most of the infants die. Those who survive may develop the conditions mentioned above if they are not already so afflicted. Infected infants shed the virus and may infect others; they pose a special threat to the unborn infants of nonimmune pregnant women working in the nursery.

RUBELLA

Rubella, or German measles, is caused by a virus that usually produces a mild disease characterized by a rash. However, if a pregnant woman gets this disease during the first 12 weeks of gestation, the virus may cause congenital malformations in the infant. Such malformations include cataracts, heart lesions, deaf-mutism, and mental defects. At present, the value of giving γ-globulin to pregnant women as a prophylactic measure against rubella is questionable.

SEXUALLY TRANSMITTED DISEASES

Syphilis and gonorrhea. Syphilis and gonorrhea are diseases transmitted by sexual intercourse. In recent years the incidence of these diseases has increased to epidemic proportions in some areas. This may be due in part to the increased use of drugs, which has caused many women to turn to prostitution as a means of supporting their habit, and to the easy accessibility of contraceptives, which has made sexual activity outside of marriage less likely to result in pregnancy but may have caused a higher degree of exposure to venereal disease.

Untreated syphilis can cause infection and death of the fetus (see Chap. 20). Expectant mothers who receive antepartal care will receive appropriate treatment. The problem arises with those who do not receive care.

Gonorrhea can cause infection in the uterus and fallopian tubes, resulting in sterility due to mechanical blocking of the tubes. If pregnancy occurs in a woman who has gonorrhea, she may abort or the pregnancy may continue to term with no apparent problems attributable to the disease. Untreated or inadequately treated gonorrhea may result in gonorrheal infection of the infant's eyes (ophthalmia neonatorum) at birth. This may cause blindness unless prevented (see Chap. 11). Gonorrhea may spread rapidly in the mother following delivery because the organism can enter even slight tears in the cervix and vagina. It may then develop into puerperal fever. As with syphilis, the treatment of gonorrhea consists of adequate doses of penicillin or other antibiotics.

Herpesvirus hominis. There are two antigenic types of herpes virus: type I, which is responsible for most nongenital infections, and type II, which is responsible for most genital tract herpes infections. Type II is probably transmitted by sexual contact in most instances. Herpesvirus hominis type II is presently the second most common venereal disease (gonorrhea is the most common).

Herpesvirus hominis lesions are vesicular, ulcerative papules surrounded by a red areola. They may grow together and form large ulcerative blisters. The lesions may appear on the vulva, vaginal mucosa, or cervix. The incubation period is 3 to 7 days. The lesions usually last 3 to 6 weeks. In addition to the lesions, other symptoms the patient may have include dysuria, dyspareunia, pain, itching, and bilateral inguinal lymphadenopathy. The pain may radiate to the groin, buttocks, and thighs. These symptoms may be accompanied by chills, fever, headache, and general malaise.

When herpesvirus hominis type II occurs early in pregnancy, spontaneous abortion is likely. Infection of the infant *in utero* or at birth frequently results in death. If death does not occur, the infant usually has serious ocular and central nervous system damage. Because treatment of infected infants has been unsuccessful, great care must be taken to prevent exposure to the herpes virus. For this reason, cesarean section is being employed by many obstetricians in cases where the lesions are present on the cervix, vagina, or vulva and the membranes are still intact. If the membranes are ruptured, the chances are great that the infant has already been exposed to the herpes virus, and delivery by cesarean section would not be effective in prevention.

✓**AIDS.** One of the newer sexually transmitted diseases is the acquired immunodeficiency syndrome (AIDS). AIDS is a deadly disease for which there is no known cure at this time. It is caused by the human immunodeficiency virus (HIV). HIV stimulates the production of antibodies that can be detected in the blood of an infected person. The virus is passed from one person to another through blood and through body secretions: semen, saliva, vaginal secretions, drainage from open lesions, and the like. The virus destroys the body's immune system. Because the immune system is the body's main defense against infection, when it is weakened or destroyed, organisms can invade and destroy the body.

Anyone can get AIDS, but those at greatest risk are homosexual males, intravenous drug users, and, until recently, recipients of blood transfusions. A new process to treat blood and blood products has reduced the risk of getting AIDS by receiving blood and blood products. Others at risk for AIDS are heterosexuals with many sex partners and those who have only one sex partner, but that partner is an active bisexual. Women with AIDS can transmit it to the infant *in utero,* during birth, and after birth.

Use of condoms by homosexuals, bisexuals, and heterosexuals with multiple sex partners or maintaining a single-partner heterosexual lifestyle are recommended to avoid AIDS. When caring for AIDS patients, the nurse can protect herself and others by frequent handwashing and by giving special attention to the drainage and secretions of the patient as well as to contaminated needles and syringes. The nurse should further protect herself by wearing gloves when drawing or handling blood or body secretions such as urine.

PYELONEPHRITIS

During pregnancy hormonal action and pressure from the enlarging uterus cause dilatation of the renal calices, pelves, and ureters. The decreased tone and peristalsis of these structures which then occurs causes stasis of urine. Stasis of urine increases the susceptibility to infection. Consequently, pyelonephritis is one of the most common medical complications of pregnancy.

Symptoms of pyelonephritis include chills, fever, urinary frequency, dysuria and pain, and tenderness in the kidney region. Uterine irritability frequently accompanies these symptoms and may be mistaken for premature labor unless urine cultures are done. Women with these symptoms are usually hospitalized for treatment. A clean catch urine sample is obtained for culture and sensitivity so that an appropriate antimicrobial agent can be prescribed to combat the causative organism. *Escherichia coli* is the organism most often cultured from the urine. An accurate record of the patient's fluid intake and output is kept so that she receives the necessary fluids which are essential to her recovery. If she is unable to retain fluids by mouth, parenteral administration is necessary.

Although recovery usually occurs with appropriate therapy, infection may recur at any time since the conditions favoring it persist throughout pregnancy. Conditions favorable to urinary tract infection are also present during the puerperium as a result of trauma to the bladder base during labor and delivery and because the capacity of the bladder increases following delivery while its tone is temporarily decreased. The increased capacity and decreased tone can result in urinary retention and residual urine, which promote stasis of urine.

HEPATITIS

Hepatitis may be caused by ingestion or parenteral administration of material infected by the two distinct viruses that cause this disease. These viruses, commonly referred to as hepatitis A and hepatitis B, may also be transmitted by kissing and sexual contact. Another virus, called hepatitis

C by some, has been found to be the most common cause of hepatitis in persons receiving multiple transfusions of blood or blood products.

Immune globulin preparations for preventing type A and type B hepatitis are available and are recommended for pregnant women who are exposed to hepatitis or who must travel in places where the disease is epidemic. Infants born to mothers with hepatitis should be given immune globulin appropriate for the virus immediately after birth to prevent them from developing the disease. Infants of mothers with hepatitis should not be breast-fed, since the virus can be transmitted through the milk and through serum from cracks in the nipples.

Early diagnosis and prompt treatment of hepatitis in pregnancy are necessary to protect the life and health of mother and fetus. This is not easy in early pregnancy, however, since nausea and vomiting, which are the early symptoms of hepatitis, may be mistakenly thought to be due to the pregnancy. The treatment of hepatitis consists of hospitalization, bed rest, a good diet, and, if vomiting is a problem, intravenous administration of fluids, electrolytes and calories.

Abortion, prematurity, maternal mortality, and the risk of the infant's becoming infected *in utero*, at birth, or following birth are possibilities when hepatitis occurs during pregnancy.

✓ INFLUENZA AND PNEUMONIA

In uncomplicated influenza during pregnancy the prognosis is good. If pneumonia develops, the condition immediately becomes serious. Antibiotics are not effective against the virus of influenza but are beneficial in treating bacterial pneumonia. When an epidemic of influenza due to a specific strain of virus is anticipated, immunization of the pregnant woman with a killed or attenuated virus vaccine is recommended.

TUBERCULOSIS

Authorities differ in their opinions regarding the effect pregnancy has on tuberculosis. Some believe that pregnancy has no effect while others believe that it aggravates the disease and therefore should not be considered except by patients in whom the condition is arrested. The effect tuberculosis has on pregnancy is considered minimal since abortion, prematurity, and stillbirths are rarely caused by it and it is seldom acquired by the fetus *in utero*.

Careful medical and obstetric supervision is indicated during pregnancy whether the disease is active or latent. This is so treatment can be initiated if latent lesions become active. In active tuberculosis, treatment can usually be on an outpatient basis using the antituberculosis drugs streptomycin, isoniazid (INH), and para-aminosalicylic acid (PAS). Usually labor and delivery can be conducted normally for tuberculosis patients, although inhalation anesthesia is not used. Breast-feeding is not recommended even in inactive cases.

The physician caring for pregnant women is in a key position to detect tuberculosis since he sees people who otherwise might not be visiting a physician. Many obstetricians prescribe tuberculin skin tests for their patients as a means of tuberculosis screening. Positive tests are followed by chest x-ray studies.

OTHER PROBLEMS

PREMATURE LABOR

The spontaneous termination of pregnancy after the age of viability but before term is known as premature labor. Among the known causes of premature labor are hypertensive vascular disease, abruptio placentae, placenta previa, untreated syphilis, multiple pregnancy, and congenital abnormalities. In about one half of premature labors; the cause is unknown. Premature birth is the leading cause of death among newborns during the first 4 weeks of life.

Nursing interventions. The nurse caring for the mother in premature labor should spend as much time with her as possible. She should make the mother as comfortable as possible and help her to relax; this will reduce her need for medication for pain relief, which is important, since the doctor usually does not want a mother in premature labor to have analgesia. Analgesic medication could cause the baby to have difficulty breathing at birth. It may be necessary for the nurse to explain this to the mother. The mother is usually cooperative when she understands why she is not given medication for pain relief, especially if she knows that all possible measures are being taken to promote her comfort.

By staying with the mother, the nurse provides opportunity for her to express her feelings and to ask questions. Because she does not understand what has caused her to have premature labor, the mother may blame herself, thinking it is due to something she has done, and her husband may also share these feelings. The guilt feelings that result can often be relieved by simple explanation by an intelligent and understanding nurse. These mothers are usually concerned for the welfare of the baby; the nurse, naturally, wants to reassure them, but she must be careful not to hold out false hopes.

When a mother is admitted in premature labor, the nursery should be notified so that preparations can be made to take care of the baby.

HYPEREMESIS GRAVIDARUM

Many pregnant women experience nausea and vomiting upon arising in the morning during the early weeks of pregnancy. Vomiting that persists and occurs several times a day is called *hyperemesis gravidarum* or pernicious vomiting. The causes are believed to be both organic and psychic. The organic causes include the endocrine and metabolic changes normally brought about by pregnancy and the decreased motility of the stomach. Fragments of chorionic villi that get into the mother's circulation might also cause nausea and vomiting. Psychically, hyperemesis may be a form of neurosis; that is, it may be due to a functional disturbance of the patient's psyche caused by a mental and emotional upset at the realization that she is pregnant.

Severe cases of hyperemesis are rare. Vomiting that persists over a prolonged period may cause symptoms of dehydration, such as decreased urinary output, dry skin, rapid pulse, and low-grade fever. Symptoms of starvation may also develop. These include a weight loss of 10 to 20 lb, the presence of acetone and diacetic acid in the urine, an increase of nonprotein nitrogen, uric acid, and urea in the blood, and a decrease in the chlorides in the blood. These changes in the urine and blood chemistry are due to incomplete combustion of fat products, which occurs when fat is burned in the absence of carbohydrate. The body burns its reserves of fat when it lacks carbohydrates and other nutrients.

Treatment. The treatment of hyperemesis consists of hospitalizing the patient; restricting visitors, including the husband, for 24 hours to remove any unfavorable environmental influences; omitting food and fluids by mouth for 24 hours to provide rest for the gastrointestinal system; providing intravenous fluids and electrolytes to prevent dehydration and to maintain electrolyte balance; and providing sedatives and psychotherapy to combat the neurosis.

After 24 hours, small feedings of dry toast, crackers, or cereal are given every 2 or 3 hours; small amounts of fluids, such as hot tea or ginger ale, are given on alternate hours. If vomiting does not occur, the feedings are gradually increased until a regular, high-vitamin diet is being given.

Nursing interventions. The nurse caring for the patient with hyperemesis should maintain a cheerful, optimistic attitude and exercise patience, tact, and understanding. She must never let the patient feel that she thinks it is "all in her head." The nurse must keep an accurate record of the intake of fluids and the output of vomitus and urine. Discussion of food should be avoided, because this may nauseate the patient. For the same reason, it is usually best to keep the emesis basin out of sight.

RH INCOMPATIBILITY

As part of antepartal care, every pregnant woman should be tested to determine her Rh factor (see Chap. 8). If she is Rh negative, her husband's Rh should be determined also. If he is Rh negative as well, there will be no problem because all of their children will be Rh negative. If he is Rh positive, there is a possibility that some of their children will be Rh negative and some will be Rh positive, since each parent carries two genes for the Rh factor. The Rh-positive gene is dominant; the Rh-negative gene is recessive. Consequently, any time there is an Rh-positive gene present, the individual is Rh positive even though he may also have one

Rh-negative gene. To be considered Rh-negative, both genes for the Rh factor must be negative.

When an individual has two of the same kind of genes for a trait, such as two Rh-negative genes, he is *homozygous* for that trait. When he has one dominant and one recessive gene for a certain trait, he is *heterozygous*. The offspring of one Rh-negative parent (homozygous recessive) and one parent homozygous Rh-positive will be heterozygous Rh positive (that is, they will have one dominant Rh-positive gene and one recessive Rh-negative gene). However, the offspring of one Rh-negative parent and one heterozygous Rh-positive parent will have a 50:50 chance of being Rh positive and a 50:50 chance of being Rh negative.

The possibility of a problem due to Rh incompatibility arises only when an Rh-negative woman married to an Rh-positive man carries an Rh-positive fetus. The problem arises because some of the Rh-positive red blood cells from the fetus cross the placental barrier and enter the maternal circulation. These Rh-positive red blood cells become antigens and stimulate the formation of antibodies against Rh-positive cells. Since these Rh-positive cells from the fetus usually do not enter the mother's bloodstream until the end of pregnancy or at birth when the placenta is delivered, and because it takes time for a sufficient quantity of antibodies to be produced to cause a problem, the first child is usually not affected.

Once antibodies are produced in the mother's bloodstream, she always has them. In subsequent pregnancies with Rh-positive fetuses, some of these antibodies cross the placental barrier and enter the circulation of the fetus. There they attack and destroy the red blood cells of the fetus. This destruction of fetal red blood cells can result in anemia, and, in severe cases, in death of the fetus. When these conditions occur as a result of Rh incompatibility, the infant is said to have *erythroblastosis fetalis* (see Chap. 20).

An Rh-negative woman who has produced antibodies against Rh-positive red blood cells is said to be *sensitized* or *isoimmunized*. (She may also become sensitized by receiving a blood transfusion with Rh-positive blood.) Not all Rh-negative women who have given birth to an Rh-positive infant produce antibodies against Rh-positive red blood cells. However, because of the grave danger to the child when she does, each Rh-negative woman who has given birth to an Rh-positive child should be tested in each subsequent pregnancy for the detection of antibodies. This antibody titer test is usually done early in pregnancy and repeated at intervals if it shows the titer rising. If the titer shows that no antibodies are being produced, there is no danger to the fetus. If the titer shows that antibodies are being produced at a rapid rate, the physician may wish to terminate the pregnancy in order to save the baby unless the baby is considered too immature to survive outside the uterus. In that case he may elect to continue the pregnancy and give the infant a transfusion while it is still in the uterus.

Before an intrauterine transfusion is given, samples of amniotic fluid are withdrawn through a trocar inserted through the mother's abdomen into the uterus (amniocentesis). This fluid is studied to find out how severely the fetus is affected. If indicated, transfusion is then accomplished by passing Rh-negative packed cells through a fine tubing that has been passed through the mother's abdomen and uterus into the peritoneal cavity of the fetus. The fetus absorbs the packed cells from the peritoneal cavity into the bloodstream (Fig. 16-6).

Prevention of sensitization. Following the birth of an Rh-positive infant, the unsensitized Rh-negative mother is given a 1-ml intramuscular dose of *Rh$_o$ (D) immune globulin (human)*, a specially prepared γ-globulin that contains a concentration of Rh-positive antibodies. This product is marketed under several trade names, including RhoGAM, Gamulin Rh, and D-Immune. It acts by combining with, and thereby neutralizing, any Rh-positive red blood cells that may have crossed over from the fetal circulation into the maternal circulation. Neutralizing the antigen (Rh-positive cells) prevents the formation of antibodies against Rh-positive cells, and the danger of the next fetus having Rh incompatibility with subsequent erythroblastosis is eliminated. To be effective, the injection must be given within 72 hours after birth so that any Rh-positive cells that may have entered the mother's circulation will not have had time to stimulate antibody formation in the mother.

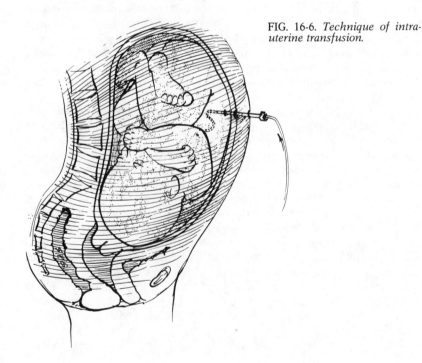

FIG. 16-6. *Technique of intrauterine transfusion.*

Although the usual dosage is 1 ml, on very rare occasions larger doses are indicated because of a transplacental hemorrhage of fetal blood into the mother's circulation. When this occurs, special tests are done to determine the amount of fetal cells in the maternal circulation, and dosage is then calculated accordingly.

This product is of no benefit to Rh-negative women who are already sensitized, and it is effective for only one pregnancy at a time. This means it must be given following *each* pregnancy in which an Rh-positive infant is born to an unsensitized Rh-negative mother. It should also be given to unsensitized Rh-negative women following abortions, ectopic pregnancies, and stillbirths, even though the Rh of the fetus may not be known. It is anticipated that by this means, problems arising from Rh incompatibility will eventually be nonexistent. Current research in this area is directed toward the development of a vaccine that need be given only once to afford protection against Rh incompatibility in all pregnancies of the same woman.

DIABETES

There are two general classifications of diabetes depending on the time of onset: *juvenile* diabetes, with onset during the growing years before the age of 20; and *adult* diabetes, with onset after age 20. The most widely used classification of diabetes is according to age at onset, duration, and vascular involvement.

Diabetes Classification

Class A Glucose tolerance test diabetics

Class B Onset: after age 20
      Duration: 0 to 9 years
      Vascular disease: none

Class C Onset: age 10 to 19 years
      Duration: 10 to 19 years
      Vascular disease: none

Class D Onset: before age 10
      Duration: 20 + years
      Vascular disease: calcification in legs, retinitis

Class E Patients with calcified pelvic vessels

Class F Patients with nephritis

There is also a diabetes classification specific to pregnancy: *gestational* diabetics are those whose diabetes is first diagnosed during pregnancy, and *pregestational* diabetics are those who were known diabetics before becoming pregnant.

Care during pregnancy. Pregnancy affects diabetes, and diabetes affects pregnancy. The care pregnant diabetics receive is vital to the health and life of the mother and fetus. This care is usually provided by a health team composed of the obstetrician, internist, nurse, nutritionist, and pediatrician. Until the 28th week, the pregnant diabetic patient is seen every 2 weeks by her obstetrician and every 2 weeks by her internist. The visits are scheduled alternately so that she is seen every week by one or the other. After the 28th week she is seen every week by both physicians.

Control of diabetes during pregnancy may be accomplished by diet alone, as in some gestational diabetics, or by administration of insulin. Oral medication to control diabetes is not recommended during pregnancy since its effect on the fetus has not been determined. During the first 2 or 3 months of pregnancy, when the fetus is utilizing much of the maternal glucose, the insulin dosage may remain the same as it was before pregnancy. As pregnancy progresses, the insulin dosage usually increases, often by as much as four times the prepregnancy dose. When a large dose is required, it is usually divided so that part is given in the morning and part in the evening.

The diet of the pregnant diabetic is of great importance, since she must receive adequate nutrients for herself and the fetus and at the same time keep the diabetes under control. The nurse and nutritionist need to obtain the cooperation of the patient in planning her diet so that she will follow it. The patient's weight and activities must be considered in assessing her caloric needs. Generally a 2,200-calorie diet with 1 to 1.5 g of protein per kg of body weight is adequate for a patient of average weight.

The length of time a patient has had diabetes and how well the diabetes is controlled appear to be the most important factors in determining the effect diabetes has on the pregnancy. The longer a patient has been a diabetic and the less controlled the diabetes, the more severely affected the pregnancy will be. Gestational diabetics and controlled mild, adult diabetics (Classes A and B) may go through pregnancy with few or no complications.

Fetal effects.   Diabetes tends to affect the vascular system, particularly the small blood vessels. When the vessels in the placenta are affected, placental insufficiency may result. When the placental insufficiency is marked, fetal death may occur. Although diabetics generally have large for gestational age (LGA) babies, those born to mothers with vascular involvement may be small for gestational age (SGA). Fetal death may also result from fetal acidosis due to ketosis in uncontrolled maternal diabetes. In uncontrolled diabetics, PIH and hydramnios (excessive amount of amniotic fluid) are frequent complications. Some 15% to 20% of the babies born to these mothers are either born dead or die within the first 4 weeks of life. Congenital abnormalities are common among offspring of diabetics whose diabetes is poorly controlled.

Management of delivery.   The timing and method of delivery of the diabetic mother are decisions the physicians on the team must make. The timing of delivery depends on such factors as the severity of the diabetes, the condition of the fetus, and whether the patient has a history of a previous fetal death *in utero.* Many gestational diabetics and others who are well controlled may be allowed to continue to term if there are no fetal indications for delivery. Uncontrolled or poorly controlled diabetics may need to be delivered as soon as the lecithin/sphingomyelin (L/S) ratio indicates fetal pulmonary maturity. This is usually between 36 and 38 weeks' gestation but may be as early as 32 to 34 weeks. The oxytocin challenge test (OCT) and estriol levels are done at frequent intervals to determine the well-being of the fetus (see Chap. 9). A positive OCT accompanied by falling estriol levels indicates that the fetus is in jeopardy and delivery should be accomplished. If a patient has a history of fetal death *in utero*, the physician may elect to terminate this pregnancy several days prior to the gestational age of the previous fetal loss.

The method of delivery for diabetic mothers depends on:

Whether she had a cesarean section previously
The condition of the fetus
The size of the baby and the mother's pelvis
Whether the cervix is favorable

If the patient has had a previous cesarean section, or if the fetus is in distress or is too large for the mother's pelvis, delivery will be by cesarean section. If these conditions do not exist and the cervix is favorable, that is, soft and partially or completely effaced, the physician may decide to induce labor and deliver the baby vaginally.

HEART DISEASE

About 1% of pregnant women have some form of heart disease. Congenital heart disease is currently the leading type of heart disease seen among pregnant women. It replaces rheumatic heart disease, which was the leading type for years but which now, as a result of effective treatment of rheumatic fever, is seen less frequently.

The pregnant woman with heart disease should be under the care of a cardiologist as well as an obstetrician. She should see her obstetrician every 2 weeks throughout her pregnancy so that signs of early heart failure can be detected immediately. She must get plenty of rest and avoid activities that can cause shortness of breath and fatigue. This means at least 10 hours of sleep each night and a half-hour nap after each meal. She should not lift heavy objects or climb stairs. Someone else may have to do the housework and care for the children so that the mother can get the needed rest.

Respiratory infections are very dangerous for the pregnant woman with heart disease. Therefore, she should avoid exposure to persons with colds and sore throats. If she gets a cold or sore throat, the doctor should be notified so that treatment can be started at once. Excessive weight also places an additional strain on the heart, so it is important that the mother follow a carefully planned dietary program, which may include limiting the amount of salt used in her diet.

Nursing assessment. During labor, the patient with heart disease should be observed closely. Her pulse and respirations should be counted every half hour during first stage labor, and every 10 minutes during the second stage. A pulse rate of 100 or higher, accompanied by rapid respirations, while the patient is resting in bed, should be reported to the doctor. Oxygen should be readily available. To minimize the exertion of pushing during second stage labor, the baby is usually delivered by low forceps. Following delivery, the mother usually remains in bed for several days. She resumes her normal activities gradually as her condition permits.

CLINICAL REVIEW

ASSESSMENT. Mrs. W. is a 23-year-old gravida 5. Her four children range in age from 6½ years to 13 months. Early one morning, during her eighth month of pregnancy she was admitted to the hospital because of bleeding. Her husband accompanied her. She stated that she had been awakened by a sudden gush of fluid. She thought her "water had broken" but when she got out of bed she discovered it was blood. She called her doctor and he told her to come to the hospital. There had been no bleeding since the firsh gush. Mrs. W. was in the hospital 3 days, during which time there was no bleeding. Then she was discharged.

Two weeks later, about noon, she was readmitted with another episode of bleeding. She seemed very upset. She stated she had been unable to contact her husband, who was at work, so she had asked a neighbor to bring her to the hospital. The bleeding had started while she was preparing lunch for her children. She hoped the neighbor would feed the children and look after them until her husband could be reached. He would take the children across town to her mother.

The two pads she wore were saturated with bright blood. The doctor ordered blood typed and cross-matched, hematocrit, and complete bed rest. Her hematocrit was 35%. The nurse checked her blood pressure, pulse, and fetal heart tones every hour. The nurse noted that Mrs. W. was saturating a pad every half hour. She reported this to the doctor. He decided to do a cesarean section as soon as the operating room was ready. Mr. W. arrived a few minutes before Mrs. W. was delivered, by cesarean section, of a 5-lb (2268-g) baby girl. The doctor stated that Mrs. W.'s bleeding was due to a complete placenta previa. Mother and baby did well.

1. Using the above information, prepare a care plan for Mrs. W., including nursing diagnoses, goals, and interventions.
2. Why did the doctor order blood typed and cross-matched? Why is it important to find out the hematocrit?
3. How might the nurse know if the baby was affected by the bleeding?
4. What changes in the blood pressure and pulse should be reported to the doctor?

BIBLIOGRAPHY

Bahr JE: Herpesvirus hominis type 2 in women and newborns. Am J Maternal-Child Nurs 3:16, 1978
Bush JJB: Protocol for tuberculosis screening in pregnancy. J Obstet Gynecol Neonatal Nurs 15:225, 1986

DeVore N, Baldwin K.: Ectopic pregnancy on the rise. AJN 86(6):674–678, 1986

Jensen MD, Bobak IM: Maternity Care: The Nurse & The Family, 3rd ed, pp 148–165, 887–903, 946–963. St. Louis, CV Mosby, 1985

Loveman A, Colburn V, Dobin A: AIDS in pregnancy. J Obstet Gynecol Neonatal Nurs 15:91, 1986

Neidhardt A: Why me? Second trimester abortion. AJN 86(10):1133–1135, 1986

Pritchard JA, MacDonald PC, Gant NF: Williams Obstetrics, 17th ed, pp 389–433, 467–488, 525–556, 580–584, 589–604, 613–614, 622–630. New York, Appleton-Century-Crofts, 1985

Reeder SR, Martin LL: Maternity Nursing, 16th ed, pp 731–805. Philadelphia, JB Lippincott, 1987

White P: Pregnancy and diabetes, medical aspects. Med Clin North Am 49:1019, 1965

high-risk parents 17 and infants

BEHAVIORAL When the goals of this chapter are reached, the student will
OBJECTIVES be able to:

o *Define "high risk."*

o *Explain how the age, socioeconomic status, and marital status of an expectant mother can qualify her as high risk.*

o *Discuss the significance of antepartal care in relation to high risk.*

o *Select three or four disease conditions and explain how they can endanger the health or life of the mother or fetus.*

o *Explain how each of the following may jeopardize pregnancy outcome: PIH, Rh incompatibility, genetic abnormalities, hemorrhagic complications.*

o *List three or four problems that may be associated with high parity.*

o *Describe a high-risk situation in which both parents are involved.*

o *Discuss three or four ways of approaching a solution to the problem of high risk.*

o *Discuss the recommendations of the American Medical Association and the American College of Obstetricians and Gynecologists for the detection and care of high-risk parents and infants.*

In the past several years, "high risk" has become a familiar phrase in maternity care. The use of this term alerts personnel to the existence of a real or potential problem that could endanger the life, health, or well-being of the infant, mother, or father. Among the general population of parents and infants, certain groups have been identified as having a higher incidence of morbidity and mortality. Certain conditions have also been recognized as posing a threat to life and health. When any one of these is present, the term "high risk" is applied. Some risk situations refer to the mother, others apply to both parents. Several scoring systems have been devised that use information from the patient's history and pregnancy to establish a risk likelihood. However, the most frequently used system has been that developed by Hobel and co-workers (Table 17-1).

INDICATIONS OF HIGH RISK

EPIDEMIOLOGIC FACTORS

Age

The age of the mother at the time of conception has an effect on her own health and well-being and that of her unborn child. Reproductive safety seems to be greatest when the mother is between 20 and 24 years of age. Maternal death rates and perinatal mortality are higher when the mother is younger than 20 years, and both rise steadily as the age of the mother increases beyond 24 years. Maternal mortality for women giving birth when they are between 40 and 45 years of age is six times greater than for women who are 20 to 24 years old. In addition, women over 40 years of age have a higher incidence of infants born with abnormalities, particularly Down's syndrome. The perinatal death rate is highest in mothers who are 15 to 19 or over 35 years of age.

Socioeconomic status

The socioeconomic status is of tremendous importance as a major social condition affecting the total being and environment of individuals and families. It influences the nutrition, education, housing, and parity of expectant mothers as well as their attitudes toward medical care. Since adult height and physique may depend on the nutrition and socioeconomic environment of individuals during the gestational and childhood periods, the importance of socioeconomic status of families is apparent. Women of short stature in the low-income group have been found to have more preeclampsia, more cesarean sections, a higher rate of prematurity, and higher perinatal death rates. Women from the low-income group usually have completed fewer grades in school, are more likely to live in substandard housing and to have higher parity, and are less likely to seek medical care during pregnancy than women from the higher income

TABLE 17-1 PREGNANCY RISK FACTORS

A. PRENATAL FACTORS	SCORE
1. Moderate to severe PIH	10
2. Chronic hypertension	10
3. Moderate to severe renal disease	10
4. Severe heart disease, Class II–IV	10
5. History of eclampsia	5
6. History of pyelitis	5
7. Class I heart disease	5
8. Mild toxemia	5
9. Acute pyelonephritis	5
10. History of cystitis	1
11. Acute cystitis	1
12. History of PIH	1

B. INTRAPARTUM FACTORS	SCORE
1. Moderate to severe PIH	10
2. Hydramnios or oligohydramnios	10
3. Amnionitis	10
4. Uterine rupture	10
5. Mild PIH	5
6. Premature rupture of membrane > 12 hr	5
7. Primary dysfunctional labor	5
8. Secondary arrest of dilation	5
9. Demerol > 300 mg	5
10. $MgSO_4$ > 25 g	5
11. Labor > 20 hr	5
12. Second stage > 2½ hr	5
13. Clinical small pelvis	5
14. Medical induction	5
15. Precipitous labor < 3 hr	5
16. Primary cesarean section	5
17. Repeat cesarean section	5
18. Elective induction	1
19. Prolonged latent phase	1
20. Uterine tetany	1
21. Pitocin augmentation	1

C. NEONATAL FACTORS	SCORE
1. Prematurity < 2000 g	10
2. Apgar at 5 min < 5	10
3. Resuscitation at birth	10
4. Fetal anomalies	10
5. Dysmaturity	5
6. Prematurity 2000–2500 g	5
7. Apgar at 1 min < 5	5
8. Feeding problem	1
9. Multiple birth	1

(Avery GB: Neonatology, 2nd ed. Philadelphia, JB Lippincott, 1981. Adapted from Hobel DH, et al: Am J Obstet Gynecol 117:1, 1973.)

groups. Women from the low socioeconomic group are not accustomed to seeking medical care for nonemergency conditions. Since pregnancy is a common occurrence among them, they do not realize the need for medical attention unless a severe problem develops. Consequently, problem pregnancies with higher maternal and perinatal death rates are common in this group.

Marital status

Although many "high-risk" mothers are married, the marital status of the unwed mother is usually reason enough to classify her as "high risk." This classification is made because unwed mothers receive less antepartal care, have more complications of pregnancy, and have a higher rate of prematurity with a greater risk of death than married mothers. Many of these problems are likely associated with factors such as low income and untreated medical conditions. The stigma attached to pregnancy out of wedlock may be a factor in preventing some unwed primigravidas from seeking antepartal care; ignorance of the need, as well as inability to pay, may also be contributing factors. Since most unwed mothers are from the low-income group, the antepartal care they do receive is usually provided by clinics and hospitals rather than by private physicians.

Antepartal care

Expectant mothers who receive little or no antepartal care may be considered "high risk." Antepartal care at the beginning of the pregnancy is important so that any problems present can be corrected or treated to prevent them from becoming greater as the pregnancy progresses. Continuous medical care and supervision throughout pregnancy are important to the early detection and treatment of problems that may develop. Expectant mothers who do not receive early and adequate antepartal care tend to have a higher incidence of maternal and perinatal mortality.

MEDICAL CONDITIONS

Disease

During pregnancy certain demands are made on the health reserves of the mother. In addition to these normal demands of pregnancy, the expectant woman is subject to all the disease conditions of the nonpregnant woman. Therefore, when pregnancy occurs in a woman who already has a disease condition, or when a disease condition is discovered during pregnancy, the additional strain may endanger the health or life of the mother or the unborn child. This is especially true if the mother's health reserves are already limited by a lack of such essentials as adequate nutrition, housing, recreation, and medical care. Anemia, infection, diabetes, chronic hypertensive vascular disease, and heart complications are examples of disease conditions that may affect the course or outcome of pregnancy.

Anemia during pregnancy is most likely to be found among women from the low-income group whose general nutrition is poor. The pregnant woman who has anemia may be in a constant state of fatigue. She is also more susceptible to infections, since her resistance is lowered. Her infant may be born with anemia and may be small for gestational age.

Infections may affect the course or outcome of the pregnancy. A classic example is *rubella* (German measles) which, when contracted by the expectant mother during the first 12 weeks of pregnancy, may cause congenital abnormalities in the newborn. The earlier in pregnancy the mother gets this infection, the greater the chances of abnormalities in the infant; after 12 weeks' gestation the danger is minimal. Rubella during the first weeks of pregnancy is sometimes an indication for therapeutic abortion. Premature rupture of the membranes also presents a dangerous threat to the fetus unless labor begins very soon thereafter. The longer the time between the rupture of the membranes and the onset of labor, the greater the chance of intrauterine infection.

Diabetes may be present and recognized before pregnancy (pregestational) or it may become apparent only during pregnancy (gestational). In either instance, it affects both mother (Chap. 16) and fetus (Chap. 20). Pregnancy increases the severity of the diabetes so that there is an increase in the insulin requirements. Also, the pregnant diabetic is more likely to develop acidosis. Compared to the nondiabetic expectant mother, the pregnant diabetic is more likely to develop pregnancy-induced hypertension (PIH) and hydramnios.

Infants born to diabetic mothers are usually very large (10 lb or more) and are likely to develop hypoglycemia, hyperbilirubinemia, hypocalcemia, unexplained cyanotic attacks, and respiratory distress syndrome. There is a higher incidence of congenital malformations as well as a higher incidence of intrauterine deaths after 36 weeks of gestation and a higher neonatal mortality rate than among the general population.

Chronic hypertensive vascular disease occurs most often in multiparas who are over 30 years of age. Approximately 15% of the women who have this condition develop preeclampsia (Chap. 16), which carries a 20% risk of death for the fetus and an increased risk of maternal mortality of 1% or 2%. In a small percentage of patients with chronic hypertensive vascular disease, the hypertension may be so severe that involvement of the kidneys, heart, or retina may be cause for termination of the pregnancy by abortion.

Heart complications may be severely aggravated by pregnancy (see Chap. 16). Thus, the mother and fetus may be placed in jeopardy. Serious heart conditions may necessitate termination of the pregnancy by therapeutic abortion or may result in premature labor or death of the fetus. Unless the mother receives early and continuous antepartal care, mild or severe heart conditions may cause invalidism or even death of the mother.

Problem pregnancies

Problems that may develop as a result of conditions directly related to the pregnancy include PIH, Rh incompatibility, genetic abnormalities, and hemorrhagic complications such as abortion, placenta previa, and abruptio placentae. When any one of these conditions is present in one pregnancy, it may recur in subsequent pregnancies.

Pregnancy-induced hypertension (Chap. 16) is one of the three leading causes of maternal mortality in this country, being responsible for about 1,000 maternal deaths each year. In addition, it causes at least 30,000 stillbirths and neonatal deaths each year. PIH occurs in about 6% to 7% of all pregnant women. Approximately 10% of all preeclamptic and 5% of all eclamptic mothers are left with permanent, chronic hypertension. About 50% of preeclamptic and 30% of eclamptic patients develop PIH in subsequent pregnancies.

Rh incompatibility (Chap. 16), if untreated, may have varying degrees of effect on the fetus. In its mild form it may produce no symptoms or only inconsequential anemia or jaundice. In its severe form, known as erythroblastosis fetalis (Chap. 20), it may cause serious anemia, resulting in heart failure and death to the fetus or marked jaundice leading to brain damage (kernicterus) or death. Erythroblastosis fetalis usually recurs in subsequent pregnancies.

Genetic abnormalities tend to increase as the mother's age increases. These abnormalities may be so gross as to cause intrauterine or neonatal death, or the infant may, with special care, survive for a few years but be mentally retarded.

Hemorrhagic complications of pregnancy (Chap. 16) constitute a threat to the life of both mother and fetus. In the case of abortion, the life of the fetus is lost and, depending on the circumstances, the life of the mother may be endangered. Approximately 10% of all pregnancies end in spontaneous abortion. Some women who desire children very much have spontaneous abortions with repeated pregnancies. These habitual aborters are classified as "high-risk" patients. In addition, induced abortions performed outside of approved medical facilities have often caused illness and death of the woman.

Placenta previa and abruptio placentae may endanger the mother because of hemorrhage. Also, hemorrhage from these conditions may decrease the oxygen supply to the fetus, resulting in damage to or death of the fetus. Or the infant may be born prematurely because the hemorrhage makes termination of the pregnancy before term imperative.

High parity

High parity alone may cause a pregnant woman to be classified as "high risk." She is at even greater risk if, with her high parity, she has a history of problem pregnancies. As the number of pregnancies increases so also do problems involving hemorrhage, uterine inertia and abnormal presentations (Chap. 18), and excessively large babies. If, in addition, the pregnancies have come so close together that the mother has had little or no time between them to build up her health reserves, she may be in a constant state of fatigue and malnutrition so that she is more susceptible to disease and problem conditions than she otherwise would be.

OTHER RISK FACTORS

Emotional disturbance

Pregnancy and birth may be very traumatic to the emotionally disturbed person, creating stress beyond the ability to cope. If the pregnancy is permitted to continue to term, the parents may be unable to relate in a meaningful manner to the child. Unrestrained outbursts of violent behavior by the parents may cause severe physical injury or death of the child, while the inability to form close attachments with the child may cause permanent damage to emotional and mental development. The emotionally disturbed parent may have periods of deep depression during which she forgets that she has a child. Neglect of nutritional needs may result in malnutrition, while lack of stimulation and parental-child attachment may result in mental retardation and failure to thrive.

Drug addiction

Drug addicts often are malnourished, and infants born to them are likely to be small for gestational age. Because these parents usually do not seek prenatal care, and because many of them support their habit through prostitution, they and their infants may have sexually transmissible disease. Infants born to these parents often are unwanted and unloved. Drugs may so deaden the sensitivities of the parents that they are unresponsive to the needs of their infants or unaware of them. Parent-infant bonding and attachment may be inadequate or lacking altogether; the infant may be considered more of an object than a human being with feelings and needs. As a result, parents may abuse the child or leave the child alone for long periods of time while they seek to satisfy their own needs. Infants born to addicted parents may be addicted themselves at birth and may die from withdrawal symptoms soon after birth unless the symptoms are recognized and treated (see Chap. 20).

Alcoholism

Alcoholic parents, like drug-addicted parents, are often more interested in meeting their own needs than those of their child. Because alcoholism interferes with the absorption and utilization of nutrients and with protein synthesis, newborns of alcoholic mothers may be malnourished, small for their gestational age, mentally retarded, or afflicted with *fetal alcohol syndrome*, a condition characterized by craniofacial, limb, and cardiovascular defects. After birth the child may fail to thrive because of deprivation of parental attention and because of the parents' periodic disregard for the child's physical needs. In their drunken state, alcoholic parents may abuse or neglect their child.

Heavy smoking

Mothers who are heavy smokers are more likely to give birth to infants who are small for gestational age than are nonsmokers or light smokers. This may be due to the lower food intake of the mother, whose appetite may be decreased by her smoking. It may also be due to the decreased blood supply to the uterus because of nicotine-induced vasoconstriction. Smoking by the parents—or anyone else in the room—during labor may add to the stress on the fetus by decreasing its available oxygen. This can be hazardous to an infant who is already in jeopardy because of uteroplacental insufficiency or prematurity. After birth, heavy smoking by the parents can make the infant susceptible to respiratory problems.

Child abuse

Child abuse may occur in any home. Although the abuse most often is inflicted by the natural or stepparents, it may be inflicted by foster parents, grandparents, baby-sitters, nurses, or anyone else with access to the child. It appears to occur most often in lonely, isolated, frustrated people who probably received inadequate parental care in their own formative years and were themselves abused. Children born out-of-wedlock or into families with marital discord are frequently victims. Parents who are emotionally disturbed, drug-addicted, alcoholic, or teenagers are frequently the abusers. Child abuse is also more likely to occur when there has been forced separation of the infant from the parents at birth as occurs, for example, in cesarean section, premature birth, and traumatic birth.

Children are abused for many reasons: the abuser may not love or want the child or may be annoyed by the child's crying or nagging; the child's needs may conflict with the abuser's needs; the parent may be overworked and exhausted and may take out his or her frustrations on the child; the parent may have unrealistic expectations of the child and may be angry when the child does not fulfill them; the parent may not know what behavior is appropriate for different stages of development and may think the child is misbehaving deliberately when he is actually performing normally for his age.

Child abuse may be in the form of physical or verbal assault or it may be in the form of neglect. Physical assault may consist of burns, beatings, violent shaking, or sexual abuse. Beatings and burns usually leave obvious signs of injury such as bruises, fractures, bleeding, or soft tissue swelling, while violent shaking may cause brain hemorrhage resulting in coma, convulsions, or death with no external signs of injury. Sexual abuse, such as incest, may cause deep and lasting emotional trauma. Verbal assault is demeaning and can result in embarrassment and development within the child of negative feelings concerning self-worth. Neglect can result in malnutrition and physical deterioration as well as stunting of emotional and mental development.

To prevent child abuse it is necessary to detect potential abusers. Obstetricians and pediatricians, their office staffs, and hospital maternity staffs are in a key position to observe attitudes and behavior that might lead to child abuse. For example, the obstetrician or nurse can sometimes detect the woman who does not want a pregnancy but delays making a decision for abortion until it is too late. They are also able to obtain information about the family's socioeconomic status and the presence of health or emotional problems. Pediatricians and their staffs see parents and children under stress, and can evaluate their interactions and how they relate in these situations. They can observe and listen to the parents as they discuss their child and can be alert to parents who have only negative things to say about the child. Hospital maternity staffs can observe the attitudes of parents toward labor, birth, and the infant at birth and during the first few days. They can see how the parents feel about the child and how parents and child react to and relate with one another.

MEASURES THAT MAY BE HELPFUL IN PREVENTING CHILD ABUSE

- o Arrange for the obstetrician and pediatrician to get to know both parents during the prenatal period and allow both parents to discuss their fears, wishes, and anxieties regarding pregnancy, labor, birth, and the child
- o Provide educational programs in parenting so that parents can develop skills and learn what behavior is normal for the different stages of the child's development
- o Provide opportunity and encouragement for both parents to see, touch, hold, caress, and establish eye contact with their infant during the first hour after birth and to provide care within a few hours after birth
- o Provide positive reinforcement of their parenting skills by commending them for their care
- o Help parents recognize that the child is an individual with a distinct personality by bringing to their attention such things as the infant's response to the sound of their voices and touch within a short time after birth

Keeping in touch with parents who do not appear to form attachments to the child during the hospital stay may be very important in preventing child abuse. This may be done by having someone, such as an obstetric nurse, a public health nurse, or a health visitor, make periodic visits to the home following birth. This person could answer questions, evaluate the home environment and interaction between parents and child, and provide support to the parents. Parents can also be helped to find nonprofessional positive support systems, such as relatives, friends, or neighbors, who can come to their rescue by taking the child for a while when they are tempted to take out their frustrations on the child. Providing a 24-hour phone service so that stressed parents can call and discuss their problems with an interested, caring person may also be helpful in preventing child abuse.

Child abuse is a serious problem with no easy solution. With general awareness of predisposing conditions and attitudes, health care workers may be able to identify and help potential abusers before they have committed the act.

RECOMMENDATIONS

Obviously, if all the conditions that place the expectant mother and her infant at high risk could be eliminated or controlled, this problem would be solved. Because this is not possible in our society the next best solution must be considered. This calls for:

Sex education of young people

Education of the public regarding the safest age for childbearing

Education of the low-income group from early childhood regarding the necessity for *preventive* as well as emergency medical care

Education of the public in family-planning and family-limiting methods, and making these methods available to all groups

Provision of early and continuous antepartal care by highly qualified personnel to *all* expectant mothers

The problem of high-risk parents and infants has been recognized for some time by both the American Medical Association and the American College of Obstetricians and Gynecologists. These organizations have made recommendations regarding programs for the identification and care of high-risk mothers and infants. Stated briefly, they call for

Specially staffed and equipped, centrally located community or regional hospitals with newborn intensive care units

Programs for the detection of high-risk mothers in time for them to deliver in the hospitals with newborn intensive care units

Programs for the early postnatal detection of high-risk infants that were not detected during pregnancy and for their prompt transfer to a hospital with a newborn intensive care unit.

These recommendations are based on the recognition that training of personnel will be necessary to adequately staff these hospitals and conduct the detection programs, and that facilities will have to be made available and properly equipped. In addition, continuing research will be necessary into the causes of high risk and into methods to improve the medical management. Furthermore, this approach to handling the problem of high risk will need to be continually evaluated. It is anticipated that through this approach there can be a marked reduction in maternal and perinatal mortality.

ROLE OF NURSES

Nursing assessment. Often it is the nurse who first detects the signs and symptoms that indicate a mother or infant is high risk. Clues that suggest a woman may be at high risk are listed in the box below.

CLUES TO POTENTIALLY HIGH-RISK PREGNANCY

○ **Obstetric or medical history.** Were there problems with a previous pregnancy or with this pregnancy early in its course? Has she had many pregnancies? An ectopic pregnancy? Miscarriages? Does she have medical problems (diabetes, heart disease, infections) that could jeopardize the pregnancy?

○ **Social status.** Is she a teenager? Is she in her late childbearing years? Is she single? Is she uneducated? Is she in the lower socioeconomic group?

○ **Emotional status.** Does she have a good support system—family, friends? How does she handle stress?

○ **Nutritional status.** Is she overweight? Underweight? Does she have poor eating habits?

○ **Other habits.** Is she a drug abuser? Smoker? Alcoholic?

○ **Laboratory studies.** Does she have sugar or albumin in her urine? Positive cultures for sexually transmitted diseases? Low hemoglobin and hematocrit?

○ **Physical examination.** Does she have an elevated blood pressure? Swelling of her face, hands, or feet?

A high-risk expectant woman is not likely to have a smooth pregnancy course. PIH, infections, hemorrhage, and other problems can require bed rest at home or hospitalizations that disrupt the family life and cause stress. If there are small children in the family, arrangements will need to be made for their care while the mother is receiving care. If the mother works and the family depends on her salary, loss of income creates stress. Restriction of her activities at home can create stress so that she does not obtain the rest she needs even though she stays in bed. She may become bored when on bed rest or when hospitalized for long periods, and this can be stressful to her. She may feel guilty because she is unable to perform her normal role as caregiver for her family. This can be damaging to her self-esteem. Illness and hospitalizations during pregnancy can interfere with the mother's ability to complete the developmental tasks of pregnancy.

Whatever affects the mother is likely to affect the rest of the family also. Stress can strain relationships. The nurse must be aware of the stresses that may be present in a high-risk situation and how the mother and the family are coping with the situation. Are they being realistic and working through the problem together? Are they denying the pregnancy or failing to become emotionally attached to the infant because they are afraid it will not survive? The nurse needs to listen to the high-risk mother and to observe her carefully in order to identify inadequate or potentially negative coping mechanisms and to assist her and her family in developing positive ways of coping.

The nurse also needs to find out what the mother and the family know about the problem. Lack of knowledge, wrong information, or misconceptions can sometimes influence the degree of effort and cooperation they are willing to expend in carrying out the treatments necessary.

Nursing interventions.   The nurse can help the high-risk mother and her family obtain correct, appropriate information regarding the high-risk problem in language they understand. Since the problem can be stressful to them, she should also include information about possible treatment, with an emphasis on positive outcomes. She should reinforce what the physician has told them. Although she must be realistic (not all high-risk pregnancies have a happy outcome), she can offer a degree of hope because of the advances in diagnosis and treatment that have improved the outcomes in high-risk pregnancies in recent years.

The nurse can encourage the mother and family to touch the mother's abdomen and feel the baby move, to listen to the baby's heartbeat, to discuss plans for the baby, to talk of possible names for the baby, to make preparations for the baby (select clothing, etc.). In this way she can help them to accept the pregnancy as real and to develop emotional attachments to the infant. She can also encourage them to discuss their feelings and fantasies about the infant.

The nurse should be aware of resources that are available to help families with high-risk pregnancies so that she can refer them, after consultation with the physician, to appropriate professionals who can help them. These might include home-maker services, social workers, nutritionists, and the like.

CLINICAL REVIEW

ASSESSMENT. Mr. and Mrs. S. are the parents of six children: four daughters ages 9, 7½, 3, and 1½ years and two sons ages 6 and 4. Mr. S. is 35 years old and his wife is 26. Neither parent has completed elementary school. The family lives in a three-room house constructed of rough, unpainted lumber. It is situated on a hillside in a coal-mining area. One room serves as a kitchen-dining room; the other two are used for bedrooms. Each room opens onto a porch that extends the length of the house in front. The house has electricity but no plumbing. The cookstove burns wood or coal and is the only source of heat. Water is obtained from a pump in the backyard. They have no automobile. Their transportation usually entails riding in a pickup truck of a neighbor or occasionally "catching" a ride to the nearest town on the school bus.

Mr. S. was employed at the local coal mine until he became unable to work because of a lung disease common among miners. Since then he has been on Social Security. Mr. and Mrs. S. supplement their meager income by growing a garden on the small plot of tillable ground behind their house; they also have a few chickens.

Mrs S. is pregnant for the seventh time. She "felt life" for the first time with this pregnancy about a month ago. She has never had any problems with her pregnancies and the births were easy. All of her babies weighed around 5 or 6 lb (2268 or 2722 g) at birth. Mrs. S. is eligible for free antenatal care at the clinic at the miners' hospital, which is about 15 miles from her home. However, she did not go for care with her other pregnancies and she has not seen a doctor during this pregnancy. She does plan to deliver at the hospital.

1. What social factors in this situation would cause Mrs. S. to be classified as high risk?

2. What medical factors would justify this classification?

3. What conditions probably prevent Mrs. S. from seeking prenatal care even though it is provided by the hospital?

4. What do you consider to be the most pressing problems of this family? How would you suggest they be solved?

5. What do you consider the most effective means of preventing the children in this family from having, as adults, the same problems their parents are having? Be realistic.

BIBLIOGRAPHY

Bishop B: A guide to assessing parenting capabilities. Am J Nurs 76:1784, 1976

Brazelton TB: Anticipatory guidance. Pediatr Clin North Am 22:533, 1975

Cupoli JM, Newberger EH: Optimism or pessimism for the victim of child abuse? Pediatrics 59:1311, 1977

Dubois DR: Indications of an unhealthy relationship between parents and premature infants. J Obstet Gynecol Neonatal Nurs 4:21, 1975

Kaplun D, Reich R: The murdered child and his killers. Am J Psychiatry 133:809, 1976

Kempe CH: Approaches to preventing child abuse: The health visitors concepts. Am J Dis Child 130:941, 1976

Kemp VH, Page CK: The psychosocial impact of a high-risk pregnancy on the family. J Obstet Gynecol Neonatal Nurs 15:232–236, 1986

Klaus MH, Kennell JH: Maternal-Infant Bonding. St. Louis, CV Mosby, 1976

Luke B: Guide to better evaluation of antepartum nutrition. J Obstet Gynecol Neonatal Nurs 5:37, 1976

Maternal alcoholism and fetal alcohol syndrome. Am J Nurs 77:1924, 1977

Mogielnicki RP, et al: Impending child abuse: Psychosomatic symptoms in adults as a clue. JAMA 237:1109, 1977

Williams ML: Long-term hospitalization of women with high-risk pregnancies: A nurse's viewpoint. J Obstet Gynecol Neonatal Nurs 15:17–21, 1986

variations of normal 18 labor and delivery

BEHAVIORAL OBJECTIVES When the goals of this chapter are reached, the student will be able to:

○ *Describe how forceps are used.*

○ *Describe vacuum extraction.*

○ *Describe version.*

○ *Give the two most common indications for cesarean section.*

○ *Discuss the emotional reaction of a couple when they are told the wife has to have a cesarean section when they had anticipated vaginal delivery.*

○ *List three indications for induction of labor.*

○ *Describe the two-bottle or "piggyback" method of oxytocin infusion.*

○ *Distinguish between hypertonic and hypotonic uterine dysfunction, describe the treatment of each, and discuss the nursing functions involved.*

○ *Explain what is meant by persistent occiput posterior position and describe the type of labor characteristic of this condition.*

○ *Name and describe the three types of breech presentations.*

○ *Describe two dangers associated with breech presentations.*

○ *Explain what is meant by CPD, and tell how the diagnosis is confirmed and how delivery is accomplished.*

○ *Give three or four possible complications of multiple pregnancy.*

○ *Define: complete rupture of the uterus, incomplete rupture of the uterus, hydramnios.*

○ *Give the symptoms, cause, and treatment of supine hypotensive syndrome.*

OPERATIVE OBSTETRICS

It is sometimes necessary for the obstetrician to assist the mother during labor and delivery through the use of certain techniques. These techniques are classified as *operative obstetrics*.

FORCEPS

Forceps are instruments used by the doctor to deliver the baby. The forceps are applied to the baby's head and traction is exerted. When forceps are used, the second stage of labor is shortened. Forceps are also used to rotate the baby's head from an undesirable position to a desirable one.

√ Each pair of forceps has a right and a left blade. Most forceps have an opening in the blades (*e.g.,* Simpson or Elliott forceps); a few are solid (*e.g.,* Tucker-McLean forceps) (Fig. 18-1). The blades of forceps are curved to fit the curvature of the baby's head and of the mother's pelvis.

In a *low* or *outlet* forceps delivery, the forceps are applied after the baby's head is visible, or almost visible, at the vaginal opening. In a *midforceps* delivery, the forceps are applied when the baby's head is level with the ischial spines. In a *high* forceps delivery, the forceps are applied before the baby's head is engaged. Applying forceps to the head before it

FIG. 18-1. *Various forceps may be used in delivery such as (Left to right) Piper, Tucker–McLean, Simpson, or Elliott.*

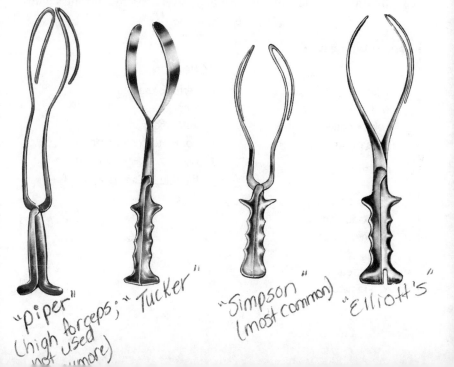

is known whether the head will fit through the pelvis carries with it grave risks to the fetus. High forceps application is very difficult and can cause injury to the woman's soft tissue. Because of the dangers associated with this type of delivery, it is rarely done anymore. Cesarean section is safer for mother and infant and is usually employed instead of high forceps delivery.

Indications. Forceps delivery can be performed for either maternal or fetal indications. Maternal indications include pregnancy-induced hypertension (PIH), heart disease, and inability to push because of exhaustion or conduction anesthesia. Fetal distress suspected from a slow, irregular fetal heart rate is the most common fetal indication for forceps delivery. Forceps are frequently used to deliver premature infants to prevent undue pressure on the fragile fetal skull by the perineum. Some obstetricians routinely use forceps to deliver primigravidas because they feel it spares the patient the exhaustion of a long second stage of pushing and because it prevents unnecessary pressure on the baby's head.

Procedure. Forceps are never applied to any part of the fetus except the head. The woman's bladder should be empty before forceps are used to allow more room for the forceps and to reduce the danger of trauma to the bladder. The membranes should be ruptured, the cervix completely dilated, the head at or below the ischial spines, and the position of the head known before forceps are applied (Fig. 18-2). After one blade of the forceps is applied to each side of the baby's head, the handles of the forceps should fit together easily. During each contraction, traction is exerted downward until the occiput has cleared the symphysis pubis; then the traction is directed upward and forward. Between contractions

FORCEPS DELIVERY

TYPES

- High
- Mid
- Low or outlet

INDICATIONS

- Maternal:
  - PIH
  - Heart disease
  - Exhaustion
  - Anesthetized
- Fetal:
  - Distress
  - Prematurity

CONDITIONS

- Vertex presentation
- Empty bladder
- Ruptured membranes
- Completely dilated cervix
- Head at or below ischial spines
- Position of head known

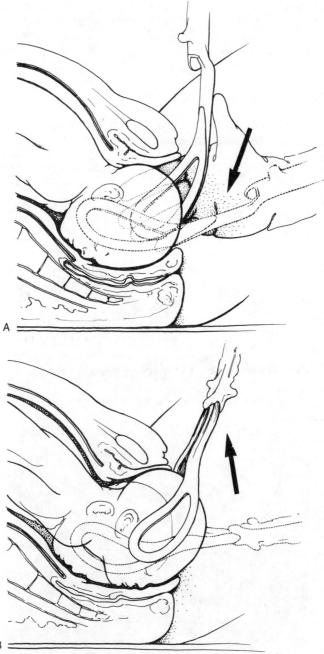

FIG. 18-2. *(A) Insertion of forceps blade and (B) applied forceps and direction of traction.*

traction is not applied and the handles of the forceps are separated to relieve the pressure of the blades against the head. Forceps delivery is usually safe for mother and infant when these conditions are present. Forceps often leave a superficial mark on either side of the infant's face; the mark disappears within a few hours.

√ VACUUM EXTRACTION

Vacuum extraction involves applying a metal cup, called a vacuum extractor, to the fetal head, creating a vacuum to secure the cup to the scalp, and then exerting traction to deliver the head. The cups come in various sizes and the largest one that can be applied easily is used. After the cup is in place, vacuum is created slowly by withdrawal of air by a pump. When the cup is firmly attached, traction is exerted to deliver the head. This procedure is an alternative to forceps delivery (Fig. 18-3)(*infer*)

VERSION

In version, the baby in the uterus is turned from an undesirable presentation to a desirable one. When the turning is accomplished from the outside through the abdominal and uterine walls, it is called *external version*. External version is done to change a breech presentation to a vertex presentation to avoid the risks involved in breech delivery. This type of version is most successful when done about a month before term. Sometimes the baby cannot be turned, and sometimes it reverts to a breech *or transverse lie (poss. small pelvis)*

FIG. 18-3. *Application of the vacuum extractor and delivery of the fetal head.*

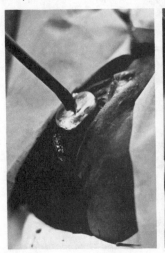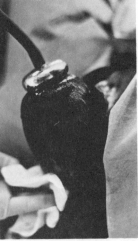

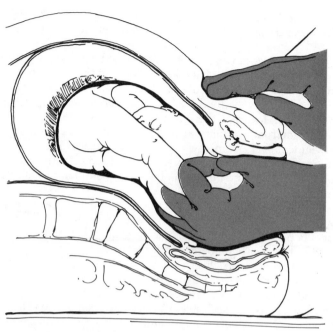

FIG. 18-4. *Internal podalic version.*

position following the version. Some obstetricians do not approve of external version.

Internal version, also called *internal podalic version*, is a procedure in which the presentation, whatever it is, is changed to a breech presentation. The physician does this by inserting one whole hand through a completely dilated cervix high into the uterus, grasping one or both feet and pulling downward toward the birth canal. At the same time the other hand is used externally to push the head upward (Fig. 18-4). Internal version is usually followed by breech extraction. This procedure is seldom used except in multiple pregnancy in which birth of the second twin is delayed or the second twin is in a transverse lie.

used c̄ more than 1 fetus. Danger: placenta rupture

CESAREAN SECTION

Cesarean section is a surgical operation in which the baby is delivered through an incision made in the abdomen and uterus of the mother. In a *classic* cesarean section, the incision is made into the body of the uterus. It can be done quickly; therefore it is usually done when an emergency exists, such as with a hemorrhage or prolapsed cord. In a *low cervical* section, the incision is made in the lower part of the uterus, thus reducing the possibility of infected material entering the peritoneal

uterus

body of uterus, classic, indices

uterus

low cervical > blood vessels smaller, closed

cavity. Therefore, a low cervical is preferred for a mother who has been in labor for several hours or who has had ruptured membranes for several hours.

Indications. A cesarean section is performed when vaginal delivery is not possible or is not safe. Many doctors believe that a mother who has had one cesarean section should have cesarean sections in subsequent pregnancies, because of the danger of the uterine scar rupturing if she goes into labor. However, there has been no documentation in the literature of maternal mortality attributed directly to rupture of a lower uterine segment scar. Women who have had a cesarean section with one pregnancy and who wish to have a vaginal delivery with a subsequent pregnancy need to locate the hospital nearest them that has the staff and facilities to manage their high-risk labor.

The most common indications for a cesarean section are cephalopelvic disproportion (see below) and previous cesarean section. Other indications are placenta previa, abruptio placentae, fetal distress, abnormal presentations, and some cases of diabetes and PIH. An *emergency* cesarean section is done when immediate delivery is necessary to save the life of the baby and/or mother or to prevent damage to them. An *elective* cesarean section is decided upon in advance because it is known that vaginal delivery is not possible or is not desirable. Elective cesarean sections are usually scheduled 1 to 2 weeks before the estimated date of confinement so that labor does not start first.

Preoperative care. The preoperative care of a mother who is to have a cesarean section is similar to that for any patient having abdominal surgery. In addition, a retention catheter is inserted to keep the bladder empty during the operation. The fetal heart tones are checked before surgery. The preoperative medication is limited to a drying agent, such as atropine or scopolamine. The mother is not given a narcotic before surgery because it might cause the baby's respirations to be depressed when born. Because she is not given a narcotic, the mother is more alert, and may be more tense and apprehensive than other preoperative patients. For this reason, the nurse may need to stay with her and give her support and encouragement.

Parental concerns. When a couple has anticipated a normal delivery but conditions arise that require that a cesarean section be done, they may become quite apprehensive and concerned about the outcome for the wife and baby. If they had planned on having natural childbirth, they may also be keenly disappointed. In such instances, the nurse can give them emotional support by explaining the procedures that will be done, and why, and by arranging for the husband to be with his wife as much as possible until she goes to the operating room. The nurse should inform the husband where he can wait and assure him that he will be notified as soon as he can see his wife and baby. Some hospitals permit the husband to be present during scheduled or emergency cesarean sections if he has attended childbirth preparation classes. Then, if the baby's condition is good, he is able to get acquainted with it soon after birth. If the wife has spinal anesthesia, she too can see and touch the baby in the operating room.

Anesthesia.   The type of anesthesia used for cesarean section depends somewhat on the skills and experience of the anesthesiologist as well as the wishes of the patient. In addition, the possible adverse effects of the anesthesia on the infant and mother must be considered. In most instances either spinal anesthesia or general anesthesia is used.

CESAREAN SECTION BIRTH *(major abdominal surgery)*

TYPES

○ Emergency—immediate delivery necessary

○ Elective—scheduled in advance

METHODS

○ Classic—incision in body of uterus

○ Low cervical—incision into lower uterine segment

INDICATIONS

○ Vaginal delivery not safe or not possible

○ Cephalopelvic disproportion

○ Previous cesarean section

○ Hemorrhage

○ Fetal distress

○ Abnormal presentations

○ Some cases of diabetes and pregnancy-induced hypertension

PREOPERATIVE PREPARATION

○ Same as for other abdominal surgery except narcotic not given preop

○ Foley catheter inserted

ANESTHESIA

○ Spinal
  • Risk: maternal hypotension with fetal hypoxia; maternal headache

○ General—prep and drape prior to administering
  • Risk: infant—respiratory depression
  • maternal—vomiting with aspiration

NEWBORN CARE

○ Pediatrician present and initiates care; shows infant to father

○ Nurse does eye care and identification procedures; if mother is awake, lets her see and touch infant

POSTOPERATIVE CARE

○ Same as for other abdominal surgery plus postpartum care

Spinal anesthesia can cause maternal hypotension, which, if untreated, may cause respiratory depression in the infant at birth. Elevation of the mother's legs, administration of oxygen, and intravenous infusion of glucose are helpful in combating anesthesia-induced hypotension. Also, severe headaches are occasionally experienced by patients who have had spinal anesthesia.

One of the most serious problems encountered in the use of *general anesthesia* is aspiration of vomitus by the patient while anesthetized. This danger is especially great in an emergency cesarean section when the patient has not been properly prepared by a period of fasting prior to the operation. There is also the possibility that the baby will be depressed at birth as a result of receiving the anesthetic. When general anesthesia is used for cesarean section, the patient is prepped and draped, and everything is made ready for the incision before the anesthetic is given. This reduces the risk of respiratory depression in the infant by minimizing the time between administration of the anesthetic and birth of the baby.

Positioning. The importance of an adequate uteroplacental blood flow prior to birth of the baby is stressed by other measures employed during cesarean section operations. These measures are directed toward prevention of maternal hypotension and subsequent fetal hypoxia and acidosis, which could delay initiation of spontaneous respirations in the newborn at birth.

Prevention of supine hypotension is accomplished by use of the left lateral recumbent position during transfer of the mother to the operating room. Then the operating table is tilted slightly to the left and the uterus is supported with a triangular foam rubber wedge until the baby is born. Thus, pressure on the vena cava is avoided.

Newborn care. The pediatrician is usually present to take care of the baby when a cesarean section is done. The delivery nurse has ready a heated crib or incubator, as well as oxygen and resuscitative equipment. She also assists the pediatrician as necessary. She instills the eye medication and sees that the baby is properly identified before being taken to the nursery. If the mother is awake following the birth, she can be shown the baby. As soon as the baby is in the nursery the father can see it and be reassured about his wife's condition.

Postoperative care. The postoperative care of the mother following a cesarean section is the same as that for any other patient having abdominal surgery. In addition, the mother needs postpartum care. She is observed closely for vaginal bleeding and for bleeding from the incision. The fundus is usually not massaged to control bleeding because of the discomfort to the mother. Instead, excessive bleeding is controlled by giving her an oxytocic such as ergonovine (Ergotrate) or methylergonovine (Methergine). A mother who has planned to breast-feed her baby may do so even though she has had a cesarean section.

✓INDUCTION OF LABOR   *Easy way to induce labor ARom*

Indications. *Induction of labor* is the intentional starting of labor by mechanical or medical means. Induction of labor is usually done because of obstetric or medical problems that make immediate delivery of the baby necessary or desirable. Inductions may also be done for the convenience of the mother or the doctor. Obstetric problems that may be indications for induction of labor include preeclampsia and Rh incompatibility. Diabetes is an example of a medical problem for which induction may be done.

Methods. Artificial rupture of the membranes is frequently the method of induction chosen by the doctor. Occasionally, 1 or 2 oz of castor oil may be ordered, followed an hour later by a high, hot enema. Oxytocin (Pitocin, Syntocinon) in small doses may be given intramuscularly, or a dilute solution of oxytocin may be given intravenously. When attended by the doctor, an intravenous infusion of a dilute solution of oxytocin is considered to be the safest way to use oxytocin for induction, since the infusion can be easily regulated and controlled.

When induction is to be accomplished by using an oxytocin infusion, the two-bottle, or "piggyback," method is usually employed (Fig. 18-5). In this method, a liter of solution, usually 5% glucose in water or 5% glucose in Ringer's lactate, is started intravenously. This is bottle No. 1. Bottle No. 2 is usually a liter of the same solution to which 5 units or 10 units of oxytocin have been added. Bottle No. 2 is connected, or added "piggyback," to the IV tubing of bottle No. 1. Thus, by clamping the tubing on bottle No. 2 and opening the tubing on bottle No. 1, the attendant can temporarily or permanently discontinue the oxytocin infusion while maintaining the IV.

It is important that the oxytocin infusion be regulated so as to maintain the labor contractions at the desired frequency and intensity. It is not always easy to maintain the desired rate of flow, however, since it can be influenced by the position of the patient's hand or arm; the tubing can get kinked; or the tubing can get under the patient and become occluded. To overcome these difficulties, certain manufacturers have developed infusion pumps that not only precisely control the rate of flow of the infusion, regardless of the position of the patient's hand or arm, but also have an alarm system with flashing red lights and an audible beep that

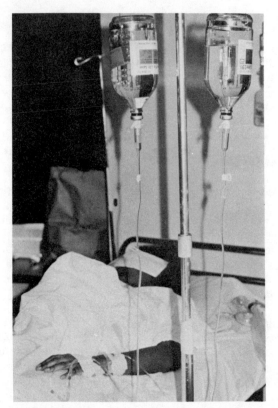

FIG. 18-5. *Administration of oxytocin (Pitocin) pit drip, with piggyback technique.*

alerts the attendant when the tubing contains air or is occluded or the infusion bottle is empty.

Complications. Rupture of the uterus, premature separation of the placenta, and fetal hypoxia may result from an improperly administered induction of labor using oxytocin.

Patient monitoring. When possible, continuous electronic monitoring of the fetal heart rate and the uterine contractions should be employed during induction of labor. Use of an electronic monitor should not lessen the watchfulness of the physician or nurse, however. When electronic monitors are not available, the monitoring must be done by the doctor or nurse, who stays at the bedside and feels the contractions and listens to the fetal heart tones during and after each contraction. The patient's blood pressure is taken at frequent intervals and recorded.

The infusion is slowed or stopped if the contractions last longer than a minute and a half, if the mother's blood pressure rises and remains

OB law suit
R/T improper
use/care of
oxytocin

elevated between contractions, or if the fetal heart rate indicates fetal distress.

Parental concerns. The mother who is to have labor induced may feel uneasy even though she understands why it is being done, and even though she may have persuaded the doctor to do it. Unless the doctor has explained to her in some detail how he plans to induce labor, she may wonder how it will be done. She is likely to want to know if her labor will be longer, harder, or more painful because it is induced. If the induction is being done for her convenience or because of a problem that could affect the baby, she may worry about the outcome. She is likely to seek assurance that the induction will be effective, and if it is not, she may be very disappointed.

PROBLEMS DURING LABOR

DYSTOCIA (DIFFICULT LABOR)

The fetus is often referred to as the *passenger* in the birth process while the uterine contractions are the *forces* and the birth canal is the *passage*. When dystocia, or difficult labor, occurs, the cause rests with either the passenger, the passage, or the forces. The passenger may be too big to enter and pass through the pelvis or it may have an abnormality, such as hydrocephalus, which causes the problem. Dystocia attributable to the passenger can also be caused by malpresentations or malpositions of the fetus.

The passage can cause dystocia if it is too small or if it offers any obstacles, such as tumors or unusual configurations, that interfere with the descent, rotations, or expulsion of the fetus.

When the forces that are supposed to bring about dilation of the cervix fail to do so, or do so much slower than normal so that labor is prolonged and difficult, the condition is known as uterine dysfunction.

Dystocia can be a serious complication causing injury to or death of the fetus and exhaustion and dehydration in the woman. In addition, the couple may develop lasting negative feelings regarding childbirth so that they are less inclined to have another child.

Uterine dysfunction

Formerly, *uterine inertia* was used to describe dystocia in which the forces were ineffective. Weak, ineffective contractions occurring at the beginning of labor were called *primary inertia,* while those occurring after several hours of labor were called *secondary inertia.* The current trend is toward using the term dysfunction in place of inertia. When the term inertia is used, primary inertia refers to prolongation of the latent phase of labor and secondary inertia to prolongation of the active phase.

hypertonic - morphine sulfate ?

hypotonic - pitoccin 0

Before a diagnosis of uterine dysfunction can be made, the contractions must be evaluated to find out if the woman is in true labor. Toward the end of pregnancy the woman may become very conscious of Braxton Hicks contractions and may mistake them for true labor. Although these contractions may cause her some discomfort and may appear to her to be strong and regular, they produce no changes in the cervix and there is no bloody show with them. In the absence of cervical changes these contractions, though uncomfortable, must be considered false labor. A diagnosis of dystocia is made only after effacement and dilatation of the cervix have started and progressed for a while and then slowed or stopped. There are two types of uterine dysfunction: hypertonic and hypotonic.

Hypertonic uterine dysfunction. In normal, effective uterine contractions, the fundus and upper segment contract while the lower segment (isthmus and cervix) relaxes. In hypertonic uterine dysfunction, incoordinate uterine action occurs, with both segments of the uterus contracting at the same time. This distorts the normal distribution of the forces so that the contractions, though very painful to the woman, are ineffective in producing dilatation. Between contractions the uterine muscles maintain a higher degree of tension than normal.

To determine whether the contractions are as strong as the woman's reaction to them would indicate or whether her reaction is due to a low pain threshold, the nurse must be able to accurately assess the intensity of contractions. This is done by trying to indent the fundus of the uterus with the fingertips at the peak of contractions. At the peak of a strong contraction it is impossible to indent the uterine wall; at the peak of a moderately strong contraction the uterine wall can be indented a little; at the peak of a mild or poor quality contraction the uterine wall can be indented easily.

Treatment of hypertonic uterine dysfunction consists of rest and fluids. Often the physician will prescribe an injection of morphine to stop the abnormal contractions and a short-acting barbiturate to help the woman get some needed rest. An intravenous infusion to maintain hydration and electrolyte balance is usually prescribed at the same time. The woman is usually able to sleep 4 to 6 hours, after which normal labor resumes.

Fetal distress may appear early in labor when hypertonic uterine dysfunction is present. Therefore, close monitoring of the fetal heart and observing for meconium-stained amniotic fluid are important. If the membranes are ruptured or if the woman has been in labor for more than 24 hours, her temperature should be taken every 2 hours.

Hypotonic uterine dysfunction. Hypotonic uterine dysfunction is a condition in which synchronous uterine contractions have been effective in dilating the cervix to at least 3 cm. Then the contractions decrease in strength and fail to dilate the cervix further. The contractions may become farther apart and irregular as well as of poor quality.

When hypotonic uterine dysfunction is suspected, the doctor will probably order x-ray pelvimetry to see if cephalopelvic disproportion, abnormal fetal position, or abnormalities are involved. If any one of these is present, a cesarean section is done. If none of these is present, labor is stimulated, either by artificial rupture of the membranes, if they are still intact, or by an intravenous infusion of an oxytocin solution. When an oxytocin infusion is prescribed, the woman's labor and the fetal heart must be monitored constantly so that adequate contractions are maintained to accomplish dilatation while avoiding a tetanic (continuous) contraction, which can be harmful to both the woman and fetus (see Induction of Labor, above).

In cases of uterine dysfunction, the woman and her husband may become quite tired, discouraged, and worried because labor is taking so long. They need to know what is happening and what can be done for it. The nurse must know the type of contractions the woman is having and must keep the physician informed of the progress or lack of progress of labor. By doing so, she can often spare the woman an unnecessarily long, drawn-out labor.

Persistent occiput posterior positions

In approximately 25% of vertex presentations, the baby's head is situated in the mother's pelvis in such a way that the occiput is toward the back of the pelvis instead of toward the front. When this occurs, labor is usually harder and longer and the mother experiences severe backache. As labor progresses, the occiput may rotate to the anterior part of the pelvis or it may remain in the posterior position. If it rotates, the backache is relieved and delivery is accomplished without difficulty. If it persists in the posterior position (persistent occiput posterior, or POP), delivery may be slow and difficult.

The mother whose baby is in the posterior position needs much encouragement to keep pushing in second stage labor, since her efforts seem ineffective. Having the mother push while lying on her side may help the baby rotate to an anterior position. Backrubs are appreciated by the mother during first stage labor.

Breech presentations

In approximately 3% of all deliveries, the presenting part is breech (Fig. 18-6). There are three kinds of breech presentations:

Footling breech, in which one foot or both feet present

Frank breech, in which the buttocks present and the legs are extended up over the abdomen and chest

Complete breech, in which the buttocks and feet present and the legs are flexed

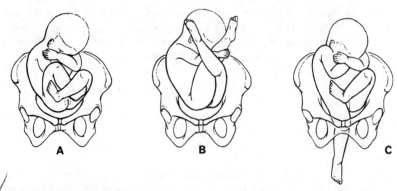

FIG. 18-6. *Breech presentations may be (A) complete breech, (B) frank breech, and (C) footling breech.*

In a breech presentation the fetal heart tones are usually heard higher in the abdomen than they are in vertex presentations, because the baby's chest is located higher in the abdomen.

There is great danger of a prolapsed cord when the membranes rupture in a breech presentation, since the presenting part is small and does not fit snugly into the pelvis. For this reason, the fetal heart tones are listened to at frequent intervals until the baby is born. If prolapse of the cord occurs, the nurse must take immediate action to relieve pressure on it. At the same time, someone else should notify the obstetrician so that preparations for immediate delivery can be started. There are several ways to relieve pressure on the cord:

Have the patient assume the knee-chest position.

Lower the head of the bed, elevate the foot, and place the patient's buttocks on an inverted bedpan. ᴛrendelenberg ↕ relieve pressure

Insert a sterile gloved hand into the vagina and cervix and push the presenting part back from the cord. 🔺will rupt

⎯ Instill electrolyte solution ᵉ push cord up (since its floating now

If the cord is protruding out of the vagina, it should not be replaced inside the cervix. Unless the cervix is completely dilated and vaginal delivery can be accomplished sooner, delivery is by cesarean section.

The amniotic fluid commonly contains meconium because of pressure exerted on the buttocks as the baby comes down the birth canal. There is also danger that the head, which does not have opportunity to mold itself to fit the birth canal, may be too large to be born. Because of this possibility, primigravidas with breech presentations are usually x-rayed to see if the mother's pelvis is large enough for passage of the baby's head.

Labor may be longer with breech presentations, but not always. Some doctors do not want the mother to have very much medication for pain relief because it may depress the baby's respirations at birth. The nurse *never* tells the mother the baby is breech, as this can be most upsetting to her.

Cephalopelvic disproportion

Cephalopelvic disproportion (CPD) is a condition in which the baby's head is too large for the mother's pelvis or the mother's pelvis is too small for the baby's head. This condition is suspected when the baby's head does not descend even though the woman is in good labor and the cervix is dilating.

The excessive size of the fetus may be due to maternal diabetes, to large parental size, or to multiparity.

When one or more diameters of the inlet, midpelvis, or outlet are shortened, the pelvis is said to be *contracted.* A contracted pelvis is the most frequent cause of cephalopelvic disproportion. Contracted pelves occur in all degrees. Whether or not an infant is able to pass through a contracted pelvis depends on many factors, including the degree of contraction, the size of the infant, and the presentation and position of the infant. For this reason, the doctor may give a woman who has been found prenatally to have a contracted pelvis a "trial labor" of 4 to 6 hours of good contractions to see if the head will pass through the pelvis. If adequate progress is not made during this time, delivery is by cesarean section. In cases of severe pelvic contraction, cesarean section delivery is done without a trial labor.

MULTIPLE PREGNANCY

The more embryos that develop in the uterus at the same time, the greater the risk to their survival and the greater the discomforts of and risk to the woman. Multiple pregnancy is suspected when the uterus is larger than usual for the period of gestation. The diagnosis can be confirmed by hearing two or more distinct fetal heart rates and by ultrasound. When a multiple pregnancy is diagnosed, the woman is observed closely for preeclampsia and premature labor, complications that frequently develop. Uterine dysfunction during labor and postpartum hemorrhage are not unusual.

The latter weeks of pregnancy may be miserable for the woman because of heaviness in the lower abdomen, back pain, swelling of the feet and ankles, shortness of breath, and inability to sleep.

During labor, the woman with a multiple pregnancy is given little or no analgesia since this may cause respiratory depression in the infants at birth. An intravenous infusion of glucose, given through a needle large enough to permit administration of blood, is started during labor. Oxytocin can be added to the solution after delivery to control bleeding. The fetal heart rates should be closely monitored throughout labor.

Since multiple pregnancies usually terminate 2 or more weeks before the estimated date of confinement, the infants are likely to be premature. Therefore, when delivery is anticipated, a pediatrician and other specially prepared personnel should be available to care for the infants as soon

Amnionitis - infection after
Rom @ 24°

as they are born. Although as little anesthesia as possible is used for the delivery, the supplies and personnel for administering general anesthesia should be readily available in case the second or subsequent infants require manipulative procedures by the doctor for birth to be accomplished.

Not all multiple pregnancies are diagnosed before the first infant is born. When this happens, the risk to all infants, including the first one, is increased because the woman may have been given sufficient analgesia or anesthesia to cause problems and because the special team to provide their immediate care is not available. The second and subsequent infants and the woman may suffer if general anesthesia is not available to help make performance of the necessary procedures, such as version and extraction, quick and comfortable.

RUPTURE OF THE UTERUS

This rare but very serious complication of obstetrics occurs when more strain than can be borne is placed on the uterine musculature. The rupture may be complete or incomplete. In complete rupture of the uterus, regular contractions stop because the torn muscles cannot contract. Blood escapes into the abdominal cavity and sometimes into the vagina. As a result, the woman goes into shock. In incomplete rupture of the uterus, the contractions may continue and the signs of shock may develop more gradually since the blood loss is slower.

The most common cause of rupture of the uterus is rupture of the scar of a previous cesarean section. For this reason, patients who have had a cesarean section are often scheduled for a repeat cesarean section a week or so before the estimated date of confinement so that they will not go into labor. Uterine rupture can also occur when oxytocin is used carelessly or unwisely during labor and in prolonged or obstructed labor, malpresentations, multiparity, and traumatic delivery, such as version and extraction.

Immediate hysterectomy is the treatment for rupture of the uterus. Blood transfusions are often necessary to replace blood loss, and antibiotics are prescribed for infection. Uterine rupture places the lives of both mother and infant in jeopardy, so early diagnosis and prompt treatment are extremely important.

HYDRAMNIOS

In hydramnios there is an excessive amount of amniotic fluid. Hydramnios is often present when congenital anomalies exist, particularly those of the gastrointestinal tract. It is a frequent complication of pregnancy in uncontrolled diabetics. When hydramnios develops, the uterus enlarges more rapidly than normal for the period of gestation. Overdistention of the pregnant uterus due to hydramnios may cause a loss of tone of the uterine muscles resulting in postpartum hemorrhage unless the woman is watched closely.

TABLE 18-1 NURSING-CARE PLAN FOR MOTHER WITH AN ABNORMAL LABOR/DELIVERY

ASSESSMENTS	POTENTIAL NURSING DIAGNOSES	INTERVENTIONS	EXPECTED OUTCOME
Determine the progress of labor	Potential for injury, lack of progress of labor related to position, presentation of baby; ineffective contractions; CPD; etc.	Examine patient; note frequency, duration, intensity of contractions; notify physician of lack of progress	Early detection of problems
	Knowledge deficit related to what is happening	Explain what seems to be happening and what is being done about it	Patient expresses understanding of what is happening
Observe physical response of patient to the prolonged labor; monitor fetal heart rate; observe for meconium in amniotic fluid	Alterations in comfort: pain related to prolonged labor	Rub patient's back; position her for comfort; medicate as ordered if she desires; report abnormal fetal heart rate; report meconium in fluid	Patient as comfortable as possible
Monitor intake and output	Actual fluid volume deficit related to low fluid intake	Give intravenous fluids as ordered	Patient receives fluids needed
Observe psychological/emotional response of patient (couple) to prolonged labor	Ineffective individual coping related to fatigue and discouragement because of prolonged labor	Listen to couple; keep them informed of what is happening; explain procedures; reassure them; stay with them; assist doctor with exams; prepare for delivery: vaginal or cesarean section	Couple able to verbalize feelings; receive support they need and are able to cope
	Fear related to safety of mother and infant		Birth is accomplished safely for mother and infant
	Disturbance in self-concept related to inability to have method of childbirth desired		Patient verbalizes feelings; accepts that she was not to blame

✓ SUPINE HYPOTENSIVE SYNDROME

During the latter weeks of pregnancy and during labor, the expectant mother may feel as though she is going to faint when she lies on her back. This is caused by the heavy uterus putting pressure on the inferior vena cava, interfering with the return flow of blood from the pelvis and the legs. The condition can be corrected quickly and simply by having the mother turn onto her side.

A nursing care plan for a mother with an abnormal labor/delivery is presented in Table 18-1.

CLINICAL REVIEW

ASSESSMENT. Mrs. E., a primigravida, was admitted at 4 A.M. in early labor. The cervix was completely effaced and 2 cm dilated. The presenting part was vertex and was at −1 station. Her membranes were intact. By 7 A.M. Mrs. E. was having moderately strong contractions at 3- to 4-minute intervals which lasted 45 to 50 seconds. Her cervix was 5 cm dilated and the presenting part was at −1 station. At this time she was given 50 mg of Demerol and 25 mg of Atarax. At 9 A.M. the doctor examined Mrs. E. and found that the presenting part was at −1 station and the cervix was 7 cm dilated. He ordered x-ray pelvimetry. The x-ray confirmed the doctor's suspicion that Mrs. E.'s pelvis was too small to permit the baby to pass through it. At 10:45 A.M., after being given a spinal anesthetic, Mrs. E. was delivered by cesarean section of an 8 lb 12 oz (3969 g) boy.

1. What is the condition called in which the mother's pelvis is too small for the baby to pass through it?
2. In what way did Mrs. E.'s labor not progress normally?
3. How would the preoperative and postoperative care given to Mrs. E. differ from that given another patient having abdominal surgery? Why?
4. What problems may be associated with spinal anesthesia? If Mrs. E. had been given general anesthesia, what precautions would have been taken to prevent respiratory depression in the infant?
5. What are the delivery nurse's responsibilities when a cesarean section is done?

BIBLIOGRAPHY

Jensen MD, Bobak IM: Maternity Care: The Nurse & The Family, 3rd ed, pp 1043–1069. St. Louis, CV Mosby, 1985
Reeder SR, Martin LL: Maternity Nursing, 16th ed, pp 807–879. Philadelphia, JB Lippincott, 1987

problems during the 19 puerperium

BEHAVIORAL OBJECTIVES When the goals of this chapter are reached, the student will be able to:

○ Define: *postpartum hemorrhage, puerperal infection, endometritis, parametritis, thrombophlebitis, puerperal morbidity, mastitis, cystitis, pulmonary embolism.*

○ *List the three main causes of postpartum hemorrhage.*

○ *Describe the symptoms and treatment of postpartum hemorrhage.*

○ *List three or four duties of the nurse in cases of postpartum hemorrhage.*

○ *Explain how organisms causing puerperal infection may be transmitted to the mother.*

○ *Describe the symptoms of puerperal infection.*

○ *List five or six measures that can be taken to prevent puerperal infection.*

○ *Explain why each of the following may be prescribed for patients with puerperal infection: antibiotics; bed rest; high-calorie, high-vitamin diet.*

○ *Describe the purpose of the position of the bed in endometritis and femoral thrombophlebitis.*

○ *Explain why the affected leg of a mother with thrombophlebitis is never massaged.*

○ *Explain why anticoagulants may be prescribed for patients with thrombophlebitis and tell what observation the nurse should make when they are prescribed.*

○ *Discuss the nursing care of the patient with a puerperal infection.*

○ *Describe the symptoms and treatment of mastitis.*

○ *List two ways to prevent mastitis.*

○ *Describe the symptoms and treatment of cystitis.*

○ *Describe the symptoms and treatment of pulmonary embolism.*

○ *List four or five possible causes of postpartum psychosis.*

✓POSTPARTUM HEMORRHAGE

It has been estimated that, near term, approximately 600 ml of maternal blood flows through the spaces within the cotyledons of the placenta each minute. When the placenta separates during third stage labor, the many arteries and veins that carry this blood to and from these spaces are suddenly left open. Massive hemorrhage can occur unless these vessels are controlled immediately. Ordinarily, two spontaneous internal mechanisms are involved in controlling bleeding (hemostasis) in the body. These are contraction of the vessel wall (vasospasm) and formation of a blood clot. However, the mechanisms more important to hemostasis at the placental site are contraction and retraction of the uterine muscle (myometrium). These mechanisms compress the vessels and close their lumina. Anything that interferes with contraction and retraction of the myometrium can result in postpartum hemorrhage.

Definition. The amount of blood lost following the third stage of labor varies, with the average being about 300 ml. Because of the increase in the blood supply during pregnancy, the body is prepared to tolerate this loss without undesirable effects. Blood loss of 500 ml or more is considered a *postpartum hemorrhage*, because the body may be affected by such a loss.

Causes. The three main causes of postpartum hemorrhage are:

✓Uterine atony
✓Lacerations of the cervix or birth canal
✓Retained pieces of placental tissue or membranes

In *uterine atony*, the uterus does not have good muscle tone. Instead of contracting and compressing the large blood vessels at the placental site, the uterus relaxes and the large vessels bleed freely. The blood may accumulate inside the uterus, where it forms clots and causes the uterus to balloon out, or it may flow out through the vagina in excessive amounts.

One of the most common causes of uterine atony is excessive stretching of the uterine muscle, such as occurs when a mother has a very large baby, twins, or hydramnios (Chap. 18). As the number of pregnancies increases, the likelihood of uterine atony also increases because the uterus loses some of its tone with each pregnancy. Also, a mother who had uterine dysfunction (inertia) (Chap. 18) or placenta previa or abruptio placentae (Chap. 16) may have uterine atony following delivery.

Lacerations of the cervix or birth canal are suspected when bleeding is excessive even though the uterus remains well contracted (Chap. 10). Lacerations are more likely to be present after a forceps delivery.

Retained tissue. Occasionally, a piece of membrane or placental tissue remains embedded in the uterine lining when the placenta is expelled. If the piece is large, such as a whole cotyledon, it can prevent the uterus from contracting down on the blood vessels at the placental site, and hemorrhage results shortly after the third stage of labor ends. If the piece is small, hemorrhage may not occur for a week or more after delivery, when the piece of tissue sloughs away from the lining of the uterus, leaving open vessels at the site where it was attached.

Symptoms.   Postpartum hemorrhage may occur in a matter of minutes as a heavy flow of blood with clots, or over a period of 2 or more hours as a small trickle of blood. Because a large amount of bleeding is startling, immediate steps are taken to stop it. When a large amount of blood is lost, the pulse becomes rapid and thready, the blood pressure drops, and the skin becomes pale, cold, and clammy. The mother may become very apprehensive and may complain of difficulty breathing due to air hunger. The constant trickle of blood is less startling and is therefore less likely to attract attention until symptoms of shock are present or the mother is near death.

Treatment.   The treatment of postpartum hemorrhage depends on its cause. When the cause is uterine atony, the uterus must be made to contract. First the uterus is massaged until it is firm, then it is compressed to expel all blood and clots that have collected inside of it. Oxytocics are usually prescribed by the doctor to keep the uterus contracted; these may be given intramuscularly or in an intravenous infusion. Lacerations of the cervix or birth canal must be repaired when they are the cause of postpartum hemorrhage. When retained pieces of placental tissue or membranes are the cause of hemorrhage, a D&C may be done to remove them.

When bleeding has been severe, transfusions are given to replace the blood lost. The doctor may also prescribe antibiotics to prevent infection, since the mother's resistance is lowered by hemorrhage.

Nursing assessment and interventions.   The nurse caring for the mother during the first few hours postpartum must be mindful of her responsibility for detecting excessive bleeding early. She must not ignore the small trickle of blood, nor should she ignore heavier bleeding simply because the uterus is firmly contracted. She should keep an accurate record of the number of pads the mother saturates in a given length of time.

When the nurse notes that bleeding is heavy or that the uterus is relaxed, she should massage the uterus until it is firm. Then she should press on the uterus to empty it of blood and clots. She should continue to massage the uterus as necessary to keep it contracted; however, over-massage should be avoided, since it tends to tire the uterine muscle and may lead to further relaxation with more blood loss.

The doctor must be notified of hemorrhage immediately. Meanwhile, necessary measures should be taken to combat shock, such as elevating the foot of the bed and keeping the mother warm. The mother, and the father if he is present, need to be told why it is necessary to massage the uterus and to take the other necessary measures—this should be done carefully so as not to alarm them. The mother is usually cooperative if she knows why the nurse is massaging her uterus, even though this may be very uncomfortable for her.

The doctor usually orders blood typed and cross-matched for transfusion and an intravenous infusion of glucose solution. The intravenous can be started with an 18- or 19-gauge needle so that a blood transfusion can be added if necessary. The doctor may order oxytocics added to the intravenous solution if the uterus does not stay contracted. In cases of severe hemorrhage, it may be necessary to administer oxygen to the mother. The nurse should stay with the mother until the hemorrhage is controlled, after which she must observe closely to be sure that the bleeding remains controlled (Table 19-1).

PUERPERAL INFECTION

Definition.   After delivery, the area in the lining of the uterus where the placenta was implanted is left raw and bleeding. It is possible for disease-producing organisms that enter and travel up the birth canal before or during labor or during the puerperium to invade the placental site. Here they find a favorable environment in which to grow and multiply. When invasion of the reproductive tract by pathogenic organisms occurs, the mother has *puerperal infection.*

Puerperal infection may be local, such as an infected stitch in the episiotomy, or it may be general, such as in *septicemia,* in which the organisms invade the bloodstream. When the lining of the uterus is infected, the condition is known as *endometritis;* in *parametritis* the connective tissue around the uterus is infected. *Thrombophlebitis* is an inflammation of the pelvic or femoral veins. It is believed to result from infected thrombi at the placental site and as such is classified as a puerperal infection. Femoral thrombophlebitis is also called "milk-leg" because it was once believed due to collection of milk in the leg.

Causes.   Most puerperal infections are caused by the streptococcus, but other organisms, such as the staphylococcus, the colon bacillus (*Escherichia coli*), and the gonococcus, may also be causes. These organisms are very easily transferred to the mother from the hands of the doctor and nurse unless careful handwashing is practiced; they can also be carried into the birth canal on contaminated gloves or instruments used by the doctor. Unless precautions are taken, organisms from the nasopharynx of doctors and nurses with upper respiratory infections are easily spread to the mother as she is being cared for by them.

Symptoms.   The symptoms of puerperal infection depend somewhat on the area involved. Generally, however, the symptoms include elevated temperature, rapid pulse, chills, headache, a general feeling of tiredness and listlessness, and pain and tenderness in the area involved. In endometritis there may be an increased amount of lochia that has a very foul odor.

During the postpartum period, a mother may develop other infections that cause her temperature to become elevated, but most temperature elevations during the puerperium are caused by puerperal infection. Ac-

TABLE 19-1 NURSING-CARE PLAN FOR PATIENT WITH POSTPARTUM HEMORRHAGE

ASSESSMENTS	POTENTIAL NURSING DIAGNOSES	INTERVENTIONS	EXPECTED OUTCOME
Observe amount and nature of bleeding	Knowledge deficit related to her condition	Remain calm; explain to patient (couple) what is happening and what will be done	Patient verbalizes understanding of her condition
Check height and tone of fundus	Alterations in comfort: pain related to massage of uterus	Massage fundus until firm	Patient tolerates discomfort
Check blood pressure and pulse frequently	Potential injury and hemorrhage related to relaxed uterus, retained placental fragments, and lacerations of birth canal	Compress uterus to empty blood and clots; start or maintain IV line for fluids; empty bladder; notify physician; administer oxytocics as ordered	Blood loss controlled and corrected
Palpate bladder			
	Fear related to her well-being	Keep patient warm; administer oxygen if indicated	Fear relieved
	Fear related to AIDS if blood transfusion is necessary	Administer blood transfusion if ordered; explain that blood for transfusions is tested for AIDS	Fear relieved
		Prepare for D&C if anticipated	

cording to the Joint Committee on Maternal Welfare, any woman who has a temperature of 100.4 °F (38 °C) or higher on two consecutive days during the first 10 days after delivery, excluding the first 24 hours, is considered to have puerperal infection. This temperature elevation is also called *puerperal morbidity*.

Prevention. The prevention of puerperal infection is the responsibility of all who have a part in the care of the mother. One of the most important preventive measures is frequent and thorough handwashing; maintaining strict asepsis in the delivery room is another important measure. To prevent droplet infection, everyone caring for the mother during delivery must wear a mask covering both nose and mouth. Anyone with an infection should be excluded from caring for the mother.

When the perineal area is cleansed, the area must be washed from front to back to avoid bringing organisms from the rectum to the episiotomy and vagina. Each mother must have her own equipment, which must be cleansed and autoclaved before being used by another mother. A mother with an infection must be isolated, preferably off the maternity unit. A nurse who cares for a mother with an infection should not care for other maternity patients.

Treatment. Samples of the drainage or blood are usually cultured to determine what kind of organism is responsible for the infection. The doctor is then able to prescribe the most effective antibiotic or sulfonamide drug. Since the mother needs all the rest she can get, the doctor usually orders bed rest. The mother's fluid intake is increased and a high-calorie, high-vitamin diet is prescribed to help build up her resistance. Analgesics are ordered to help keep her free of discomfort. In endometritis the doctor may prescribe ergonovine (Ergotrate) to keep the uterus well contracted and thus prevent the spread of the infection to the surrounding areas. Also, the head of the bed may be elevated to promote drainage from the uterus.

In femoral thrombophlebitis, the feet and legs are elevated 30° to 45° while the rest of the bed is kept flat, to aid return circulation from the feet and legs. Moist or dry heat may be prescribed to help decrease the size of the thrombus. Because of the danger of dislodging the thrombus and causing an embolism, neither the nurse nor the mother should ever massage the affected leg (see Pulmonary Embolism, below). Anticoagulants such as heparin or dicumarol may be prescribed by the doctor to prevent formation of additional thrombi. Because these drugs interfere with normal clotting of the blood, the nurse must observe the mother closely for hemorrhage from the uterus when they are used.

Nursing assessment and interventions. The mother who develops puerperal infection usually feels tired and listless and generally uncomfortable. She becomes easily discouraged and depressed. If she has been breast-feeding her baby, this may have to be discontinued temporarily in order to conserve the mother's energy and to protect the baby. Although she may understand why this is necessary, it may add to her discouragement. Being isolated from other patients may help her to get more rest, but it may also make her feel depressed.

The nurse should do all that she can to make the mother comfortable and to conserve her strength. She should help the mother to get as much rest and sleep as possible. She can encourage her to eat and to take plenty of fluids. In all of her contacts with the mother, the nurse should be pleasant and sensitive to the mother's needs.

Potential nursing diagnoses:

Knowledge deficit related to her condition

Anxiety related to her condition and the added expense of prolonged hospitalization

Anxiety related to the effect of her illness on the infant and her inability to care for the infant

Alterations in comfort: pain related to the disease process

Sleep pattern disturbance related to her illness

✓MASTITIS

Mastitis is an inflammation of the breast. It is caused most commonly by *Staphylococcus aureus,* but may also be due to hemolytic streptococcus organisms. The organism may be carried to the breasts on the hands of the mother or on the hands of the nurse who examines the breasts each morning. If the baby has acquired the staphylococcus organism in the nursery, the infection may be carried to the breasts during nursing. The organism can easily enter the breasts through cracks in the nipples.

Symptoms. Chills and fever are among the first symptoms experienced by the mother who is developing mastitis. In addition, the lobe of the breast involved becomes reddened and painful and feels hard to the touch.

Prevention. It is important that the mother and the nurse wash their hands well with soap and water before touching the breasts. The first sign of cracked nipples must be reported to the doctor immediately so that treatment can be started.

Treatment. Antibiotics are usually prescribed in treating mastitis. Icebags may be applied to the affected breast to relieve the discomfort and to slow the infection. To make the mother more comfortable, the breasts should be supported well with a snug breast binder or with a well-fitting bra. The doctor decides whether breast-feeding is to continue or not, but even if it is to be continued, the baby is placed on formula temporarily until the infection is healed. With prompt treatment the symptoms subside in one or two days and abscess formation seldom occurs.

CYSTITIS

Cystitis is an inflammation of the bladder caused by bacteria. It is likely to occur in a mother whose bladder is allowed to become overdistended or who is unable to empty her bladder completely when she urinates. The urine that remains in the bladder after a voiding is called *residual* urine. Usually, a mother who voids frequent, small amounts has residual urine; stagnant residual urine is an excellent medium for bacteria. During catheterization, bacteria may be carried from the vulva into the bladder if there is a lapse in aseptic technique.

When a mother is tested for residual urine, catheterization must be done within 5 minutes after the last voiding to be accurate. If 60 ml or more of urine is obtained, the mother is not emptying her bladder completely and residual urine is present.

Symptoms. A mother with cystitis has chills and fever, frequent, painful urination, and a feeling of not having emptied her bladder. She may also complain of pain in her lower abdomen. A urine culture reveals bacteria in the urine.

Treatment. The treatment of cystitis consists of antibiotics, increased fluid intake, and complete emptying of the bladder. An indwelling catheter may be ordered to keep the bladder empty until the infection is cured.

PULMONARY EMBOLISM

Pulmonary embolism is a serious complication that can occur at any time during the puerperium. In this condition, the blood flow to the lungs is partially or completely blocked by a part of a thrombus that has broken loose and been carried along the bloodstream to the right side of the heart, where it occludes the pulmonary artery. If the clot is large enough to completely block the blood flow to the lungs, the woman may die of asphyxia within a few minutes. If the clot is small, she may survive the first attack, but repeated attacks may prove fatal.

Often the thrombus originates in a uterine or a pelvic vein, although it may originate in another vessel. Pulmonary embolism may occur after infection, thrombosis, or severe hemorrhage or shock. Measures that are effective in preventing these conditions can also be helpful in preventing pulmonary embolism. Such measures include careful attention to surgical asepsis, proper management of labor and delivery, and early ambulation after delivery.

Symptoms. The first symptoms the woman with a pulmonary embolism experiences are a sudden, severe pain over her heart and severe difficulty breathing. These are quickly followed by extreme apprehension, syncope, pallor or cyanosis, and an irregular, feeble, or imperceptible pulse. If the clot completely occludes the pulmonary artery, the symptoms may consist of a sudden outcry followed by coma and death.

Treatment. In pulmonary embolism, oxygen must be administered immediately to combat anoxia and shock. The woman should be kept quiet and on her back because any movement could result in death. Morphine is usually given to relieve apprehension and pain, and anticoagulants are prescribed to prevent thrombus formation. If the woman survives for a few hours, it is likely that she may recover. Absolute bed rest is maintained after the initial crisis is over in the hope that the clot will be reabsorbed. Anticoagulant therapy is continued and the woman is kept quiet, warm, and as comfortable as possible. A light, nourishing diet is usually given when she is able to take it.

POSTPARTUM PSYCHOSIS

The postpartum period is a time of adjustments for the woman as she recuperates from labor and birth and begins to assume responsibility for the care of her infant. Most women are able to make these adjustments with little difficulty, probably because of their own mental health and physical and emotional reserves and because of the support they receive from a caring husband, relatives, and friends. Occasionally a woman is unable to make these adjustments and develops a true postpartum psychosis.

Following the birth, the woman needs periods of uninterrupted rest so that she can replenish her depleted energy supply, which is vital to her ability to cope. When this need is ignored, either by the woman, by her husband, family, and friends in their eagerness to celebrate the birth, or by hospital personnel who adhere to rigid schedules of care for the woman and her infant, she may continue to experience fatigue and exhaustion, which diminish her coping capacity. If, in addition, the woman's ability to cope is lessened by other factors, such as a lack of support from her partner and significant others, conflicts between her own desires and the expectations of others, insecurity regarding her ability to provide care for her infant, disappointment because the realities regarding her role of mother are so different from her fantasies, and failure of the birth of the infant to reestablish a desired relationship with her partner, her anxiety and depression may so increase that a postpartum psychosis is the result.

CLINICAL REVIEW

ASSESSMENT. The delivery nurse transferred Mrs. J. to the recovery room at 2:40 P.M. She gave the following report to the recovery nurse: Mrs. J. had a spontaneous delivery of a 9 lb 2 oz (4139 g) baby boy at 2:10 P.M. This is her seventh child. She was given a pudendal block and a midline episiotomy was done. After the placenta was expelled Mrs. J. was given oxytocin 10 units and Methergine 0.2 mg IM. She plans to breast-feed her baby. Her blood pressure is 110/70, her pulse is 80, and her fundus is firm and one fingerbreadth above the umbilicus.

1. From the information obtained in this report, the recovery nurse should observe Mrs. J. for a problem of:
   a. Postpartum hemorrhage
   b. Puerperal infection
   c. Mastitis
   d. Cystitis

2. The most likely cause of this problem is:
   a. *Staphylococcus aureus*
   b. Hemolytic streptococcus
   c. Uterine atony
   d. Residual urine

3. The recovery nurse should suspect this problem if:
   a. Mrs. J.'s lochia is heavy and contains clots
   b. Mrs. J.'s breasts are red and hard and painful.
   c. Mrs. J. has frequent, painful urination
   d. Mrs. J. has a temperature of 100.4 °F (38 °C)

4. If this problem develops, the recovery nurse should:
   a. Have Mrs. J. drink plenty of fluids
   b. Isolate Mrs. J.
   c. Support Mrs. J.'s breasts with a snug-fitting breast binder
   d. Massage Mrs. J's uterus until it is firm.

5. For this problem, the doctor usually prescribes:
   a. Antibiotics
   b. Oxytocics
   c. Icebags to the breasts
   d. Indwelling catheter

BIBLIOGRAPHY

Pritchard JA, MacDonald PC, Gant NF: Williams Obstetrics, 17th ed, pp 719–742. New York, Appleton-Century-Crofts, 1985
Reeder SR, Martin LL: Maternity Nursing, 16th ed, pp 880–900. Philadelphia, JB Lippincott, 1987

problems
of the 20
newborn

BEHAVIORAL When the goals of this chapter are reached, the student will
OBJECTIVES be able to:

○ *Define: asphyxia neonatorum, narcosis, atelectasis, phocomelia, hydrocephalus, tracheoesophageal fistula, pyloric stenosis, omphalocele, cryptorchidism, kernicterus, phototherapy.*

○ *Discuss the feelings and attitudes that parents may exhibit when confronted with the information that their infant is dead or has a problem.*

○ *Describe the care of the infant with asphyxia neonatorum.*

○ *Discuss the treatment of respiratory distress syndrome.*

○ *Describe the symptoms of an infant with pneumonia.*

○ *Explain the cyanosis that may be present in congenital heart defects.*

○ *Discuss the feeding of an infant with cleft lip and cleft palate.*

○ *Discuss nursing problems involving the infant with hydrocephalus.*

○ *Differentiate between spina bifida with meningocele and with meningomyelocele.*

○ *List responsibilities of the nurse caring for an infant whose clubfoot is in a cast.*

○ *Describe the infant with Down's syndrome.*

○ *Explain the cause, detection, and treatment of phenylketonuria.*

○ *List three ways an exchange transfusion benefits the erythroblastotic infant.*

○ *Describe the origin, symptoms, and treatment of thrush.*

○ *Describe the lesions of congenital syphilis.*

○ *List four or five withdrawal symptoms of a drug-addicted infant.*

○ *Discuss the effects of diabetes on the fetus.*

○ *Name and discuss three kinds of birth injuries.*

Most pregnancies end happily with the birth of a healthy, normal infant. Occasionally, however, problems develop during pregnancy, labor, birth, or shortly after birth that result in death or threaten or damage the physical or mental health of the infant. Many of these problems can be cured by appropriate treatment or corrected by surgery. Others can be improved so that the infant can survive and live an almost normal life. A few cannot be treated or improved and, although the infant may survive, a normal life may be impossible.

PARENTAL REACTIONS

The parents of a newborn with a problem are usually deeply affected. How they react to knowing that their child has a problem may be influenced by:

When and how they are informed of the problem

The seriousness of the problem and whether or not it is correctable by surgery or other means

Whether it may occur again with future pregnancies

Their emotional and spiritual maturity

It is usually the responsibility of the doctor to tell the parents that their infant is dead or has a problem. Generally it is considered better to tell them as soon as possible, so that they do not assume that all is well and build up false hopes. The parents may become quite anxious if they are not told what is wrong and yet are not allowed to see the infant. The nurse should be present when the doctor informs the parents, or she should find out from him what information he has given them, so that she can give the parents support and answer their questions intelligently.

Parents are shocked and grieved when they are first informed that their newborn infant is dead or has a problem. They may react by being very talkative: if the child has a disorder, they may ask many questions about the cause, treatment, prevention, cure, and so forth; or they may be silent. They may shed tears or express resentment that this has happened to them, or they may show no emotion. They may wish to be alone or they may appreciate having the doctor or nurse with them. The nurse should try to sense the desires of the parents and should respect their wishes. If they want her with them she should be a good listener and let them express their feelings. While they are deeply involved in their own grief, they usually do not appreciate hearing of other people who have had a similar experience.

The family's pastor, priest, or rabbi or the hospital chaplain may provide support in this situation and should be contacted if the parents wish it. If the infant is in imminent danger of dying, the subject of baptism should be discussed with the parents so that their wishes can be carried out. This is very important to members of the Roman Catholic church and to members of some Protestant denominations.

Some parents never adapt to having a child who is less than normal. These parents' mental health, marriage, and relationship with the child are in jeopardy. A higher divorce rate and an increase in child abuse are found among parents of premature or sick infants. Support groups are effective in helping these parents cope and thereby reduce these undesirable outcomes. However, even parents who are able to cope find that their lives are permanently affected, emotionally and economically, by the birth of a severely ill or anomalous infant who survives.

The nursing-care plan for the family of a dead or severely ill infant is presented in Table 20-1.

PROBLEMS AFFECTING RESPIRATION

ASPHYXIA NEONATORUM

If the infant does not breathe within 30 to 60 seconds after birth, the condition is known as *asphyxia neonatorum*. In asphyxia the oxygen supply to the body is decreased and the carbon dioxide is increased. A brief period of asphyxia may do no harm, but prolonged asphyxia may result in permanent brain damage or death.

Any condition of the mother, such as pregnancy-induced hypertension (PIH), placenta previa, and abruptio placentae, that may interfere with the oxygen supply to the fetus can cause asphyxia. However, the most common causes are:

Interference with oxygen supply before birth (anoxia), such as when prolapse of the cord occurs

Injury to the brain, which can occur during a long, difficult labor or a difficult delivery

Too much analgesia or anesthesia given to the mother during labor and delivery (narcosis)

Nursing interventions. The infant with asphyxia should be kept warm and handled gently. Resuscitative measures include clearing the air passages of mucus and fluid and administering oxygen. It is the responsibility of the nurse to have the needed supplies and equipment ready for use when this emergency develops (Fig. 20-1).

RESPIRATORY DISTRESS SYNDROME

Respiratory distress syndrome (RDS) is a condition in which a hyaline membrane forms in the lining of the alveoli of the lungs. This membrane prevents the normal exchange of carbon dioxide and oxygen in the part of the lung where it forms. As a result, collapse (atelectasis) of that part of the lung occurs, and the unaffected part of the lung must work harder to provide enough oxygen for the body. For this reason, the breathing of the infant with RDS is rapid and labored. Respirations may be accompanied

TABLE 20-1 NURSING-CARE PLAN FOR THE GRIEVING FAMILY

ASSESSMENTS	POTENTIAL NURSING DIAGNOSES	INTERVENTIONS	EXPECTED OUTCOME
Identify the family experiencing loss of an infant or birth of an infant with an anomaly or a life-threatening illness	Anticipatory or dysfunctional grieving	Encourage family to verbalize feelings; allow family time with dead or sick infant as soon as possible; prepare family by describing how infant looks before showing him to them; prepare infant so that he looks as normal as possible before showing him	Family works through grief
	Knowledge deficit related to cause of death, anomaly, or illness; prognosis for sick infant; probability for recurrence in future pregnancy	Provide information family seeks; answer questions; give family photograph and crib card with measurements if they desire; obtain written consent for autopsy according to hospital policy	Family verbalizes understanding of cause, prognosis, or probability of recurrence
Determine religious affiliation		Notify clergy; see that infant is baptized if parents desire	
Find out what family support systems are available	Ineffective individual or family coping	Inform parents of community support groups, social worker, counseling available; assign patient a room away from mothers with healthy infants; encourage family to visit nursery and to touch, hold, feed, and cuddle ill infant as his condition permits	Family members supportive of each other
Determine effect the experience is having on the family structure		Be realistic regarding prognosis; explain equipment used in care of infant; provide follow-up care as needed	Individuals and family able to cope successfully; family structure strengthened

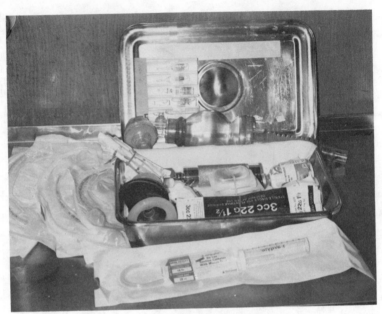

FIG. 20-1. *Resuscitation equipment tray.*

by a grunting sound, flaring of the nostrils, and pulling in (retraction) of the chest wall. When breathing is extremely difficult, the abdomen rises and the chest sinks on inspiration, and the chest rises and the abdomen sinks on expiration; this is known as seesaw breathing (Fig. 20-2). If unable to get sufficient oxygen, the infant becomes cyanotic. What causes the hyaline membrane to form is not known.

RDS may develop within a few minutes after birth or it may not appear until several hours later. It is the leading cause of death among premature infants and occurs in about 50% of infants of diabetic mothers and those who had vaginal bleeding during pregnancy. It is also found in infants born by cesarean section, although the incidence is not believed

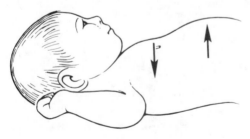

FIG. 20-2. *Seesaw respirations. (Oehler JM: Family-Centered Neonatal Nursing Care. Philadelphia, JB Lippincott, 1981)*

to be higher in full-term infants born by cesarean section with no other complications.

Some conditions that cause higher cortisol levels in the fetus may lessen the risk of RDS by stimulating earlier lung maturity. Among these conditions are premature rupture of the membranes, partial abruptio placentae, intrauterine infections, and maternal hypertensive disease. When betamethasone, a synthetic steroidal hormone, is given to a pregnant woman a few days before her expected premature delivery, it stimulates maturation of the fetal lungs and may be helpful in preventing RDS in the small premature infant.

Nursing assessment and interventions. The nurse must observe all newborn infants closely for signs of respiratory distress during the first few hours following birth. The first signs of difficult breathing must be reported to the doctor so that treatment can be started at once (Table 20-2).

Infants with RDS are placed in an incubator with oxygen and humidity administered as prescribed by the doctor. The additional oxygen and the humidity make breathing easier, and the humidity also helps to maintain an even temperature in the incubator. The infant's respirations, color, and temperature are observed closely. To facilitate observation of respirations, the infant is undressed except for a diaper. The nurse regulates the temperature of the incubator to meet the body temperature needs of the infant. The baby's position is changed frequently and mucus is suctioned as necessary.

Some babies recover quite rapidly from RDS, but others do not survive.

TREATMENT OF RESPIRATORY DISTRESS SYNDROME

○ Adequate oxygenation
○ Correction of acid-base imbalance
○ Adequate caloric and fluid intake
○ Protection against heat loss
○ Rest
○ Assisted ventilation if necessary

PNEUMONIA

Nursing assessment and interventions. The nurse's observations of newborns' respirations, color, cry, activity or lack of it, and how they take their feedings are very important to the early detection of problems. This is especially true in the detection of pneumonia, which causes approximately 10% of the deaths among newborns. An infant with pneumonia has rapid respirations, is pale or cyanotic, eats poorly or refuses to eat, is listless, and may have a temperature higher or lower than normal.

TABLE 20-2 CLINICAL MANIFESTATIONS OF RESPIRATORY DISTRESS SYNDROME

OBSERVATIONS	AUSCULTATION	ARTERIAL BLOOD GASES	X-RAY FINDINGS
Tachypnea	Diminution of breath	Hypoxia	Reticulogranular
Nasal flaring	sounds	Hypercarbia	pattern
Retractions		Acidosis—respiratory	Ground glass
Paradoxical (seesaw)		and often	appearance
respirations		metabolic	Perihilar streaking
Grunting			Air bronchogram
Cyanosis			Atelectasis
Generalized edema			
Pitting edema of hands			
and feet			
Flaccid, hypotonic			
posture			

An infant may be born with pneumonia as a result of bacteria entering the uterus during a prolonged labor or after early rupture of the membranes. Pneumonia may develop as a result of the infant aspirating fluid during birth or after a feeding. It may also be caused by bacteria and viruses coming in contact with the infant in the nursery. The mother with prematurely ruptured membranes may be given antibiotics to protect her and her infant from infection. At birth, efforts are made to prevent aspiration of fluid into the lungs by clearing the airway before the infant begins to breathe. In the newborn nursery, the infant is placed on one side after a feeding so that regurgitated fluid can roll out of the mouth instead of being aspirated. The infant who has a problem with regurgitation may be helped by having the head of the crib elevated for a while after each feeding. To protect the infant against bacteria and viruses, personnel with infections are excluded from the nursery. If the mother has a cold, she is given a clean mask to wear each time the baby is taken to her.

Treatment. Infants with pneumonia are isolated and given oxygen and antibiotics. The oxygen makes breathing easier and improves the infant's color, and the antibiotics combat the infection. Intravenous or subcutaneous fluids may also be given to maintain hydration and to provide nourishment until the baby is eating well again (Table 20-3).

DEVELOPMENTAL AND HEREDITARY PROBLEMS

Developmental and hereditary problems may manifest in any part of the body. They may be obvious at birth, or skilled observation may be required to detect them. Some of these problems can be corrected by surgery; others cause handicaps but permit survival. Still other problems are so extensive or so involve vital organs that the infant cannot survive outside the uterus. The nurse caring for the newborn must be on the alert to detect signs of problems early.

TABLE 20-3 NURSING-CARE PLAN FOR INFANT WITH RESPIRATORY DISTRESS SYNDROME

ASSESSMENTS	POTENTIAL NURSING DIAGNOSES	INTERVENTIONS	EXPECTED OUTCOME
Observe for rapid, labored, seesaw breathing; cyanosis; nasal flaring; grunting; retractions; edema; flaccid, hypotonic state; dehydration or fluid overload; electrolyte imbalance	Impaired gas exchange related to lack of lung surfactant	Give oxygen as needed; record oxygen concentration every hour	Infant with problem identified immediately
	Ineffective airway clearance related to increased secretions and decreased ability to cough	Suction as needed; change position frequently; restrain infant as necessary	Breathes easily with assistance
	Fluid volume and electrolyte imbalance related to RDS, fluid loss, and use of parenteral fluids	Give intravenous fluids as ordered; maintain correct rate; feed with high calorie formula; gavage feed if needed to conserve energy; elevate head after feeding; record weight	Fluid and electrolyte balance attained and maintained
	Alterations in nutrition, less than body requirements related to higher caloric usage than intake	daily; maintain appropriate temperature of infant and incubator; record and report infant's response to treatment	Infant gains weight steadily, responds to treatment

CONGENITAL HEART DEFECT

Congenital heart defect causes more deaths during the first year of life than any other defect. Among the more common defects are a patent ductus arteriosus, in which the opening between the aorta and the pulmonary artery does not close after birth; and a patent foramen ovale, in which the opening between the right auricle and the left auricle does not close (see Fig. 7-5). In these instances, the venous blood mixes with the arterial blood and the infant is cyanotic or a grayish color. In other heart defects, where there is no mixing of venous and arterial blood, cyanosis may not be present. Breathing is usually rapid and labored when congenital heart defects exist; the infant may also eat poorly. Some congenital heart defects can be corrected by surgery.

CLEFT LIP AND CLEFT PALATE

Cleft lip is a condition in which there is a separation of the upper lip on one or both sides of the midline. When the separation is on one side only, it is a unilateral cleft lip; when it is on both sides, it is a bilateral cleft lip. The separation may be small or may extend into the nostril. A cleft lip may exist alone or may be accompanied by a cleft palate, which is a separation down the middle of the roof of the mouth. A cleft palate may be present without a cleft lip (Fig. 20-3).

Nursing interventions. Infants with a cleft lip and/or a cleft palate need to be suctioned frequently because they have more mucus and are less able to cope with it than normal newborns. An ointment or oil is rubbed on the lip to keep it from becoming dry.

Feeding is a major problem with infants who have a cleft lip and cleft palate. They may be fed by nipple, with a rubber-tipped medicine dropper, with an Asepto syringe, or with a cup (Fig. 20-4). They should be held in an upright position while being fed so that gravity can aid in swallowing.

FIG. 20-3. *This baby has a cleft lip and complete cleft palate.*

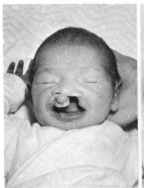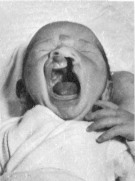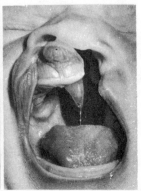

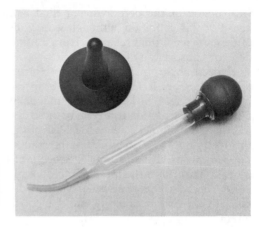

FIG. 20-4. *Lamb's nipple and Chetwood feeder. (Oehler JM: Family-Centered Neonatal Nursing Care. Philadelphia, JB Lippincott, 1981)*

Babies with this condition usually swallow a lot of air during a feeding and must be burped often. Mothers are taught to feed their babies before taking them home.

Treatment.   Surgery is performed on the lip when the baby's condition permits, usually when a weight of 8 to 10 lb (3629 to 4536 g) is reached. Many doctors prefer to keep these infants in the hospital until surgery is done, to prevent them from being exposed to infections and also to avoid shocking other children in the family by the sight of the unrepaired cleft lip.

The cleft palate is repaired as soon as the infant's mouth is large enough for the surgeon to work in, usually by 18 months of age. Many doctors prefer to repair the cleft palate before the child begins to talk so that a nasal tone of the speech does not develop.

PHOCOMELIA

An infant with phocomelia is born without arms or legs or with only stumps where the limbs should have developed. One cause of this abnormality is the drug thalidomide, if taken by the mother during the early part of pregnancy. Since many drugs are known to be harmful to the fetus and the effects of many others are not known, the pregnant woman is cautioned against taking drugs not considered by her doctor to be essential to her health.

The child born with phocomelia can be fitted with artificial limbs at one of the many child amputee centers located throughout this country.

HYDROCEPHALUS

In hydrocephalus an excessive amount of cerebrospinal fluid is generated in the ventricles of the brain. This causes an increase in the size of the infant's head proportional to the amount of excess fluid present.

Obstruction of the cerebrospinal fluid pathways is the most common cause of this condition, although it may also be due to overproduction of cerebrospinal fluid resulting from a tumor of the choroid plexus or to defective absorption of the fluid.

Hydrocephalus may develop before birth or it may not be evident until after birth. When it develops before birth and the head is greatly enlarged, labor is long and difficult, and normal delivery is difficult or impossible. Often the presentation is breech in these cases, since the head is too large to fit into the mother's pelvis. Because of the cephalopelvic disproportion, the doctor may have to puncture the cranial vault and aspirate enough of the cerebrospinal fluid to make delivery of the head possible; this is not in itself harmful to the infant. Fetal mortality in cases of hydrocephalus is 70%. Both parents need much support during the prolonged labor and difficult delivery because of the risk to the mother and danger to the infant.

Treatment. Treatment of hydrocephalus usually entails inserting a shunt that bypasses the obstruction and drains the excess fluid into a body cavity. This treatment is not curative, but it helps to prevent further enlargement of the head so that care of the infant is easier. Although an occasional case of hydrocephalus is self-limiting and becomes arrested before pressure causes brain damage, curative surgical procedures have been devised for only certain rare types of hydrocephalus.

Nursing interventions. The infant with hydrocephalus has the same need to be held and loved as any other infant, although the size of the head may make this difficult. Holding the infant during a feeding may be very tiring unless the chair has an arm on which the elbow can rest while supporting the infant's heavy head. Burping the infant may also be difficult because of the heavy head. Vomiting may be a problem if brain damage has occurred. In addition to keeping the infant warm, clean, and dry, the nurse or mother must prevent breakdown of the skin on the head by frequent changes of position. The nurse or mother caring for the infant with hydrocephalus can convey love and comfort by a gentle touch and soothing voice.

SPINA BIFIDA

Spina bifida is a defect of the spine in which the bony part of the spinal canal fails to close. The membranes (meninges) of the spinal cord may protrude through the opening or they may remain in the spinal canal. If they remain in the spinal canal, the spina bifida may present no problems. When the membranes bulge through the opening, they form a soft sac that fills with cerebrospinal fluid; this is known as a meningocele. If nerve fibers as well as membranes protrude, the condition is called meningomyelocele (or myelomeningocele) (Fig. 20-5). When either of these is present, the sac may rupture and the infant may develop meningitis. Hydrocephalus frequently accompanies either meningocele

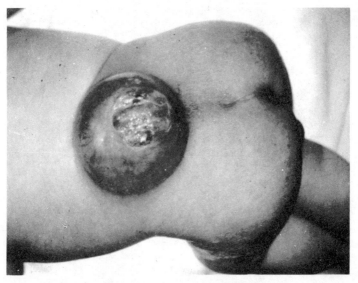

FIG. 20-5. *Myelomeningocele.*

or meningomyelocele. Paralysis of the trunk, legs, and bowel and bladder sphincters may be present in meningomyelocele. Surgical correction of spina bifida is possible, although it may accelerate the development of hydrocephalus; the paralysis in meningomyelocele is likely to persist in spite of surgery.

CLUBFOOT

Clubfoot (talipes) is a deformity in which there is an abnormal turning of one or both feet (Fig. 20-6). It is caused by an unequal pull of muscles that may result from hereditary factors, or from muscle imbalance or intrauterine position.

Treatment. Treatment depends on the severity of the condition. Nonsurgical measures include passive overcorrection of the foot by the nurse or mother several times a day or application of plaster casts. In passive overcorrection, the leg is well supported under the calf and the knee is flexed while the entire foot is pulled as far as possible in the opposite direction and held for 1 minute. Supporting the leg and flexing the knee protect the lateral ligaments of the knee and the epiphysis of the tibia from strain.

When treated with a plaster cast, the foot is held in a position as near to normal as possible, without forcing it, while the cast is applied over the foot, ankle, and leg to midthigh; the knee is flexed.

Surgical correction of clubfoot may be necessary when nonsurgical

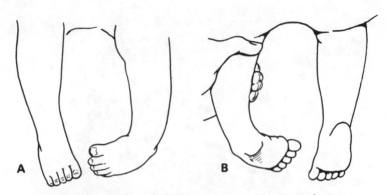

FIG. 20-6. *Unilateral clubfoot. (A) Front view. (B) Back view.*

correction is not feasible. Surgical correction usually entails lengthening the Achilles tendon, capsulotomy of the ankle joint, or release of medial structures.

Nursing assessment and interventions. When a cast is applied, the nurse must prevent denting of the cast before it dries. Frequent observations of the infant's toes and thighs are necessary to detect signs of circulatory impairment, such as swelling, coldness, and discoloration. If these signs appear, the doctor should be notified at once. He should also be notified if the infant seems unusually restless, because this could indicate that the cast is causing undue irritation. The cast is changed every 1 to 3 weeks to provide gradual correction and to allow for growth. The mother may need to be reassured that the cast does not hurt the baby and that she will be able to care for the baby properly while the cast is on. Arranging for her to care for the baby in the hospital before she and the baby go home is an effective way to give her this reassurance.

TRACHEOESOPHAGEAL FISTULA

A tracheoesophageal fistula consists of a tubelike passage between the esophagus and the trachea. It is often present when the esophagus ends in a blind pouch instead of continuing to the stomach. Anything the infant tries to swallow, including milk and his own secretions, overflows from the blind pouch into the trachea. This causes coughing, gagging, cyanosis, and expulsion of the milk through the nose during feedings. Because he is unable to manage his secretions, the infant appears to have excessive drooling. Frequent suctioning and elevation of the infant's head 30° or more are necessary to prevent aspiration.

The nurse should report the symptoms promptly so that the condition can be corrected before complications from aspiration or inadequate hydration and nutrition develop. The diagnosis is confirmed with radiography and the defect is corrected by surgery. After surgery the infant is placed in an incubator for warmth, humidity, and oxygen. His color and vital signs are monitored closely. Frequent nasopharyngeal suctioning is done to maintain a clear airway. Parenteral fluids are usually given until the infant is able to take oral feedings. Antibiotics may be prescribed to prevent infection.

PYLORIC STENOSIS

The pylorus is the lower opening of the stomach connecting it with the duodenum. In pyloric stenosis, the pylorus is hypertrophied so that its opening is very narrow. This delays emptying of the stomach with the result that the stomach becomes distended. The infant with pyloric stenosis forcefully ejects the stomach contents within 30 minutes after each feeding. This forceful vomiting is called projectile vomiting and is characteristic of this condition. Another characteristic symptom consists of visible peristaltic waves that can be seen passing from left to right during and immediately after a feeding. In addition, the hypertrophied pylorus can usually be palpated as a mass about the size of an olive in the upper right quadrant.

Treatment. If the condition is not corrected, the infant soon loses weight and becomes dehydrated. Then the dehydration and electrolyte imbalance must be corrected before surgery is performed. Although surgery is the usual treatment, some doctors prefer first to try antispasmodic drugs, changes in the amount, frequency and thickness of feedings, and changes in the infant's position after feedings. If these changes produce no improvement, then surgery is performed.

Nursing assessment and interventions. After the surgery, the nurse observes the infant's color and monitors his vital signs closely. When oral feedings are begun, it is important that the doctor be kept informed of how the feedings are tolerated so that he can increase the amount and strength of them as needed. It may be necessary for the nurse to help the parents develop positive feelings regarding feedings if the parents were dismayed by the vomiting.

OMPHALOCELE

An omphalocele is a defect in the abdominal wall through which the peritoneal sac covered with amnion and filled with abdominal organs protrudes (Fig. 20-7). The defect is caused by failure of the lateral folds of the abdomen to fuse by the tenth week of fetal life.

The immediate care of the infant consists of measures to prevent rupture of the sac, if it is still intact after delivery, and to prevent infection. The sac or the exposed abdominal organs are covered with sterile towels or sponges saturated with normal saline. Then a dry towel is placed over the wet ones. Sterile gloves are worn to apply the dressings and to change them. The infant must be restrained and great care taken when

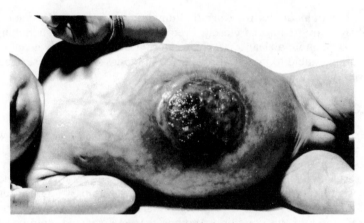

FIG. 20-7. *Omphalocele.*

positioning and turning him to prevent tension on the sac. Nasogastric suction may be necessary to prevent distention. Antibiotic therapy is instituted to protect against infection. If the sac ruptures, there is grave danger that peritonitis, sepsis, respiratory difficulty, and pneumonia may develop.

Treatment. Treatment entails replacing the abdominal organs into the abdominal cavity and surgically correcting the defect. If the defect is small, this can be done in one operation. If it is large, it may need to be done in stages. Intravenous fluids are given to maintain hydration and electrolyte balance.

Nursing interventions and assessment. The infant is kept in an incubator for warmth, humidity, and oxygen before and following surgery. His color and vital signs are monitored closely and the condition of the sac and the presence of distention are noted.

IMPERFORATE ANUS

In imperforate anus there is no opening to the anus; instead, the rectum ends in a blind pouch. The abnormality is usually discovered when the nurse attempts to take a rectal temperature, or during the doctor's examination of the infant. Immediate correction by surgery is necessary.

CRYPTORCHIDISM

Cryptorchidism denotes the failure of one testis or both testes to descend into the scrotum. It is much more prevalent in premature infants than in those born at term. Spontaneous descent occurs by puberty in most cases. If spontaneous descent does not occur, treatment may consist of a series of injections of chorionic gonadotropin, followed by surgery (orchiopexy) if the hormone therapy fails. Sterility is inevitable when the testes remain in the abdomen because the higher temperature of the abdomen retards spermatogenesis and damages the tubules.

EPISPADIAS AND HYPOSPADIAS

In these defects, the urethra does not extend the length of the penis. In epispadias, the urethral meatus is located on the dorsal surface of the penis; in hypospadias it is located on the ventral surface. When the urethra is very short, it must be extended surgically so that the meatus is located in the glans.

BIRTHMARKS

Occasionally an infant is born with a so-called birthmark. This may consist of a pigmented nevus or a vascular nevus (hemangioma). Pigmented nevi are generally of three types: (1) a smooth, flat, brown or black pigmented area; (2) a pigmented area containing downy or stiff hair; or (3) a raised, wartlike area. Pigmented nevi may create no problems, or they may be so located that they are subject to trauma or repeated irritation, or they may be large and disfiguring. Surgical excision may be indicated for cosmetic purposes or to prevent trauma or irritation.

Vascular nevi (port wine marks) are flat, red to purplish areas that are commonly seen on the face or neck. Surgery and irradiation are sometimes tried with this type of nevus but often the results are unsatisfactory. Use of cosmetic creams to cover the area may be the most satisfactory treatment. The nurse's acceptance of an infant with a disfiguring mark may help the parents accept and love him. Their acceptance and love are important to the child's psychological adjustment to his disfigurement.

DOWN'S SYNDROME

Down's syndrome, also called mongolism, is a disorder in which the infant has physical defects and is severely retarded mentally. Characteristically, the infant with Down's syndrome has slanting eyes that are close together, a small head, thick neck, flat nose, a large protruding tongue, short and thick hands with unusual creases across the palmar surfaces, flabby skin, underdeveloped muscles, and relaxed joints (Fig. 20-8). Cataracts, hernias, and heart and alimentary tract abnormalities may also be present. The infant has little resistance to infection; this may cause death at an early age.

Down's syndrome results from three types of chromosome abnormalities. Most commonly it is caused by trisomy of chromosome 21, which increases the chromosome count to 47 instead of the normal number of 46. This abnormality usually occurs in infants born to older women and is rarely familial. The second type occurs in infants born to younger women

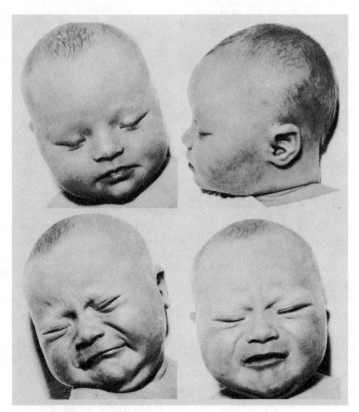

FIG. 20-8. *Newborn baby showing facial characteristics of Down's syndrome. (Potter EL: Pathology of the Fetus and the Newborn. Chicago, Year Book, 1952)*

and is familial. It results from translocation of a chromosome during cell division. In this type, which is rare, the chromosome count is 46, but two chromosomes are misplaced. The third type, due to mosaicism, is very rare. In mosaicism an individual has a different number of chromosomes in some cells than in others; for example, the blood cells may have 47 chromosomes while the skin cells have 46 chromosomes. This type is not familial and may result in fewer abnormalities than the other types.

It is a shocking experience for parents to learn that their child has Down's syndrome, and they need all the emotional support the nurse and doctor can given. The decision of whether or not to place the child in a special institution is difficult to make. The parents will also be concerned about whether any other children they may have will be born with this defect. The nurse can help by being informed about available resources to care for the child and by permitting the parents to express their feelings about the child and the future.

PHENYLKETONURIA

Phenylketonuria (PKU) is also a hereditary problem. In this condition the body is unable to metabolize the protein phenylalanine. This substance is taken into the body in certain foods, such as milk, that are high in protein. Since the phenylalanine cannot be metabolized by the body, it accumulates in the tissues and blood and eventually spills over into the urine, where it is excreted as phenylketone bodies (thus the name, phenylketonuria).

A simple blood test can detect PKU within a few days after birth. This test involves obtaining a drop or two of blood from the infant's heel to determine the phenylalanine level in the blood (Fig. 20-9). It can be done after the baby has been receiving milk feedings for at least 24 hours. Normally the blood contains 1 to 2 mg of phenylalanine per 100 ml; a finding of 8 mg/100 ml is considered an indication of PKU.

After the infant is 4 to 6 weeks old, a urine test can be done to detect PKU. A solution of ferric chloride is dropped on the wet diaper immediately after the infant voids. If the area on the diaper turns green, the test is positive.

Many hospitals are testing for PKU before newborn infants are dis-

FIG. 20-9. *A simple blood test that involves obtaining blood from the infant's heel is used to detect PKU.*

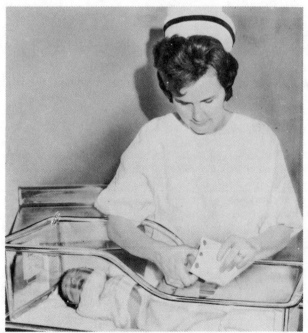

charged home. Some states have passed laws requiring that all newborns be tested by the time they are 28 days old.

Treatment. Unless PKU is detected and treated early, the infant usually becomes mentally retarded. Treatment consists of putting the infant on a special diet containing a limited amount of phenylalanine.

FAILURE TO THRIVE

Failure to thrive is characterized by malnutrition, failure to grow, and a delay in motor and social development. The child often appears very solemn and watchful and may resist physical contact. He may seem unable to establish a trusting relationship with the persons caring for him.

The cause of failure to thrive is a lack of maternal love. Separation of the infant from the mother soon after birth because of prematurity or some other problem may result in a deprivation of maternal love, or it may occur as a result of a lack of love in the home. Treatment consists of providing the infant or child with love and attention. The child improves remarkably when he feels loved and wanted.

Maternity nurses can help prevent this condition by promoting maternal-infant bonding during the first hour after birth and during the entire hospital stay. Nurses in intensive care nurseries can help by providing opportunity for the mother to touch and talk to the infant during the acute phase of the illness and to hold and cuddle him as soon as his condition permits.

PROBLEMS INVOLVING THE BLOOD

The most common problems of the newborn involving the blood are Rh incompatibility and ABO incompatibility.

RH INCOMPATIBILITY

The mechanisms responsible for Rh incompatibility and erythroblastosis fetalis are discussed in Chapter 16. The following discussion concerns primarily the detection and treatment of erythroblastosis fetalis. Varying degrees of erythroblastosis may occur in newborns. It may be so mild as to require no treatment or it may be so severe as to cause the death of the infant before or soon after birth. If the infant is born alive, the severity of the condition can usually be determined by performing tests on the cord blood and by observing the infant.

When an Rh-negative mother gives birth, a sample of umbilical cord blood is collected for the following tests: (1) blood group, (2) Rh factor, (3) hemoglobin, (4) Coombs, and (5) bilirubin. Other tests may be done if the doctor so desires. The Coombs test determines if the infant's red blood cells are coated with antibodies. A low hemoglobin level (less than

15 g/100 ml), and a high bilirubin level (more than 3 or 4 mg/100 ml) and a positive Coombs test on the cord blood of an Rh-positive infant are indications of erythroblastosis, and the infant may need treatment.

The infant of an Rh-negative mother is observed closely for jaundice. Unlike physiologic jaundice, which appears on the third or fourth day of life, jaundice due to erythroblastosis may appear within a few hours or a day or two after birth. The doctor must be notified if the infant becomes jaundiced.

Jaundice is an indication that the infant's bilirubin level is rising. Very high bilirubin levels may cause permanent brain damage known as *kernicterus*. Infants with kernicterus are lethargic, eat poorly, have a shrill cry, and, if they survive, are mentally retarded.

Treatment.   The treatment of erythroblastosis fetalis consists of replacing the infant's blood with Rh-negative blood; this is called an exchange transfusion. In an exchange transfusion, a small amount of the infant's blood is withdrawn and an equal amount of Rh-negative blood is injected. The process is continued until the desired amount of blood is exchanged. This type of transfusion removes from the infant the red blood cells that are coated with antibodies and also removes some of the bilirubin in the bloodstream. At the same time it supplies fresh hemoglobin. The infant continues to be Rh positive and to manufacture Rh-positive red blood cells, but since no more antibodies are received from the mother, the treatment is effective.

When called on to assist with an exchange transfusion, the nurse is usually responsible for having the sterile supplies and blood ready. She may also be responsible for keeping a record of the amount of blood withdrawn and the amount given. Throughout the procedure, infants are usually given oxygen as a supportive measure; they must also be kept warm. Color, respirations, and pulse are observed closely to see how the infant tolerates the procedure.

ABO INCOMPATIBILITY

When the mother's blood type is O and the baby's type is A or B, ABO incompatibility may develop. This condition is very similar to Rh incompatibility.

Although maternal and fetal blood normally do not mix, breaks in the placental barrier may occur, permitting fetal red blood cells to enter the maternal circulation, or the large gamma M or 19S antibodies from the maternal circulation to enter the fetal circulation. The smaller gamma g or 7S antibodies are able to cross the intact placental barrier. Both 19S and 7S antibodies are present in Rh disease, while 19S antibodies are present in ABO incompatibility. Because these large antibodies must gain access to the fetal circulation through breaks in the placental barrier, and because the A or B antigens present in all the infant's body cells tend to absorb excess antibodies and reduce the effect on the red cells, ABO disease is usually much milder than Rh disease. However, the infant may be born with anemia and may develop jaundice within a few hours after birth. Unlike Rh disease, the first baby born to a mother may be affected by ABO incompatibility.

Treatment. Phototherapy (treatment by exposure to light) is often used to treat or prevent jaundice in the newborn and premature infant. Some doctors advocate its use after an exchange transfusion to prevent the need for further transfusions; others recommend it as an alternative to exchange transfusion. Phototherapy may also be used in cases of hyperbilirubinemia not associated with Rh and ABO incompatibilities and in treating premature infants who, because of their immature liver enzyme systems, are unable to excrete bilirubin adequately. The purpose of phototherapy is to reduce the bilirubin levels in the blood and thus prevent brain damage from kernicterus.

Phototherapy consists of exposing the infant to light from either fluorescent or the GE daylight 20-watt bulbs. Usually fluorescent light tubes are used. The light is placed over the infant's crib or incubator at a distance of 15 to 24 inches from the baby.

The baby's eyes are covered during the treatment as a precaution against possible retinal damage from irradiation (Fig. 20-10). Eye pads may be used and held in place by a piece of stockinette. Care must be taken when covering the eyes to make sure the eyelids are closed; otherwise corneal abrasions can occur.

To provide maximum exposure of the skin during the treatment, the baby is kept uncovered and undressed, except for a diaper. The diaper is necessary in most instances because these infants tend to have loose green stools, and also as a precaution against the male infant spraying urine and possibly breaking the bulbs. The diaper also prevents one of the rare side effects of phototherapy: priapism (painful continued erection of the penis).

If a commercial light that has a safety shield is not being used, the nurse must be sure there is an adequate protector of some kind between the bulb and the infant to prevent injury should a bulb break. She should devise a method to indicate the length of time a given bulb has been in used, since the energy output of bulbs decreases rapidly after 200 hours of use and the rate of decline of the bilirubin levels would be reduced by using the same bulbs for too long a time. When a commercial light is used, the manufacturer's instructions regarding replacement of bulbs should be followed.

The nurse needs to keep close watch over infants receiving phototherapy. She must keep their eyes covered and see that their temperature does not rise. If there is an increase in temperature, they should be removed from under the light temporarily. If the temperature continues to stay up, the doctor must be notified. Because infants may have loose stools and lose excessive fluid from the tissues, the nurse should give them water to replace this loss. The infant's position should be changed every 2 hours.

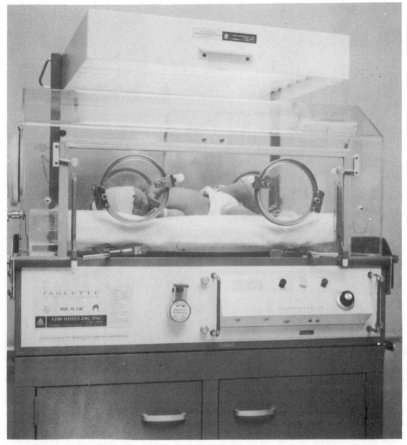

FIG. 20-10. *During phototherapy treatment the infant's eyes are covered.*

Some infants receiving phototherapy seem restless for a while when the treatment is begun. This may be due to their eyes being covered or because they are not dressed and snuggled. Usually if they are wrapped snugly with a blanket for a few minutes they will go right to sleep; then the blanket can be removed.

The nurse also needs to know that, due to capillary dilatation, the skin may take on a sunburned look. This appearance is usually transient and is not considered significant. However, the eating and sleeping patterns of the infant should be observed and changes reported to the doctor (Table 20-4).

The length of time the infant is under the light is prescribed by the doctor. Although a specific schedule is usually set, such as 12 hours under

TABLE 20-4 NURSING-CARE PLAN FOR INFANT WITH JAUNDICE DUE TO Rh OR ABO INCOMPATIBILITY

ASSESSMENTS	POTENTIAL NURSING DIAGNOSES	INTERVENTIONS	EXPECTED OUTCOME
Find out mother's and infant's Rh and ABO blood type; find out if direct Coombs' test is positive	Potential for injury, kernicterus related to elevated bilirubin levels	Give frequent feedings; record intake and output	Decreased bilirubin levels with maintenance of hydration and stable temperature
Observe for jaundice within first 24 hr	Potential for injury, dehydration, conjunctivitis, hyperthermia related to phototherapy	Give phototherapy as ordered; remove clothing except for diaper; cover infant's eyes; uncover every 4 hr for visual stimulation; report conjunctivitis	Prompt recognition of symptoms
Check infant's eyes at least every 4 hr for conjunctivitis during phototherapy; observe infant's response to visual stimulation			No conjunctivitis; infant responds to visual stimulation
Observe for diarrhea, dehydration, elevated temperature during phototherapy; monitor intake and output	Alterations in bowel elimination: diarrhea related to phototherapy	Record temperature of infant and incubator frequently; report elevated temperature of infant; change diaper as necessary; keep skin clean; change position frequently	No diaper rash
Observe infant's interaction with parents	Potential alterations in parenting related to separation caused by infant receiving phototherapy	Take infant to parents for feeding and interaction	Infant interacts normally with parents
If transfusion ordered, observe infant closely after transfusion for jaundice, apnea, jitteriness, irritability, low temperature	Potential for injury, hyperbilirubinemia, electrolyte imbalance, hypoglycemia, hypothermia related to exchange transfusion	Prepare infant for exchange transfusion; restrain infant; obtain supplies needed; keep infant warm; give oxygen as ordered; keep record of blood withdrawn and given; assist doctor as necessary; report signs of problems after transfusion	Infant tolerates transfusion without developing problems

and 12 hours out or 6 hours under and 2 hours out, most doctors feel it is important that the infant not be under the light continuously for several days. The long-range effects of the light on growth and development are not known at this time. Follow-up studies are being conducted to determine such effects.

Exactly how phototherapy acts to reduce the bilirubin level is not completely understood. It is recognized that photo-oxidation of the bilirubin occurs in the skin and not in the plasma, because parts of the body that are covered by clothing during the treatment remain jaundiced. It appears that the light converts the bilirubin into a colorless, polar, water-soluble compound that can be readily excreted in the urine.

INFECTION

STAPHYLOCOCCAL INFECTIONS

Staphylococcal organisms may be brought into the nursery through the air, in the nasopharynx of personnel, or on nursery equipment. The skin, nose, and umbilical areas of the newborn may then become reservoirs for these organisms. Staphylococcal infections may appear as pustular eruptions on the skin.

Impetigo is a staphylococcal infection in which yellow blisterlike lesions are found on moist skin surfaces, such as in the creases of the thighs and the neck and under the arms.

Cord infections may also result from invasion by staphylococci. The organisms may gain access to the body through the cord and a generalized infection may follow.

An infant with suspicious pustules or with a red, moist, foul-smelling cord should be isolated immediately, and the symptoms brought to the attention of the doctor (Table 20-5).

DIARRHEA

One of the most dangerous organisms to the newborn is *Escherichia coli* (abbreviated *E. coli*). The pathogenic strain of this organism is frequently the cause of epidemic diarrhea.

The infant with epidemic diarrhea has frequent, loose, watery, green stools. As a result, the infant quickly becomes dehydrated and loses weight rapidly. Isolation of an infant with epidemic diarrhea is of extreme importance, because the infection can spread very rapidly in the nursery. The doctor prescribes treatment according to the specific organism causing the infection. Water, glucose in water, and electrolyte fluids are given to combat the dehydration, to provide nourishment, and to maintain electrolyte balance. Usually these fluids are given intravenously or subcutaneously, but small amounts may be given orally.

TABLE 20-5 NURSING-CARE PLAN FOR INFANT WITH INFECTION

ASSESSMENTS	POTENTIAL NURSING DIAGNOSES	INTERVENTIONS	EXPECTED OUTCOME
Observe infant for skin rash, lesions, jaundice, unstable temperature, lethargy, lack of muscle tone, full or bulging fontanel, rapid respirations, apnea, retractions, grunting, cyanosis, vomiting, diarrhea, cool skin, hypotension, mottling	Potential for infection related to immature immune system, environmental factors, exposure to maternal infection, exposure to infection in nursery	Obtain lab specimen as ordered; assist with diagnostic tests; record vital signs and other symptoms; report abnormal findings; record intake and output; give intravenous fluids as ordered; give antibiotics and other medication as ordered; wash hands frequently and thoroughly; give oxygen as ordered; handle infant gently; keep infant warm; use isolation precautions according to hospital policy	Prompt detection of signs of infection
	Ineffective airway clearance related to infectious process		Breathes normally without assistance
	Alterations in bowel elimination: diarrhea related to infection		Normal stools
Check vital signs frequently			Normal vital signs
Monitor intake and output; check environmental temperature frequently	Fluid volume deficit related to diarrhea, vomiting, feeding problems		Takes adequate feedings; no vomiting; fluid volume maintained; urinates adequately
	Alterations in comfort: pain related to infectious process		Able to rest comfortably

THRUSH

Candida albicans causes an infection called thrush in the mucous membrane of the mouth of the newborn. In this condition, white, curdlike patches resembling milk are found on the gums, palate, inside the cheek, and on the tongue. When these patches are rubbed off, they leave a raw, bleeding surface.

The infant may get this infection from the mother, if she has a vaginal infection caused by the same organism, or in the nursery, unless cleanliness and strict aseptic techniques are practiced. Thrush responds well to treatment with gentian violet or nystatin.

CONGENITAL SYPHILIS

Congenital syphilis, which has become more prevalent in recent years, can be prevented by good prenatal care. Treatment of the syphilitic mother with adequate doses of penicillin is effective in protecting the fetus because penicillin readily crosses the placenta. Since treatment does not prevent future acquisition of syphilis, the woman must be observed for signs of reinfection so that she can be retreated if necessary. If possible, her partner should also be treated.

Congenital syphilis can cause stillbirths and prematurity. The infant with this disease may be born with obvious lesions, or the lesions may not appear for a few days or up to 4 months after birth. The lesions, which are highly infectious, occur on the face, buttocks, palms, and soles (Figs. 20-11

FIG. 20-11. *Congenital syphilis showing shiny erythema and desquamation of hands.*

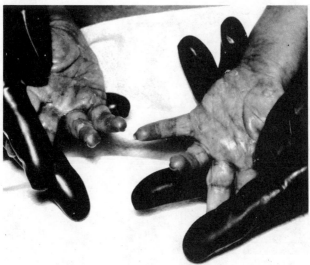

and 20-12). Mucous patches are present in the mouth and condylomas about the anus. The infant may become jaundiced and develop "snuffles" (rhinitis) and a hoarse voice. The ends of the long bones become enlarged and may become inflamed so that a pseudoparalysis is present. Loss of weight, anemia, and enlargement of the liver and spleen occur.

If the condition is untreated, severe manifestations of the disease, such as deformed teeth, bones, nose, and joints, may show up later in life. The disease may also spread to the central nervous system. Penicillin in adequate doses is effective in treating congenital syphilis.

DRUG ADDICTION

With narcotic addiction becoming more widespread, the number of infants born with addiction is also on the increase. The symptoms manifested by these infants include restlessness, tremors, shrill cry, convulsions, or twitchings of the extremities or face. Diarrhea, vomiting, anorexia, yawning, sneezing, and excessive mucus may also be present. These symptoms are due to withdrawal and should be brought to the attention of the doctor so that treatment can be started.

The doctor usually orders an increased fluid intake, supportive measures, and diminishing doses of sedatives. These measures usually result in a permanent cure since the infant is not mentally and emotionally dependent on the drug.

Research is being done to find out the effects on the offspring of mothers who have taken the drug lysergic acid (LSD-25) before or dur-

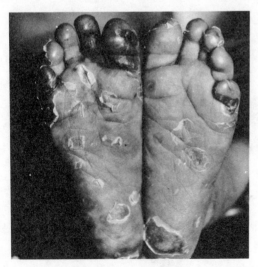

FIG. 20-12. *Congenital syphilis showing shiny erythema and desquamation of feet.*

ing pregnancy. This research has revealed that there is an increase in chromosomal abnormalities in the children born to women who took LSD-25 during pregnancy. There is also an increase in chromosomal abnormalities in the children born to women who took this drug prior to but not during pregnancy; the increase in this group, however, was not as great as it was in those who took the drug during pregnancy. It is not known yet if and how these chromosomal abnormalities will be manifested as malformations.

Maternal alcoholism is another condition that can cause problems in the newborn. These problems are reviewed in Chapter 17.

INFANTS OF DIABETIC MOTHERS

The condition of the baby born to a diabetic mother depends to a great extent on:

The duration and severity of the diabetes
How well controlled the diabetes is
Whether other complications are present
Whether the infant was delivered prematurely

In mild cases of diabetes that are well controlled and where no other complications exist, the pregnancies are usually allowed to continue to term. The infants generally are in as good condition as infants of nondiabetic mothers. If the diabetes has existed for a longer period of time and has been more difficult to control, the infant is at greater risk for problems. The more severe the diabetes and the less controlled it is, the greater the risk to the infant. The risk increases when complications or prematurity are present.

Infants born to mothers with severe or poorly controlled diabetes are usually large for gestational age (Fig. 20-13), have a higher stillbirth and neonatal death rate, and have more congenital anomalies than infants of nondiabetic mothers.

The excessive size—often 10 lb (4536 g) or more—of infants of diabetic mothers is due to hyperglycemia in the mother and hyperinsulinism in the fetus. When the mother has hyperglycemia, glucose crosses the placenta and enters the fetal circulation. There it promotes fetal growth by increasing fat deposits in the fetal tissues and enlargement of the fetal organs. It also stimulates the islets of Langerhans to increase production of insulin. Since insulin stimulates growth, this hyperinsulinism of the fetus contributes to its unusual size. Problems associated with large-for-gestational-age infants include hypoglycemia, respiratory distress syndrome, hyperbilirubinemia, and hypocalcemia (Table 20-6).

Diabetes tends to affect the vascular system. The placenta is a highly vascular organ and it is also the organ that maintains the life and health of the fetus. Vascular changes in the placenta that result from uncontrolled

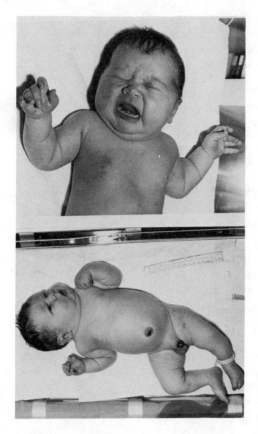

FIG. 20-13. *Infant of diabetic mother (IDM). (Avery GB: Neonatology, 2nd ed. Philadelphia, JB Lippincott, 1981)*

maternal diabetes can render it ineffective in its life-supporting functions. Thus placental insufficiency can result in fetal death. Also, a pregnant woman with severe or poorly controlled diabetes may develop ketosis, which can result in fetal acidosis and death.

The longer a woman has had diabetes, the more likely she is to give birth to an infant with congenital anomalies. Hydramnios is often associated with congenital anomalies even when the mother is not a diabetic. When the mother is a diabetic of long standing and the pregnancy is complicated by hydramnios, the infant is very likely to have anomalies. These anomalies may occur in any part of the body, although the more common ones appear to be:

Those involving the upper gastrointestinal system, such as stenosis of the esophagus or duodenum

Left colon syndrome (microcolon)

Ventricular septal defect of the heart

Sacral agenesis

TABLE 20-6 NURSING-CARE FOR INFANT OF DIABETIC MOTHER

ASSESSMENTS	POTENTIAL NURSING DIAGNOSES	INTERVENTIONS	EXPECTED OUTCOME
Identify infant of diabetic mother	Potential for injury at birth related to excessive size	Weigh and record; keep infant warm; give frequent early feedings; give oxygen as needed; give intravenous fluids as ordered; maintain correct rate; give calcium as ordered	No birth injury
Observe for metabolic problems due to hypoglycemia: jitteriness, irritability, apnea, Dextrostix less than 45	Fluid volume and electrolyte imbalance related to maternal diabetes		Fluid and electrolyte balance
Observe for metabolic problems due to hypocalcemia: tremors, convulsions, twitchings, calcium levels below 7 mg/dl			
Observe for birth injuries resulting from excessive size of infant: subdural hematoma, cephalhematoma, fracture of clavicle, nerve injury			
Observe for anomalies			

Of the deaths occurring among infants of diabetic mothers during the neonatal period, over half are due to congenital anomalies.

Babies born to diabetic mothers are observed closely and are treated as premature infants regardless of their size. These babies are often jittery, lethargic, poor eaters, and subject to frequent attacks of cyanosis; they often have a peculiar, high-pitched cry. Hypoglycemia often develops within 3 hours after birth. This is because the supply of glucose the infant has been receiving from the mother is terminated abruptly by birth and the high production of insulin by the infant cannot be stopped as quickly. Hypoglycemia is detected by using a Dextrostix to test the blood sugar immediately after birth and hourly thereafter, or as ordered by the physician. If the Dextrostix shows the blood sugar to be less than 45 mg/100 ml, the physician is notified. The hypoglycemia is corrected by an intravenous infusion of 10% glucose. An infusion pump is used so that a constant rate of flow is maintained (Fig. 20-14).

Recent developments in fetology that are helping to reduce the risk to babies of diabetic mothers include estriol determinations, ultrasound, the oxytocin challenge test, and amniocentesis (see Chap. 9).

BIRTH INJURIES

INTRACRANIAL HEMORRHAGE

Intracranial hemorrhage is bleeding anywhere within the cranial vault. Most often it occurs as a result of stretching and lacerations of the tentorium cerebelli, so that the bleeding is into the cerebellum, the pons, and the medulla oblongata. Intracranial hemorrhage is most likely to occur in difficult vaginal deliveries in which version and extraction or difficult forceps applications are involved. It may also occur as a result of excessive pressure on the fetal head in a rapid, precipitous delivery, or as a result of prolonged pressure on the head with excessive molding and overlapping of the fetal skull bones in an unusually long primiparous labor.

The onset and severity of symptoms of intracranial hemorrhage depend on the amount of bleeding present. When sudden, massive hemorrhage occurs, the infant may be born dead. If the bleeding is slow, the infant may be born in apparently good condition, with symptoms appearing a few hours or days later. The symptoms may include drowsiness, apathy, a sharp, shrill cry, pallor or cyanosis, grunty respirations, convulsions, and flaccidity or spasticity. Often *opisthotonos*, backward bowing of the head and neck and extension of the legs, accompanies spasticity.

Treatment. Treatment consists of supportive measures, including providing warmth and oxygen, gentle, minimal handling, close observation of vital signs, and gavage or intravenous feedings. The physician usually prescribes sedation for the convulsions, vitamin C and vitamin K to control

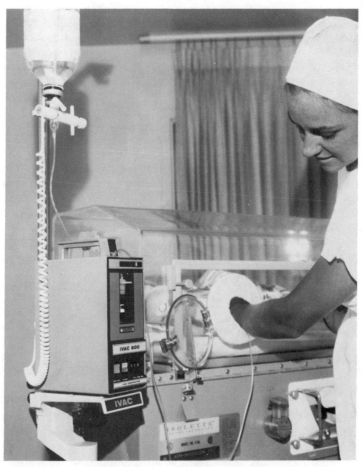

FIG. 20-14. *An infusion pump is used to control the rate of flow of intravenous fluids administered to the baby of a diabetic mother. (Photo courtesy of IVAC Corporation, San Diego, California)*

the hemorrhage, and prophylactic antibiotics. The infant should not be placed in the Trendelenburg position; rather, the head should be kept a few inches higher than the hips to lower intracranial pressure. The physician may perform a spinal tap for diagnostic purposes and to remove excess bloody fluid if a subdural hematoma is suspected.

In mild cases recovery may be complete with no residual damage. In more severe cases the outcome may be fatal. Some infants who survive may develop motor disturbances, including cerebral palsy, and mental deficiency. With cesarean section delivery replacing difficult vaginal deliveries, this injury is much less common than it once was.

The parents may need considerable support when their infant has intracranial hemorrhage. The nurse should be as realistic as possible when giving them reports on the condition of the infant so as not to encourage false hopes or cause undue concern. Although it is important that the infant be kept quiet, the parents can usually be encouraged to see it and talk to it softly and perhaps to touch it gently.

FACIAL PARALYSIS

Sometimes an infant delivered by forceps develops paralysis of the muscles on one side of the face as a result of pressure by the forceps on the facial nerve. The eye on the affected side may remain open and the mouth may be drawn to the other side, giving a distorted appearance to the face. This can cause concern to the parents, who need to be reassured that the condition is temporary and that spontaneous recovery will occur in a few days or hours. While the paralysis lasts, sucking may be a problem for the infant; the nurse should be aware of this and assist the mother with feedings as necessary.

BRACHIAL PLEXUS PALSY

The brachial plexus is a network of nerves that supplies the arm, forearm, and hand. Stretching or tearing of these nerves may occur in difficult deliveries, such as in breech delivery when there is forceful pulling of the shoulder away from the head, or in vertex delivery of a large baby with shoulder dystocia when the head is sharply flexed on the shoulders. This injury to the nerves results in paralysis of the upper arm, lower arm, or whole arm. In most instances, only the upper arm is affected, a condition known as Erb-Duchenne paralysis. The paralysis is easily detected since the affected arm hangs limply at the infant's side with the elbow extended and the hand rotated inward.

As soon as the diagnosis is made, the physician may order splinting of the arm to reduce tension on the brachial plexus and to permit edema to subside. Passive range of motion exercises are usually begun early and continued as healing occurs to prevent contractures and muscle deterioration. The parents are taught how to care for the infant with the splint and how to do the exercises before the infant is discharged.

Recovery depends on the extent of the nerve damage. If the nerves are only stretched, recovery usually occurs within a few weeks. If moderate damage has occurred, recovery may take months and may be incomplete so that reconstructive surgery may be necessary. If the nerves are completely ruptured, there may be no recovery and the muscles may gradually waste away. In severe cases where surgery is not beneficial, amputation above the elbow and fitting with a prosthesis may be accomplished during adolescence.

FRACTURES AND DISLOCATIONS

Manipulative procedures such as version, and difficult deliveries may result in fractures and dislocations in the infant. Difficult breech deliveries can result in fractures of the clavicle, humerus, femur, or cervical spine, or in dislocations of the hips, clavicle, jaw, or cervical spine. Fractures or dislocations of the cervical spine may be accompanied by spinal cord injury that causes flaccid paralysis of the trunk. Vertex delivery in which there is shoulder dystocia may result in fracture of the clavicle. Dislocation of the hip may occur as a result of defective formation of the acetabulum, which permits upward and backward movement of the femur.

A fracture may be detected because the infant refuses to move the affected arm or leg or cries when it is moved. It may also be detected because of a visual angulation or hypermobility of the bone, or because of a hematoma over the fracture. The Moro reflex is reduced on the side of the fracture. X-ray studies are used to confirm the diagnosis and aid in setting the fracture.

Fractures are set, and splints, slings, casts, and traction are used as necessary to maintain good alignment and to immobilize the part. Swaddling the infant is often helpful in immobilizing the part. Fractures usually heal quickly in the newborn infant.

Gentle manipulation is employed to reduce dislocations. This is done immediately to prevent permanent joint deformity. After the dislocation is corrected, splints may be used to maintain the desired position.

The apparatus used in treating the infant with a fracture or dislocation makes caring for him difficult. It may intimidate the parents so that they are afraid to touch him. Since the use of splints and similar devices is likely to continue after the infant goes home, the parents should become familiar with them while he is in the hospital so that they can care for him comfortably without adding to the injury. They should be encouraged to hold him even though it may be awkward, so that he does not lack love and attention.

HEARING PROBLEMS

Routine hearing testing is conducted in some newborn nurseries to detect deaf or hard-of-hearing infants. Early detection of infants with hearing problems is important so that treatment or corrective measures can be started in time to develop what hearing remains and to prevent retardation in speech as far as possible.

A nurse or other trained person tests the infant by using either of two specially designed instruments, the *Vicon Apriton* or the *Rudmose Warblet 300.* While the infant rests quietly or sleeps in the crib, the instrument is held within 4 to 10 inches of the ear. Pressing a button on the instrument causes a shrill noise of measured intensity and output to be emitted. A record is made of the date and time of the testing, the state of the infant, the infant's response, and the intensity of this response (Table 20-7). If the response to the test is normal, the date and "Cleared for hearing" are

TABLE 20-7 NEONATAL HEARING TEST*

Swedish Medical Center
Neurodiagnostic Lab
Routine Hearing Screening Program

    Anticipated date of discharge _____

High-risk register

1. Positive family history of deafness	1.	_____
2. Rubella, or other nonbacterial intrauterine fetal infection	2.	_____
3. Maxillofacial abnormalities	3.	_____
4. Intensive care nursery	4.	_____

Hearing screening test   Test Dates

1. Positive response	1.						
2. No response	2.						
3. Inappropriate state to test	3.						

Comments:_____

_____

Follow-up

    Parents advised infant passed test (Date) _____

    Parents advised follow-up at SMC _____

        Parent's name _____

        Address _____

        Phone number _____

        Date _____

Referral letter sent to doctor advising at SMC _____

Letter to parents advising follow-up at SMC _____

Follow-up letter to doctor advising test clearance _____

Parents telephoned advising follow-up at SMC _____

*Neurodiagnostic Lab, Swedish Medical Center.

stamped on the infant's chart. If there is no response, even after repeated testing, the date of the tests and "Not cleared for hearing" are stamped on the chart. The pediatrician is notified when an infant is not cleared for hearing, so that follow-up care can be given.

CLINICAL REVIEW

ASSESSMENT. Scott and Shari B. are an attractive young couple who are attending the university. Pregnancy did not seem to interfere with their education or their very active social life. When Shari became aware that she was pregnant, she and Scott began to read and inform themselves about human reproduction. They also attended a series of classes for expectant parents.

Shari was awake when she gave birth to her son. Almost immediately she noted that something was wrong with the infant's mouth. She became quite excited and demanded that the doctor tell her whether the baby had a cleft lip. Very calmly the doctor examined the infant's lip and mouth and replied that he did indeed have a bilateral cleft lip and also a cleft palate. Shari screamed, "Take it away! I don't want to see it. I'll not have it! It isn't mine!"

1. How do you feel about Shari reacting this way toward her baby?
2. Why do you think she reacted this way?
3. How do you feel about caring for Baby B.?
4. Although the doctor talked with Mr. and Mrs. B. for a long time and answered the many questions they asked about the cause, treatment, and possible recurrence in future children of cleft lip and cleft palate, they asked the nurse the same questions when she checked Shari in the recovery room. Why do you think they did this?
5. What do you think Baby B.'s greatest needs are?
6. What nursing problems is he likely to present?

Three days after her baby was born, Shari began to accept him and his problems and became very attentive to him and his needs.

BIBLIOGRAPHY

Galloway KG: Placenta evaluation studies: The procedures, their purposes, and the nursing care involved. Am J Maternal-Child Nurs 1:300, 1976
Hawkins JW: "Did we do all we could?" Am J Nurs 2:158, 1986
Jackson PL: When the baby isn't perfect. Am J Nurs 4:396–399, 1985
Jasper ML: Pregnancy complicated by diabetes. Am J Maternal-Child Nurs 1:307, 1976
Paritzky JF: Tay-Sachs: The dreaded inheritance. Am J Nurs 3:260–264, 1985
Reeder SR, Martin LL: Maternity Nursing, 16th ed, pp 982–987, 1019–1068. Philadelphia, JB Lippincott, 1987
Whitaker CM: Death before birth. Am J Nurs 2:157–158, 1986

low birth weight and **21** preterm infants

BEHAVIORAL When the goals of this chapter are reached, the student will
OBJECTIVES be able to:

○ Tell how weight and gestational age are used in classifying newborns.

○ List at least six possible classifications of an infant at birth.

○ List four or five causes of growth retardation in utero.

○ List four or five problems the preterm infant may experience, and two or three problems common to postterm infants.

○ Define: premature infant, preterm infant, low birth weight infant.

○ State the most common cause of prematurity and list two or three other causes.

○ Name the leading cause of death among preterm infants.

○ Describe the external appearance of the preterm infant.

○ Describe the breathing of the premature infant and explain why it is as it is.

○ Explain the physiological basis for each of the following problems common to the small premature infant: hemorrhage, unstable temperature, regurgitation.

○ Discuss the dangers associated with regurgitation.

○ List four or five ways the premature infant can be protected from infection.

○ Explain why the oxygen a premature infant receives is carefully controlled.

○ Discuss ways the premature infant may be fed.

○ Describe gavage feedings and tell what observations are made during such feedings.

o *List four or five observations the nurse makes of the premature infant.*

o *Discuss how the premature infant's emotional needs can be met.*

o *Discuss ways the nurse can provide support to the parents of a premature infant.*

CLASSIFICATION OF INFANTS BY SIZE AND GESTATIONAL AGE

Newborn infants were once classified simply as premature or term. A premature infant was one born before 37 weeks' gestation or one weighing 2500 g (about 5½ lb) or less. A term infant was one born after 37 weeks or one weighing more than 2500 g. The inadequacies of this classification are obvious, for many infants do not fit into either of these categories. For instance, infants of some nonwhite races may be well developed and mature although weighing less than 2500 g at term. Others, such as infants of diabetic mothers, may weigh more than 2500 g but be very immature. Infants with growth retardation may be born at 40 weeks' gestation but weigh less than 2500 g. Because of these discrepancies, this classification has been replaced by one that more accurately describes the growth and maturity of infants at birth.

In this new classification, weight is used to indicate growth, and gestational age is used to indicate maturity. Through studies and observations, weights that are appropriate to each stage of pregnancy have been established (Fig. 21-1). Infants whose weights fall into the category appropriate for their gestational age are classified as *appropriate for gestational age* (AGA); those whose weights are less than they should be for their gestational age are classified as *small for gestational age* (SGA); and those weighing more than they should for gestational age are classified as *large for gestational age* (LGA). Infants are also classified according to the gestational age. Those born before 37 weeks are *preterm*, those born between 37 and 42 weeks are *term*, and those born after 42 weeks are *postterm*. Thus, an infant born before 37 weeks' gestation and weighing less than the expected weight would be classed as preterm, SGA, while another infant born at the same time and weighing the expected weight would be classed as preterm, AGA. These classifications recognize individual growth rates and also serve to alert the health team to certain problems associated with infants who fall into the SGA and LGA categories and the preterm and postterm categories (Table 21-1).

Before these classifications can be applied, the infant's weight and gestational age at birth must be known. The weight can be determined easily by placing the infant on a scale. The gestational age can be determined by finding out the date of the mother's last menstrual period or by assessing the infant's physical and neurologic development. Signs of the physical and neurologic development normally present at various weeks of pregnancy have been arranged in chart form and assigned scores to make assessment easier (Table 21-2 and Fig. 21-2). The higher the score the greater the gestational age, and the greater the gestational age the more mature the infant.

Most small-for-date infants are born at or near term and are mature. Their growth may have been retarded early in pregnancy due to an interference with mitosis, which resulted in fewer new cells being formed. The cells that were formed, however, are normal in size. Or their growth may

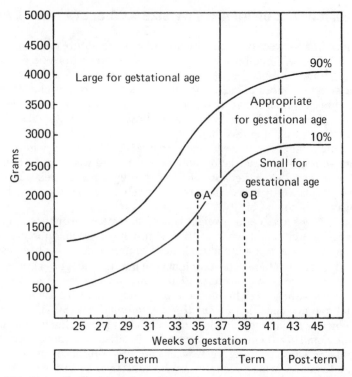

FIG. 21-1. *The birth weights of liveborn singleton Caucasian infants at gestational ages from 24 to 42 weeks.*

have been retarded later in pregnancy, so that they have a normal number of cells but these are smaller in size. It is also possible for growth to be interrupted early and for stunting to continue throughout pregnancy, so that the number of cells is decreased and the cells are small in size.

Many factors may be responsible for growth retardation, including malnutrition, genetic factors, placental insufficiency, multiple pregnancy, moderate and heavy smoking by the mother, and infections such as rubella and cytomegalic inclusion disease.

Certain problems are associated with infants who are preterm, SGA, LGA, or postterm. Preterm infants may develop hypothermia, hyperbilirubinemia, hypoglycemia, anemia, and respiratory distress syndrome. Most congenital malformations occur in SGA infants. In addition, these infants are susceptible to intrauterine infections and hypoglycemia. LGA infants are usually those of diabetic mothers (see Chap. 20). They too may encounter such problems as hypoglycemia, hypocalcemia, hyperbilirubinemia, and respiratory distress syndrome. Neonatal asphyxia, meconium as-

(*Text continues on p. 494*)

TABLE 21-1 NURSING-CARE PLAN FOR SMALL-FOR-GESTATIONAL-AGE (SGA) INFANT

ASSESSMENTS	POTENTIAL NURSING DIAGNOSES	INTERVENTIONS	EXPECTED OUTCOME
Determine gestational age	Potential for injury, asphyxia, meconium aspiration, hypoglycemia, unstable temperature related to intrauterine growth retardation	Have resuscitative equipment ready for use at birth; assist with resuscitation as necessary; assist with direct visualization and suctioning of meconium and amniotic fluid as necessary; give oxygen as necessary; keep infant warm	Normal respirations
Check weight			Normal color and activity
			Tolerates feedings
Observe for SGA characteristics: loose, dry skin; lack of subcutaneous fat; sunken abdomen; decrease in chest and abdominal circumference; thin, yellowish, dull, dry umbilical cord; sparse scalp hair			Normal temperature
Check for glucose with Dextrostix		Record Dextrostix findings; report abnormal findings	
Observe for signs of complications typical for these infants		Carry out treatment for complications as ordered	No complications, or, if complications develop, respond to treatment

TABLE 21-2 SYSTEM OF SCORING EXTERNAL PHYSICAL CHARACTERISTICS

EXTERNAL SIGN	SCORE*				
	0	1	2	3	4
Edema	Obvious edema of hands and feet; pitting over tibia	No obvious edema of hands and feet; pitting over tibia	No edema		
Skin texture	Very thin, gelatinous	Thin and smooth	Smooth; medium thickness. Rash or superficial peeling	Slight thickening Superficial cracking and peeling, especially of hands and feet	Thick and parchment-like; superficial or deep cracking
Skin color	Dark red	Uniformly pink	Pale pink; variable over body	Pale; only pink over ears, lips, palms, or soles	
Skin opacity (trunk)	Numerous veins and venules clearly seen, especially over abdomen	Veins and tributaries seen	A few large vessels clearly seen over abdomen	A few large vessels seen indistinctly over abdomen	No blood vessels seen
Lanugo (over back)	No lanugo	Abundant; long and thick over whole back	Hair thinning especially over lower back	Small amount of lanugo and bald areas	At least ½ of back devoid of lanugo
Plantar creases	No skin creases	Faint red marks over anterior half of sole	Definite red marks over > anterior ½; indentations over < anterior 1/3	Indentations over > anterior 1/3	Definite deep indentations over > anterior 1/3
Nipple formation	Nipple barely visible; no areola	Nipple well defined; areola smooth and flat, diameter < 0.75 cm	Areola stippled, edge not raised, diameter < 0.75 cm	Areola stippled, edge raised, diameter > 0.75 cm	

Breast size	No breast tissue palpable	Breast tissue on one or both sides, < 0.5 cm diameter	Breast tissue both sides; one or both 0.5 to 1.0 cm	Breast tissue both sides; one or both > 1 cm
Ear form	Pinna flat and shapeless, little or no incurving of edge	Incurving of part of edge of pinna	Partial incurving whole of upper pinna	Well-defined incurving whole of upper pinna
Ear firmness	Pinna soft, easily folded, no recoil	Pinna soft, easily folded, slow recoil	Cartilage to edge of pinna, but soft in places, ready recoil	Pinna firm, cartilage to edge; instant recoil
Genitals: Male	Neither testis in scrotum	At least one testis high in scrotum	At least one testis right down	
Genitals: Female (with hips ½ abducted)	Labia majora widely separated, labia minora protruding	Labia majora almost cover labia minora	Labia majora completely cover labia minora	

Source: Adapted by Dubowitz et al.: Clinical assessment of gestational age in the newborn infant. J Pediatr 77:1, 1970. From Farr et al.: The definition of some external characteristics used in the assessment of gestational age of the newborn infant. Dev Med Child Neurol 8:507, 1966.
*If score differs on two sides, take the mean.

FIG. 21-2. *Techniques of neurological assessment and scoring of findings. (According to Dubowitz et al from Amiel–Tison C: Neurological evaluation of the maturity of newborn infants. Arch Dis Child 43:89, 1968)*

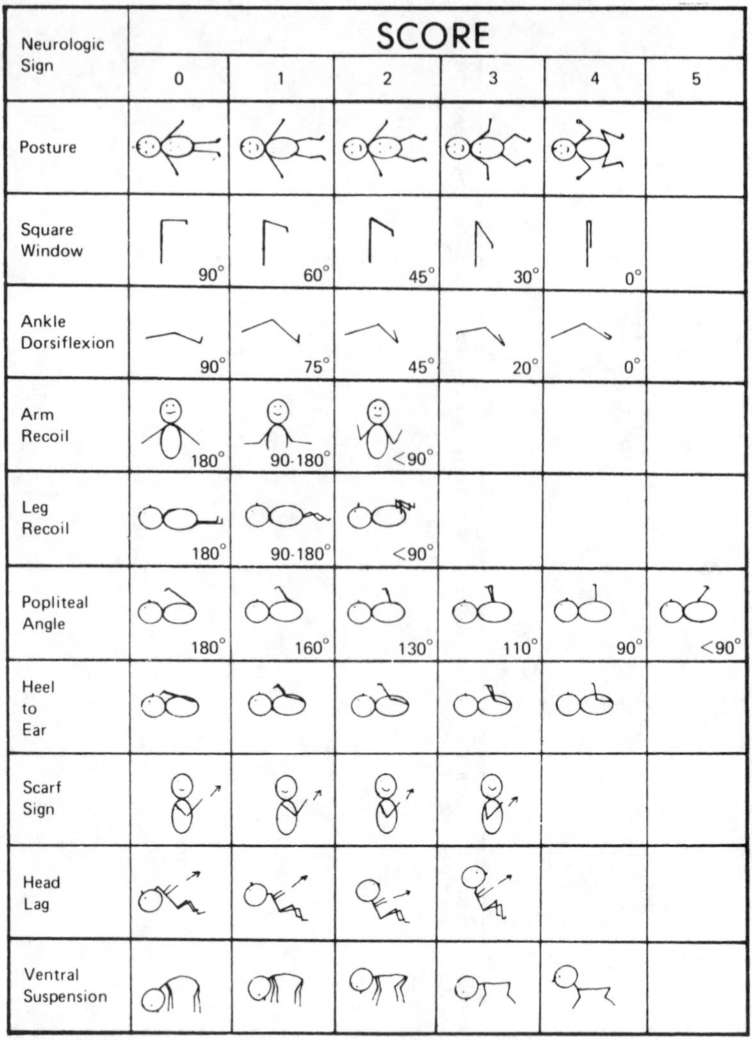

Neurologic Sign	SCORE					
	0	1	2	3	4	5
Posture						
Square Window	90°	60°	45°	30°	0°	
Ankle Dorsiflexion	90°	75°	45°	20°	0°	
Arm Recoil	180°	90-180°	<90°			
Leg Recoil	180°	90-180°	<90°			
Popliteal Angle	180°	160°	130°	110°	90°	<90°
Heel to Ear						
Scarf Sign						
Head Lag						
Ventral Suspension						

POSTURE

○ With the infant supine and quiet, score as follows:

- arms and legs extended = 0
- slight or moderate flexion of hips and knees = 1
- moderate to strong flexion of hips and knees = 2
- legs flexed and abduced, arms slightly flexed = 3
- full extension of arms and legs = 4

SQUARE WINDOW

○ Flex the hand at the wrist. Exert pressure sufficient to get as much flexion as possible. The angle between the hypothenar eminence and the anterior aspect of the forearm is measured and scored according to illustration. Do not rotate the wrist.

ANKLE DORSIFLEXION

o   Flex the foot at the ankle with sufficient pressure to get maximum change.
    The angle between the dorsum of the foot and the anterior aspect of the
    leg is measured and scored as in illustration.

ARM RECOIL

o   With the infant supine, fully flex the forearm for five seconds, then fully
    extend by pulling the hands and release. Score the reaction according to:

- remain extended or random movements   = 0
- incomplete or partial flexion   = 1
- brisk return to full flexion   = 2

LEG RECOIL

o   With the infant supine, the hips and knees are fully flexed for five seconds, then
    extended by traction on the feet and released. Score the reaction according to:

- no response or slight flexion   = 0
- partial flexion   = 1
- full flexion (less than 90° at knees and hips)   = 2

POPLITEAL ANGLE

o   With the infant supine and the pelvis flat on the examining surface, the
    leg is flexed on the thigh and the thigh fully flexed with the use of one
    hand. With the other hand the leg is then extended and the angle attained
    scored as in illustration.

HEEL TO EAR MANEUVER

o   With the infant supine, hold the infant's foot with one hand and move it
    as near to the head as possible without forcing it. Keep the pelvis flat on
    the examining surface. Score as in illustration.

SCARF SIGN

o   With the infant supine, take the infant's hand and draw it across the neck
    and as far across the opposite shoulder as possible. Assistance to the elbow
    is permissible by lifting it across the body. Score according to the location
    of the elbow:

- elbow reaches the opposite anterior axillary line   = 0
- elbow between opposite anterior axillary line and midline
  of thorax   = 1
- elbow at midline of thorax   = 2
- elbow does not reach midline of thorax   = 3

HEAD LAG

o   With the infant supine, grasp each forearm just proximal to the wrist and
    pull gently so as to bring the infant to a sitting position. Score according
    to the relationship of the head to the trunk during the maneuver:

- no evidence of head support   = 0
- some evidence of head support   = 1
- maintains head in the same anteroposterior plane as the body   = 2
- tends to hold the head forward   = 3

VENTRAL SUSPENSION

o   With the infant prone and the chest resting on the examiner's palm, lift
    the infant off the examining surface and score according to the posture
    shown in illustration.

piration, and unexplained intrauterine death are problems associated with postterm infants (Table 21-3). With the current classification, all infants fit into two categories. For example, most infants are *term* and *AGA*. Others may be preterm AGA, or postterm AGA. Infants who are preterm as well as SGA or LGA are at increased risk, since they are susceptible to problems common to infants in both categories.

DEFINITION, CAUSES, AND EFFECTS OF PREMATURITY

Prematurity means underdevelopment. With the current classification of infants, a *premature* infant is now defined as any infant born alive before 37 weeks' gestation, regardless of weight. Thus a premature infant is a preterm infant. The infant may be SGA, AGA, or LGA. A *low birth weight* infant is any live-born infant whose weight at birth is 2500 g or less.

The most common cause of prematurity is multiple pregnancy. Other causes include:

Pregnancy problems such as pregnancy-induced hypertension (PIH), placenta previa, abruptio placentae, hydramnios, and premature rupture of the membranes

Medical problems such as diabetes and acute infectious diseases

Other problems such as an inadequate diet

Excessive smoking by the mother may be a contributing factor. In many instances the cause of prematurity is not known.

The effects of prematurity depend on the degree of immaturity present. Infants born near term may show few or no signs of immaturity, even though they may weigh less than 2500 g. Many infants born prematurely, however, are too immature to survive. Prematurity is the leading cause of death among newborn infants in this country. Many premature infants die of respiratory distress syndrome. Other common causes of death are anoxia, pneumonia, infection, birth injuries, and malformations.

STOPPING PRETERM (PREMATURE) LABOR

Preterm, or premature, labor can be nature's way of dealing with a problem pregnancy in which the fetus has anomalies or a condition that makes survival outside the uterus impossible. In such instances it is unwise to try to stop the labor. However, when ultrasound studies indicate that the fetus is alive and viable (20 to 37 weeks' gestation) and there are no signs of fetal disease, and if the labor is diagnosed before the cervix is more than 50% effaced or more than 4 cm dilated, measures may be taken to try to stop labor.

If the physician decides to try to stop labor, he will either permit the mother to stay home or he will admit her to the hospital for treatment. If she stays home, she is treated with bed rest and sedation. She should be

TABLE 21-3 NURSING-CARE PLAN FOR POSTTERM INFANT

ASSESSMENTS	POTENTIAL NURSING DIAGNOSES	INTERVENTIONS	EXPECTED OUTCOME
Determine weight and gestational age	Potential for injury, birth trauma, temperature problems related to large size of infant	Have resuscitative equipment ready for use at birth; assist with resuscitation as necessary; assist with direct visualization and suctioning of meconium and amniotic fluid as necessary; keep infant warm; give oxygen as needed	Normal respirations
Observe for typical characteristics: decreased or absent vernix caseosa; dry, cracked, thin skin; yellow tint to skin, nails, cord; abundant scalp hair	Potential for injury, asphyxia, meconium aspiration, hypoglycemia, polycythemia related to aging of placenta		Normal temperature
			Tolerates feedings
Determine diabetic status of mother			
Test for glucose with Dextrostix		Record Dextrostix findings; report abnormals	
Observe for signs of birth injury and other complications		Carry out treatments for complications as ordered	No complications, or, if complications develop, respond to treatment

instructed to refrain from sexual intercourse because the prostaglandins in the semen may stimulate labor, or touching the cervix may stimulate an increase in contractions. She should be given written instructions regarding the dosage and times for taking the sedative as well as possible side effects of the medication. She should also be instructed in the importance of personal hygiene and what to do if her labor persists or her membranes rupture.

If she is admitted to the hospital, she will probably be given medications such as magnesium sulfate or ritodrine hydrochloride (Yutopar) to stop the labor. Use of these drugs require that she be observed closely. Magnesium sulfate may be given intravenously or intramuscularly; it works by relaxing smooth muscle. Since central nervous system depression occurs as a result of magnesium sulfate toxicity, it is important that her respirations be at least 16 per minute and her patellar and other reflexes be checked to see that they are present before each dose of this medication is given. Her urinary output should also be monitored and should be at least 100 ml every 4 hours while she is receiving magnesium sulfate. Depressed or absent reflexes, respirations less than 16 per minute, or a urinary output less than 100 ml per 4 hours should be reported to the doctor. Other symptoms that should be reported include complaints of feeling "hot all over," excessive thirst, flaccid paralysis, hypothermia, circulatory collapse, or depressed cardiac function. Calcium gluconate is the antidote for magnesium sulfate toxicity and should be kept at the bedside while this medication is being used.

Ritodrine hydrochloride (Yutopar) also relaxes smooth muscle, thereby decreasing uterine activity. It may be given intravenously or orally. An intravenous solution is usually started once preterm labor is diagnosed; after labor is stopped, the intravenous solution is discontinued and oral doses are given to keep labor stopped. Intravenous administration may be accomplished as the primary solution or it may be piggybacked to a primary solution. An infusion pump should be used to control the rate of flow.

Ritodrine may cause an increase in maternal and fetal heart rates, an elevation in the mother's systolic blood pressure, and a decrease in her diastolic blood pressure. Other symptoms associated with this drug include nausea, vomiting, tremors, headache, erythema, nervousness, jitteriness, and anxiety. These symptoms should be reported to the doctor, who will usually decrease the dosage or discontinue the medication.

CHARACTERISTICS OF THE PRETERM INFANT

EXTERNAL APPEARANCE

The closer to term the pregnancy is at birth, the more the infant resembles a normal newborn. The premature infant's length is under 19 inches (47.5

cm). The head is round and, compared to the body, large. The eyes are large and seem to bulge forward in the small face.

The premature infant's skin is red and wrinkled and is so delicate and thin that the underlying blood vessels are clearly visible through it. The face, arms, and back are covered with lanugo. Because of the underdeveloped muscles, the premature infant is likely to develop hernias.

INTERNAL DEVELOPMENT AND ACTIVITY

The internal organs of the premature infant may be poorly developed, making survival outside the uterus difficult or impossible.

The respiratory system is immature and the lungs are poorly expanded, which causes the breathing to be rapid, shallow, and labored. At times breathing becomes so tiring that the infant is unable to put forth the required effort and actually stops breathing temporarily, a condition known as apnea. The cry of the premature infant is often weak and whiny.

Hemorrhage can occur very easily, because the blood vessels are weak and fragile. Since the temperature-regulating mechanism is immature and very little fat is deposited under the skin, the temperature is unstable.

The stomach is narrow and upright and its sphincters are incompletely developed, so the infant tends to regurgitate food. Regurgitation can be very dangerous because the material can be aspirated into the lungs, and drowning or infection can result. The premature's tendencies to abdominal distention and to constipation are due to decreased peristalsis of the alimentary tract and to weak, poorly developed abdominal muscles. Overfeeding can cause diarrhea.

The nervous system is immature and, as a result, the gag, sucking, and swallowing reflexes may be absent, adding to the problem of feeding. The infant may also be quite listless and inactive.

NURSING ASSESSMENT AND INTERVENTIONS

When a premature birth or birth of a high-risk infant is anticipated, the mother is transferred to a regional hospital that has a premature or neonatal intensive care unit, if at all possible. Transport is usually safest if it can be accomplished while the fetus is still in the uterus, and the infant can begin immediately after birth to receive the specialized care needed for survival.

If it is not possible to transfer the mother before birth, a team of doctors and nurses from the regional center should be on hand at the time of birth so that they can begin immediate care of the infant. Transfer of the infant is then accomplished by the team (Fig. 21-3). Before and during transfer, the infant is kept warm and protected from infection. The air passages are kept free of mucus by gentle suction. Oxygen is readily available and administered as needed.

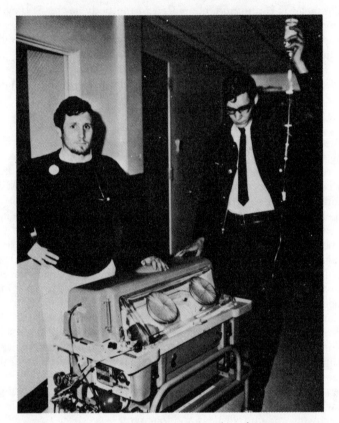

FIG. 21-3. *The premature infant is transferred to a premature center. The doctor accompanies and observes the infant.*

PREVENTION OF INFECTION

Those providing care must be aware of the premature infant's high susceptibility to infection and must do everything possible to protect against it.

> **SOME NURSING MEASURES THAT HELP PREVENT INFECTION IN THE PREMATURE INFANT**
>
> - Practicing strict asepsis
> - Limiting the number of people who come in contact with the infant
> - Suctioning mucus as necessary to prevent aspiration and subsequent lung infection

o Preventing regurgitation and aspiration of feedings by avoiding overfeeding, and by elevating the infant's head and shoulders after a feeding

o Eliminating from the premature nursery anyone who has an infection or who has recently cared for a patient with an infection

o Avoiding injury to the infant's skin

o Sterilizing all linen that comes in contact with the infant

PHYSICAL CARE

The mother who is in premature labor is given little or no medication for pain so that the baby will not be depressed when born. The labor and delivery nurse notifies the nursery when the mother is about ready to give birth, so that preparations can be made to care for the infant. These preparations include heating an incubator and getting oxygen and other supplies ready. The labor and delivery nurse also checks to be sure that the supplies needed for the baby in the delivery room are ready.

In the delivery room, the infant is handled gently and care is taken to provide warmth. Depending on the infant's condition, it may be necessary to postpone the routine procedures done in the delivery room, such as eye care, so that transfer to the nursery can take place as soon as possible.

In the nursery, the infant is placed in an incubator with the humidity and oxygen controlled as prescribed by the doctor. Not all premature babies need oxygen. When oxygen is given to a premature infant, it is in the lowest concentration possible to maintain adequate respirations and a normal color and is discontinued when it is no longer needed. Concentrations of oxygen above 40% given to a premature infant over a prolonged period can cause blindness due to a condition called *retrolental fibroplasia.* It is important, however, that the infant be given as much oxygen as needed even though the concentration may exceed 40%. Oxygen analyzers are available for measuring the concentration of oxygen in the incubator.

The incubator is regulated to maintain a constant, desirable temperature for the infant. The incubator temperature and the baby's temperature are checked at frequent intervals to avoid extreme changes in the baby's temperature. Some incubators are designed so that care can be given through hand holes in each side, thus eliminating the need for removing the infant from the environment.

The clothing the infant wears in the incubator can be limited to a diaper, which should be changed as soon as it is soiled.

Premature infants may or may not be given a bath every day, depending on their condition, and the practice in the hospital. However, the skin should be inspected daily for breaks and for signs of infection.

Because premature infants need to be kept warm, tire easily, and are susceptible to infection, they usually are not held any more than

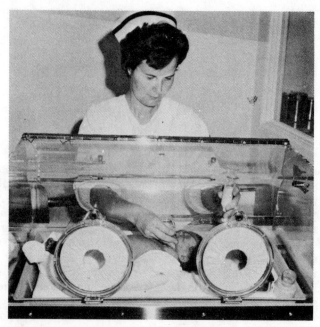

FIG. 21-4. *In gavage feeding of a premature infant in the incubator the nurse works through hand holes to maintain even temperature of the incubator.*

is absolutely necessary. Handling must be gentle to avoid injury. Their position should be changed every 2 hours to avoid lung complications.

Feeding. Premature infants are usually fed 6 to 12 hours after birth. Early feeding is beneficial in several ways. It:

Increases their chances for normal growth and development

Reduces the incidence of hyperbilirubinemia and hypoglycemia

Prevents nutritive depletion and maintains biochemical balance

The method of feeding depends on the size and condition of the infant and the ability to suck. The very small immature infant is given intravenous feedings, whereas the larger premature infant is fed by bottle or gavage. Some larger premature infants may be breast-fed. A small amount of water is usually given for the first few oral feedings because water is less likely to cause severe lung problems should the infant regurgitate and aspirate it. If the water is well tolerated, small amounts of formula are given. The feedings are gradually increased as the infant's tolerance and nutritional needs increase. Overfeeding can cause vomiting, distention, and diarrhea.

Gavage feeding involves placing a tube into the baby's stomach, attaching an Asepto syringe to the tube, and pouring the formula into the syringe (Fig. 21-4). Care is taken to avoid forcing air into the stomach. The formula in the syringe flows through the tube and into the infant's stomach. Infants are observed to see how they take feedings, whether they suck on the tube, whether they seem fatigued, and whether they seem hungry or satisfied after the feeding. This information is helpful to the doctor in deciding when to increase the feedings and when to change from gavage to bottle feedings.

Observations. The smaller the infants, the more closely they need to be observed (Table 21-4).

OBSERVATIONS OF PREMATURE INFANTS

o   Take their temperature regularly.

o   Count their pulse and respirations at frequent intervals.

o   Observe their color for cyanosis, pallor, or jaundice.

o   Note whether their cry is weak or absent.

o   Observe how they take feedings and whether they seem satisfied following the feeding.

o   Note the presence of muscular twitchings or convulsions, vomiting, abdominal distention, lethargy, or limpness.

EMOTIONAL CARE

The emotional needs of the premature infant may not be met completely at first because the physical needs take precedence. However, as soon as the mother's condition permits, she can be encouraged to touch the infant through the hand holes in the incubator (Fig. 21-5). The father should also be encouraged to touch the infant as soon as possible and to hold it when the infant's condition permits.

After the critical period is over and infants no longer need to be in the intensive care unit, they may be placed in a continuing care unit or transferred back to the nursery at the hospital in which they were born. Here their parents may be more directly involved in their care. Some hospitals are attempting environmental stimulation of premature infants by playing tape recordings of the voices of the parents and siblings for 20 minutes at feeding times. When infants are able to be out of the incubator, the parents are encouraged to hold and feed them.

PARENTS OF THE PREMATURE INFANT

The parents of the premature infant may have many worries. They may wonder if something they did or did not do caused the premature birth.

TABLE 2-1 NURSING CARE PLAN FOR PRETERM INFANT

ASSESSMENTS	POTENTIAL NURSING DIAGNOSES	INTERVENTIONS	EXPECTED OUTCOME
Determine gestational age from mother's LMP, from physical characteristics and appearance, and from neurologic behavior	Altered growth and development related to preterm birth	Handle very gently; wash hands before and after caring for infant; use individual supplies; use sterilized linens	Continues to grow and develop outside uterus
	Potential for infection related to immature immune system		No infection
Observe for signs of respiratory problems: rapid, labored breathing, retractions, grunting, nasal flaring, decreased breath sounds, apnea, cyanosis	Impaired gas exchange related to lack of surfactant	Give oxygen as indicated	Breathes normally or with ease on ventilator
	Ineffective airway clearance related to immaturity	Suction as necessary	
Observe for signs of dehydration: skin turgor, urinary output, mucous membranes	Fluid volume deficit related to insensitive water loss and inadequate fluid intake	Give type and amount of fluid ordered; record intake and output	Maintains normal fluid/electrolyte balance
Observe for skin breakdown	Potential impairment of skin integrity related to use of tape and other adhesive materials	Use as little tape as possible on skin; use op-site for skin devices	Maintains healthy, intact skin
Monitor temperature of infant and incubator	Ineffective thermoregulation related to immaturity; potential for injury and cold stress related to immature temperature-regulating mechanism	Record temperature of infant and incubator frequently; adjust incubator temperature as necessary to maintain desired temperature of infant	Temperature stable
Determine infant's ability to take feedings	Alterations in nutrition: less than body requirements related to decreased caloric intake	Feed appropriately (by gavage, nipple, etc.) according to infant's ability; record amount of feeding and how infant tolerated it; elevate head after feeding; do not overfeed; weigh daily and record; report abnormal stools	Loses minimal birth weight; gains weight steadily
Determine parents' feelings concerning infant and their ability to care for him	Parental knowledge deficit related to care of preterm infant	Teach parents care of infant; involve parents in care of infant as much as possible; encourage parents to touch, hold, feed infant; refer to public health nurse, social services, support groups for follow-up care	Parents demonstrate understanding of care of infant, able to give care; parent-infant bonding occurs, emotional needs are met

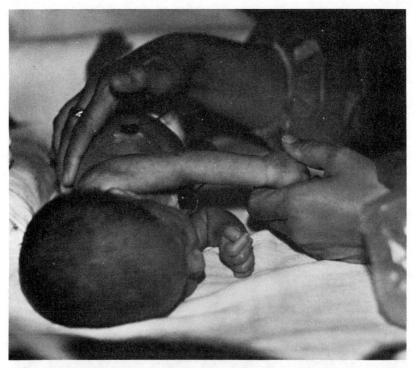

FIG. 21-5. *The mother strokes her premature infant by reaching through the hand holes of the incubator. As the infant is stroked, the infant relaxes and the mother is pleased with her mothering ability.*

They may fear that the infant will not live or be normal. They may be awed by the equipment and wonder if they will be capable of taking care of their baby at home. They may be concerned about the expense involved in the long hospitalization. The mother may find it hard to realize that she has actually given birth, because she cannot hold and feed her infant as the other mothers do. Both parents may be disappointed because they cannot take the baby home with them when the mother is discharged.

Preterm infants sleep more than full-term infants and are less predictable and responsive. This may create problems in parental-infant bonding and in the development of parental-infant relationships, particularly if the parents expect the preterm infant to behave the same as a full-term infant. They may feel that the infant's unresponsiveness reflects on their competence as parents, rather than being the typical immature behavior of the preterm infant. The nurse may need to help them understand what is normal behavior for the preterm infant so that they will not feel threatened in their parenting abilities. It is very important that a positive parent-infant relationship be developed in order to prevent abusive behavior by the parents toward the infant.

The nurse can provide extensive support to the parents of the preterm infant. She can arrange for them to see and touch or hold the infant (Fig. 21-6), she can keep them informed of his progress, she can explain the equipment used in his care, she can encourage them to feed him when his condition permits, she can teach them the care he will need after discharge, and she can assure them that someone will be available

FIG. 21-6. *Mother holding her premature infant on a ventilator. (Oehler JM: Family-Centered Neonatal Nursing Care. Philadelphia, JB Lippincott, 1981)*

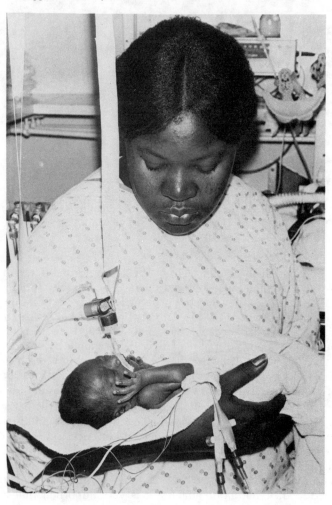

to help them and to answer their questions at all times after the infant is discharged from the hospital.

Unless complications develop, premature infants are usually ready for discharge from the hospital by the time they weigh 5 or 5½ lb (2268 or 2495 g). After obtaining the doctor's approval, the nurse can discuss with the mother the assistance available through the public health nursing service or the Visiting Nurses' Association. A nurse from these agencies visits the mother in her home before the baby is discharged from the hospital and helps in planning and preparing for the care of the infant at home. After the infant is home, the nurse visits periodically to assist the mother. The mother is usually reassured to know that this help is available. Of course, she can also contact her doctor if problems arise in the care of the infant.

CLINICAL REVIEW

1. An infant born prematurely is likely to have immaturity of certain organs and systems, which causes problems requiring specific care. In column I list the immature organ or system; in column II list the problem resulting from the immaturity of the organ or system; and in column III list the care indicated for the problem. An example is given.

I	II	III
Immature organ or system	*Problem*	*Care indicated*
A. Immature respiratory system; poor expansion of lungs	Apnea; atelectasis; rapid, labored breathing	Close observation of respirations and color; oxygen and humidity
B.		
C.		
D.		

2. Why might parents of a preterm infant have trouble developing a relationship with their infant? How can the nurse help them with this problem?

BIBLIOGRAPHY

Gennaro S: Anxiety and problem-solving ability in mothers of premature infants. J Obstet Gynecol Neonatal Nurs 15:160–164, 1986
Gill PJ, Katz M: Early detection of preterm labor: Ambulatory home monitoring of uterine activity. J Obstet Gynecol Neonatal Nurs 15:439–442, 1986
Harrison LL, Twardosz S: Teaching mothers about their preterm infants. J Obstet Gynecol Neonatal Nurs 15:165–172, 1986
Jensen MD, Bobak IM: Maternity Care: The Nurse & The Family, 3rd ed, pp 1086–1120. St. Louis, CV Mosby, 1985
Reeder SR, Martin LL: Maternity Nursing, 16th ed, pp 969–1017. Philadelphia, JB Lippincott, 1987
Scherer JC: Lippincott's Nurses' Drug Manual, pp 947–949. Philadelphia, JB Lippincott, 1985

glossary

Many of the following words have more than one meaning, either in specialized sciences or in general use. However, as listed here they refer only to maternity and related subjects.

ABCs. Abbreviation for *alternative birthing centers.*

abortion. Termination of pregnancy before the fetus is viable, that is, before it can survive outside the uterus.

abruptio placentae. Premature separation of a normally implanted placenta.

afterbirth. Placenta and structures cast off after the birth of the baby; includes membranes with placenta and umbilical cord.

afterpains. Cramplike pain in abdomen following birth; caused by contractions of the uterus as it returns to its normal size.

alternative birthing centers (ABCs). Facilities associated with a hospital or as free-standing clinics that provide a homelike atmosphere and have liberal policies regarding the presence of family and friends, labor practices, no separation of parents and infant, and early discharge.

amenorrhea. Absence of menstrual discharge.

amnesia. Loss of memory.

amniocentesis. Withdrawal of some of the fluid surrounding the fetus by inserting a sterile needle through the abdominal and uterine walls into the amniotic sac.

amnion. Inner membrane surrounding the fetus in the uterus; contains the fluid in which the fetus lives.

analgesic. Agent that relieves pain without loss of consciousness.

anoxia. Lack of oxygen; decreased amount of oxygen.

antepartal. Before birth; prenatal.

areola. Ring of pigment surrounding the nipple.

Ascheim-Zondek test. Pregnancy test. Urine from a woman suspected of being pregnant is injected into immature mice. If the test is positive, the mice develop lutein cells and hemorrhages in the ovaries within 100 hours after the urine is injected.

asphyxia neonatorum. Delayed or deficient respiration in newborn.

bag of waters. Membranes and fluid surrounding the fetus in the uterus.

ballottement. Term used in an examination in which the fetus can be pushed about in the pregnant uterus.

Bartholin's glands. Two small glands situated one on either side of the vagina.

blastodermic vesicle. Hollow space within the morula formed by the rearrangement of the cells into two layers.

Braxton Hicks sign. Painless uterine contractions occurring periodically throughout pregnancy.

breech delivery. Delivery in which the buttocks and/or one or both feet are presenting.

caput succedaneum. Swelling on the head due to pressure from the cervix during labor.

caudal anesthesia. Anesthesia resulting from the introduction of an anesthetic solution into the caudal canal.

cephalhematoma. Swelling on one or both sides of the scalp due to bleeding between the bone and the periosteum.

cervix. Lower, narrow end of the uterus.

cesarean section. Delivery of the baby through an incision in the abdominal wall and uterus.

Chadwick's sign. Purplish discoloration of the vagina, seen after the fourth week of pregnancy.

chloasma. Blotchy brown areas of pigmentation occurring on the face during pregnancy.

chorion. Outer membrane surrounding the fetus in the uterus.

chromosomes. Rodlike structures occurring in pairs within the nucleus of each cell in the body; each species of animal and plant life has a specific number of chromosomes, which remains constant and is typical for that species.

circumcision. Removal of all or part of the foreskin of the penis.

cleft lip. Separation of the upper lip on one or both sides of the midline.

cleft palate. Separation of the roof of the mouth.

clitoris. Small, elongated, erectile organ located at the upper end of the labia; comparable to the penis in the male.

colostrum. Yellowish fluid secreted by the breasts during the latter part of pregnancy and for 3 or 4 days postpartum, when it is replaced by milk.

conception (fertilization). Union of sperm from male with ovum from female; beginning of pregnancy.

corpus luteum. Yellowish body formed by the graafian follicle after the ovum is expelled.

cotyledon. Segment or subdivision of the maternal side of the placenta.

delivery. Expulsion of a child from the uterus by the mother, or its extraction by the obstetric practitioner.

ductus arteriosus. Blood vessel in the fetus connecting the pulmonary artery with the aorta.

ductus venosus. Blood vessel in the fetus leading from the umbilical vein to the inferior vena cava.

dystocia. Difficult, slow, or painful labor or delivery.

eclampsia. Severe pregnancy-induced-hypertension in which convulsions and/or coma occur.

ectoderm. Outer layer of the three germ layers of the embryo; from the ectoderm develop the skin, nervous system, nasal passages, crystalline lens of the eye, the pharynx, and the mammary and salivary glands.

ectopic. Out of place; ectopic pregnancy is a pregnancy occurring outside the uterus.

effacement. Thinning and shortening of the cervix.

ejaculation. A sudden act of expulsion, as of semen.

embryo. Developing organism during the first 5 weeks of pregnancy; after that time it is called a fetus.

endometrium. Mucous membrane lining the uterus.

engagement. Settling of the presenting part into the pelvis.

engorgement. Congestion of the breasts due to an increased blood supply and glandular activity in preparation for lactation.

entoderm. Innermost layer of the three germ layers of the embryo; from the entoderm develop the alimentary tract, respiratory tract, bladder, pancreas, and liver.

episiotomy. Surgical incision of the perineum to permit delivery of the baby without tears to the area.

erythroblastosis fetalis. Blood problem of the newborn due to Rh incompatibility.

estrogen. Female sex hormone; secreted by the ovaries and by the placenta.

fallopian tubes. Two canals extending from either side of the fundus of the uterus.

fetus. Baby in the uterus from the fifth week of gestation until birth.

fimbria. Fringe, especially the fringelike end of the fallopian tube.

fontanel. Space or "soft spot" at the junction of the bones in the baby's head; the diamond-shaped space in front of the baby's scalp is known as the anterior fontanel; the triangular-shaped space at the back of the baby's head is known as the posterior fontanel.

foramen ovale. Opening in the partition between the right and left atria in the fetus.

foreskin. Prepuce; fold of skin covering the glans penis.

fornix. Area of the vagina surrounding that part of the cervix which protrudes into the vagina.

Friedman's test. Pregnancy test. Urine from a woman suspected of being pregnant is injected into an unmated mature rabbit twice daily for two days; the test is positive if fresh corpus luteum or hemorrhage occurs in the ovaries of the rabbit.

FSH. Abbreviation for follicle-stimulating hormone.

fundus. Upper, rounded portion of the uterus.

gamete. Mature germ cell.

gavage feeding. Feeding through a tube into stomach; frequently the method of feeding premature infants.

gene. Factor in chromosomes responsible for transmitting inherited traits or characteristics of individuals.

genitalia. Reproductive organs.

gestation. Period of development of the young within the uterus.

gonadotropin. Substance having an affinity for or a stimulating effect on the gonads.

Goodell's sign. Softening of the cervix.

graafian follicle. Small spherical bodies in the ovaries, each containing an ovum.

gravida. Pregnant woman.

Hegar's sign. Softening of the lower uterine segment.

hormone. Chemical substance produced by one organ, which affects the function of another organ.

hydramnios. Excessive amount of amniotic fluid.

hymen. Membrane surrounding the opening of the vagina.

hypoxia. Decreased amount of oxygen.

implantation. Embedding of the fertilized ovum in the lining of the uterus.

inertia. Inactivity; sluggishness of uterine contractions during labor.

infant. Child under 12 to 14 months (time of erect posture).

inlet. Upper limit of the pelvic cavity.

involution. Return of the uterus to its normal size and condition after delivery.

ischium. Under part of each hip bone.

IUD. Intrauterine device, used as a contraceptive.

labia majora. Folds of skin containing fat and covered with hair which form each side of the vulva.

labia minora. Folds of delicate skin inside of the labia majora.

labor. Series of processes by which the products of conception are expelled from the mother's body.

lactation. Secretion of milk; the time or period of secreting milk.

lanugo. Fine, downy hair on the body of the fetus.

large for gestational age (LGA). An infant born at 36 weeks' gestation and weighing 3500 g (about 90th percentile for weight); LGA infants are immature but overgrown; typically born to diabetic mothers.

LGA. Abbreviation for large for gestational age.

LH. Abbreviation for luteinizing hormone.

lightening. Sensation of decreased abdominal distension produced by the descent of the uterus into the pelvic cavity, which occurs two or three weeks before the onset of labor.

linea nigra. Dark line appearing on the abdomen and extending from the pubis toward the umbilicus of the pregnant woman.

lochia. Vaginal discharge expelled following delivery and several days thereafter.

low birth weight infant. Live-born infant whose weight at birth is 5½ lb (2500 g) or less.

maturation. In biology, a process of cell division during which the number of chromosomes in the germ cells is reduced to one half the number characteristic of the species.

meconium. Dark green or black substance found in the large intestine of the fetus or newly born infant; first stool of newborn.

menstruation. Cyclic, physiologic uterine bleeding which normally occurs at approximately four-week intervals, in the absence of pregnancy, during the reproductive period.

mesoderm. Middle layer of the three germ layers of the embryo; from the mesoderm develop muscles, circulatory system, bones, reproductive system, connective tissue, kidneys, and ureters.

milia. Tiny, white spots on the skin of the nose and forehead of the newborn, usually caused by clogged oil glands or hair follicles.

miscarriage. Abortion.

molding. Shaping of the baby's head to adjust itself to the size and shape of the birth canal.

mons pubis. Mound of fatty tissue covered with hair, situated in the lower abdomen above the pubis in women.

Montgomery's tubercles. Small glands on the areolae around the nipple.

multigravida. Woman who has been pregnant several times.

multipara. Woman who has borne several children.

navel. Umbilicus.

neonatal. Newborn.

nullipara. Woman who has not borne children.

ophthalmia neonatorum. Infection of the eyes of the newborn caused by gonococcus.

os, external. External opening of the canal of the cervix.

os, internal. Internal opening of the canal of the cervix.

ovary. Female sex gland.

ovulation. Rupturing of a graafian follicle and expelling of mature ovum.

ovum. Female germ cell, or sex cell, pl. **ova.**

oxytocic. Agent which stimulates the uterus to contract.

oxytocin. Hormone secreted by the posterior lobe of the pituitary gland; stimulates uterine contractions.

palpation. Light fingertip pressure exerted by doctor on the woman's abdomen to determine outline of the fetus.

para. Refers to past pregnancies that have produced a viable infant, whether or not the infant is dead or alive at birth.

parametrium. Outer serous layer of the uterus, continuous with the peritoneum.

parturition. Process of giving birth.

pelvimetry. Measurement of the pelvis.

penis. Male organ of copulation.

perinatal. Period of time shortly before and after birth; beginning at approximately 28 weeks' gestation and ending 1 to 4 weeks after birth.

perineum. Area between the vagina and the anus.

phimosis. Tightness of the foreskin of the penis.

phototherapy. Treatment to prevent or dissipate jaundice by means of exposure to light.

Pitocin. Agent that stimulates the uterus to contract.

placenta. Circular, flat vascular organ present in the gravid uterus, which establishes communication between the fetal and the maternal blood supplies through the umbilical cord. It is a part of the afterbirth cast out following delivery.

placenta previa. Placenta implanted in the lower uterine segment so that it adjoins or covers the internal os of the cervix.

position. Relation of a certain point on the presenting part of the fetus to the mother's pelvis.

postpartum. After delivery or childbirth.

post-term infant. Infant born after 42 weeks' gestation.

preeclampsia. Disorder encountered during pregnancy or early in the puerperium characterized by elevated blood pressure, edema, and albuminuria.

pregnancy. Condition of being with child.

pregnancy-induced hypertension. Disorders encountered during pregnancy or early in the puerperium that are characterized by one or more of the following signs: elevated blood pressure, edema, albuminuria, and in severe cases, convulsions and coma.

premature infant. See *preterm infant.*

prepuce. Fold of skin that covers the glans penis in the male.

presentation. That part of the fetus lowest in the mother's pelvis.

preterm infant. Infant born before 37 weeks' gestation but after the age of viability.

primigravida. Woman who is pregnant for the first time.

primipara. Woman who has given birth to her first child.

primordial. Original or primitive; of the simplest and most undeveloped character.

progesterone. Hormone secreted by the corpus luteum, the function of which is to prepare the endometrium for the reception and development of the fertilized ovum.

prolactin. Hormone from the anterior lobe of the pituitary gland that stimulates lactation in the mammary glands.

puberty. Age at which the reproductive organs become capable of functioning.

pubis. Pubic bone forming the front of the pelvis.

pudendum. External genitalia.

puerperium. Period from delivery until the reproductive organs return to their normal condition, about 6 weeks.

quickening. First movements of fetus felt by the mother.

Rh factor. A term applied to an inherited antigen in the human blood.

rubella. German measles. May be injurious to fetus if contracted by mother in first trimester of pregnancy.

semen. A seed. The fluid secreted by the male reproductive organs.

SGA. Abbreviation for *small for gestational age.*

show. Blood-tinged mucus discharge expelled from the vagina before or during labor.

small for gestational age (SGA). Pertaining to infants whose weight falls below the tenth percentile for their gestational age. These infants have experienced growth retardation during the prenatal period and may be born close to term but weigh less than 2500 g.

spermatozoon. Male reproductive cell.

striae gravidarum. Shiny, reddish lines found upon the abdomen, thighs, and breasts during pregnancy.

symphysis pubis. Union of the pubic bones, which are connected to each other by interarticular cartilage.

term infant. Infant born between 37 and 42 weeks' gestation.

testicle (testis, testes). One of the two glands contained in the male scrotum that produce spermatozoa.

thrush. An infection of the mouth of the newborn caused by the fungus *Candida albicans.*

trimester. Three-month period; pregnancy is divided into three trimesters.

umbilical arteries. Arteries that form part of the umbilical cord; used blood is carried through them from fetus to placenta.

umbilical cord. The cord connecting the placenta with the umbilicus of the fetus; made up of the two umbilical arteries and the umbilical vein, surrounded by a mass of gelatinous tissue called "Wharton's jelly."

umbilical vein. Vessel in the umbilical cord through which oxygenated blood is carried from the placenta to the fetus.

uterus (womb). Hollow, muscular organ in the female in which the fetus is housed and nourished during its development until birth.

vagina. Canal in the female extending from the vulva to the cervix of the uterus.

vernix caseosa. Cheesy substance covering the skin of the fetus.

vertex. Top of the head.

viable. Able to live, especially relating to a fetus which has developed enough that it can live outside the uterus.

villi. Vascular projections on the chorion of the early embryo.

vulva. External genitals of the female.

Wharton's jelly. Jellylike mucous tissue surrounding the vessels in the umbilical cord.

zygote. Cell resulting from the union of two gametes.

appendix

APPROVED NURSING DIAGNOSES, NORTH AMERICAN NURSING DIAGNOSIS ASSOCIATION JUNE 1988

Activity intolerance
Activity intolerance, potential
Adjustment, impaired
Airway clearance, ineffective
Anxiety
Aspiration, potential for
Body temperature, altered,
  potential
Bowel elimination, altered:
    Constipation
  Colonic constipation
  Perceived constipation
Bowel elimination, altered:
    Diarrhea
Bowel elimination, altered:
    Incontinence
Breastfeeding, ineffective
Breathing pattern, ineffective
Cardiac output, altered:
    Decreased (specify)
Comfort, altered: Pain
Comfort, altered: Chronic pain
Communication, impaired: Verbal
Coping, family: Potential for
  growth
Coping, ineffective, family:
    Compromised
Coping, ineffective, family:
    Disabling
Coping, ineffective, individual
  Defensive coping
  Ineffective denial
Decisional conflict (specify)
Disuse syndrome, potential for
Diversional activity, deficit
Dysreflexia
Family process, altered
Fatigue
Fear

Fluid volume deficit, actual
Fluid volume deficit, potential
Fluid volume excess
Gas exchange, impaired
Grieving, anticipatory
Grieving, dysfunctional
Growth and development, altered
Health maintenance, altered
Health-seeking behaviors (specify)
Home maintenance, impaired
Hopelessness
Hyperthermia
Hypothermia
Incontinence, functional
Incontinence, reflex
Incontinence, stress
Incontinence, total
Incontinence, urge
Infection, potential for
Injury, potential for (specify):
    poisoning, suffocation,
    trauma
Knowledge deficit (specify)
Mobility, impaired physical
Noncompliance (specify)
Nutrition, altered: Less than body
    requirements
Nutrition, altered: More than body
    requirements
Nutrition, altered: Potential for
    more than body requirements
Oral mucous membrane, altered
Parental role conflict
Parenting, altered: Actual
Parenting, altered: Potential
Post trauma response
Powerlessness
Rape trauma syndrome
Role performance, altered

Self-care deficit: Feeding,
bathing/hygiene,
dressing/grooming, toileting
Self-concept, disturbance in body
image, self-esteem, role
performance, personal
identity
Self-esteem disturbance
Chronic low self-esteem
Situational low self-esteem
Sensory/perceptual alteration:
Visual, auditory, kinesthetic,
gustatory, tactile, olfactory
Sexual dysfunction
Sexuality patterns, altered
Skin integrity, impaired: Actual
Skin integrity, impaired: Potential
Sleep pattern disturbance
Social interaction, impaired

Social isolation
Spiritual distress (distress of the
human spirit)
Swallowing, impaired
Thermoregulation, ineffective
Thought processes, altered
Tissue integrity, impaired
Tissue perfusion, altered:
Cerebral, cardiopulmonary,
renal, gastrointestinal,
peripheral
Unilateral neglect
Urinary elimination, altered
patterns
Urinary retention
Violence, potential for:
Self-directed or directed at
others

index

Note: A page number followed by the letter "f" indicates a figure; a page number followed by the letter "t" indicates tabular material.